The Phenomenon of Ment al Dis

CONTRIBUTIONS TO PHENOMENOLOGY

IN COOPERATION WITH
THE CENTER FOR ADVANCED RESEARCH IN PHENOMENOLOGY

Volume 75

Scope

The purpose of the series is to serve as a vehicle for the pursuit of phenomenological research across a broad spectrum, including cross-over developments with other fields of inquiry such as the social sciences and cognitive science. Since its establishment in 1987, Contributions to Phenomenology has published nearly 60 titles on diverse themes of phenomenological philosophy. In addition to welcoming monographs and collections of papers in established areas of scholarship, the series encourages original work in phenomenology. The breadth and depth of the Series reflects the rich and varied significance of phenomenological thinking for seminal questions of human inquiry as well as the increasingly international reach of phenomenological research.

More information about this series at http://www.springer.com/series/5811

Petr Kouba

The Phenomenon of Mental Disorder

Perspectives of Heidegger's Thought
in Psychopathology

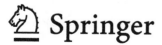 Springer

Petr Kouba
Philosophical Institute of the Czech
  Academy of Sciences
Charles University
Prague, Czech Republic

Translation from the Czech language edition (As the English version of the text has been revised in a significant way, it differs from the Czech original): Fenomén duševní poruchy. Perspektivy Heideggerova myšlení v oblasti psychopatologie by Petr Kouba © OIKOYMENH, Prague, 2006. All rights reserved

Translated by David Vichnar and Petr Kouba

FILOSOFICKÝ ÚSTAV AV ČR

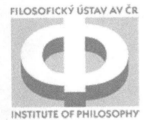

INSTITUTE OF PHILOSOPHY

Revision and translation of this monograph were financed from the research grant of the Czech Science Foundation 'Philosophical Investigations of Body Experiences: Transdisciplinary Perspectives' (GAP401/10/1164)

ISSN 0923-9545
ISBN 978-3-319-36237-3   ISBN 978-3-319-10323-5 (eBook)
DOI 10.1007/978-3-319-10323-5
Springer Cham Heidelberg New York Dordrecht London

Dedicated to Alice

Translated by David Vichnar and Petr Kouba

Acknowledgement

I would like to express my gratitude to Dr. Robin Rollinger for his careful proof reading and copy-editing of this text. His suggestions have helped me to make the text accessible to an English readership without undermining its original intentions.

I would also like to thank the Institute of Philosophy of the Czech Academy of Sciences for its institutional support. Last but not least, I am grateful to the Czech Science Foundation who's support for the research project "Philosophical Investigations of Body Experiences: Transdisciplinary Perspectives" (GAP401/10/1164) made possible translation and revision of this work.

Prague 2014

Contents

Chapter 1
Introduction

The question of whether Heidegger's thought represents the crucial turning point in the history of Western philosophy could in and of itself be a topic for a lengthy discussion. Whatever might be decided on this point, it is nonetheless clear that his thought cannot simply be neglected.

The significance of Heidegger's thought can be seen by the mere fact that its influence extends far beyond the realm of philosophy. The extraordinary fame that *Sein und Zeit* brought upon its author has been followed by the remarkable response it evoked in various specialized disciplines, the most prominent of which are those concerned with the problems of mental health and illness. Numerous psychiatrists and psychotherapists have approached Heidegger's philosophy in search of new means of analytical reasoning and, in some cases, for a new basis of medical science as such. Beginning with Ludwig Binswanger, who made use of its terminology in his study *Über Ideenflucht* only 6 years after the publication of *Sein und Zeit*, there is a long list of names (including Alfred Storch, Heinz Häfner and many others) whose fame is to some extent connected with the philosophy of being.

A qualitatively new phase of this influence was marked by Heidegger's friendship with the Swiss psychiatrist Medard Boss. Thanks to him Heidegger decided to overcome his long-standing reticence about the reception of his work within the field of medicine and to begin interacting openly with medical thought. Especially the records of his Zurich series of lectures and seminars, published under the title *Zollikoner Seminare*, bear testimony to the arduous search for a common language. There we see him – a thinker striving for the most comprehensible explication of the foundational principles of the phenomenological method, facing a committee of medical specialists whose thinking is formed especially through concepts drawn from the discourse of natural sciences. In order to bridge the gap between himself and his audience, Heidegger cannot but launch a critical examination of the primary presuppositions of contemporary natural science. Insofar as scientific rationalism shapes the concepts of health and illness in the realm of contemporary medicine, it is necessary to unmask their artificiality and reveal their underlying intellectual

© Springer International Publishing Switzerland 2015
P. Kouba, *The Phenomenon of Mental Disorder*, Contributions
to Phenomenology 75, DOI 10.1007/978-3-319-10323-5_1

constructs. However, the criticism of the natural sciences does not consist only in a negative evaluation of them. Heidegger's critique is in fact primarily constructive, for its goal remains the unveiling of new thematic possibilities and connections. Its task is to mark out a new path to the region of being which is instrumental in determining human health and illness. Regardless of how difficult this path may be, the records of the lectures and the interviews as well as the excerpts from private correspondence included in *Zollikoner Seminare* provide us with unique material for the examination of the possible value of the ontological analysis of human existence for psychopathology and psychotherapy.

Despite his avowed lack of familiarity with up-to-date results of scientific inquiry in the fields of psychopathology and psychotherapy, Heidegger attributes principal importance to the issues of these two disciplines.[1] His focus is not so much specific pathological symptoms, detailed casuistic studies, or therapeutic practices, as it is the very foundation of the medical view of human existence. Without a careful consideration of the question of the specifically human mode of existence, it is impossible to find an adequate approach to human suffering. This is the only way to establish psychopathology and psychotherapy on a foundation that systematically does away with standardized ways of treating patients. It is not enough to strive to prevent the practical attitudes of physicians and therapists from slipping into a one-sided manipulation of suffering human beings. What is at issue is primarily the question of method, not one of the prerequisites of medical ethics. Psychopathology and psychotherapy must be given clearly defined methodical guidelines. While determining its nature, Heidegger refuses to reduce human existence to a mere functioning of the psychic or somatic apparatus and tries to view human being in the whole breadth of its existence. The fact that we are imperfect and, because of our imperfection, constantly prone to losing ourselves, does not, in Heidegger's opinion, give the least credit to the approach which views the afflicted patient purely in terms of the object of scientific observation and medical treatment. Even while dealing with the most severe cases known to psychopathology, experts shouldn't give in to the impression that what they observe are mere effects of natural mechanisms rather than human existence in all of its essential features. If this impression prevails, they deprive themselves of the only possible guidelines that can positively lead to an unreduced and undistorted understanding of pathological states. Doctors who do not want to ignore the individual experience of their patients must always keep in mind that "the unifying pole in psychotherapeutic science is the existing human being."[2]

The above statement, however, says nothing about what or how human existence actually is. In order to evade the trap of Cartesian dualism in his description of the principal moments of human existence, Heidegger dismisses the distinction between *res extensa* and *res cogitans*, replacing it with being-in-the-world. To be a human

[1] Heidegger, Martin. 1987. *Zollikoner Seminare*, ed. Medard Boss.. Frankfurt am Main: Vittorio Klostermann, 299.

[2] Heidegger. *Zollikoner Seminare*, 259. English edition: Heidegger, Martin. 2001. *Zollikon Seminars* (trans. Mayr, Franz, and Askay, Richard). Evanston: Northwestern University Press, 209.

being is not to be an entity divided up into a physical and a spiritual sphere, but an indivisible whole, whose existence is characterized in *Zollikoner Seminare* as dwelling in the clearing of beings. This type of existence, however, needs to be understood correctly. It does not consist in being an entity simply situated amidst others; rather, our existence is distinguished by preserving an open realm in which beings can manifest themselves as what they are.

From what has been said here thus far, it already becomes clear that to talk about "mental" illness in connection with human existence is at least misleading, for the disturbances designated by this term are in their nature not only psycho-somatic, but involve complex relations to the world in which human existence is involved. Binswanger is well aware of this, taking in his crucial treatise on schizophrenia the phenomenological analysis of being-in-the world as his point of departure.[3] If, for the sake of convention, we have to resort to the expression "mental disorder" we shouldn't forget that what is meant thereby is a specific disturbance of being-in-the-world.

As Binswanger's analysis of various cases of schizophrenia makes clear, the disturbance of dwelling in the clearing of beings entails the disintegration of the consistency of experience. Whereas the so-called "natural" experience can indeed also integrate encounters with the unknown and the unexpected without the slightest violation of its consistency, a schizophrenic existence is destabilized to such an extent that the integral order of its experience comes undone. The inconsistency of experience in its various forms can be observed in Binswanger's casuistries, together with the resulting effort to re-establish the meaningful order of existence. The impossibility of a balanced being-in-the world, merely emphasized by the futility of repetitious attempts to stabilize itself, thrusts human existence into an impasse. The threat of disintegration of individual existence becomes manifest in the incessantly recurring inconsistency of experience, which can result in utter resignation.

Although schizophrenia represents a certain extreme in this respect, a similar disorder of being-in-the-world announces itself (albeit to a much lesser extent) also in the case of other pathological changes of human existence. Disorders of the neurotic character, obsessive states, phobias, deep depressions – none of these leads to a disintegration of consistency of experience, and yet they all reflect a disturbance in the open relation to beings, whether to things, to others, or to one's own body.

Insofar as a psychopathological disorder is a disturbance in the open relation to beings, the direction to be taken by the therapeutic process is in fact already prefigured: the primary goal of therapeutic effort can only be to help the patient to achieve an open and steady being-in-the-world. The basic presupposition of a treatment thus conceived is to avoid mistaking the disturbed being-in-the-world for a functional defect or for an objective process that occurs within the patient on the basis of its own inner determinism. While psychiatry formed on the principles of natural sciences conceives of symptoms as manifestations of a hidden illness, Binswanger strives for an interpretation of pathological experience in accordance with phenomenological insights. As opposed to a classifying diagnosis that pigeonholes the

---

[3] Binswanger, Ludwig. 1957. *Schizophrenie*. Pfullingen: Neske.

ascertained data within a certain category of the psychiatric system, what he attempts is to arrive at an understanding of psychopathological disorders that unmasks them as belonging to the essential possibilities of being-in-the-world.

If the natural scientific explanation of symptoms prevents the phenomenon of psychopathological disorder from becoming manifest at all, our inquiry should take exactly the opposite direction. The aim of this inquiry is not to find the objective causes for mental disorders or to undertake their systematic classification, but to provide an answer to the question concerning the circumstances under which the psychopathological disorder of being-in-the-world could manifest itself as a phenomenon.

Within the context of a standard social environment we encounter what common language calls "insanity" first of all in the form of abnormal, deranged behavior. However, any action ill-adjusted to given circumstances, attesting to the possibility of a pathologically disturbed existence, also tells us something about the nature of human existence as such. A first encounter with senseless behavior that has not yet been fashioned by a specific diagnosis and categorized within the clinical classifying system offers an intuitive insight into the unanchored nature of our existence. Does not the possibility of senseless behavior make evident the essential unsteadiness of human existence? Does not the extreme possibility of inconsistent experience refer to the question of the finitude of human existence?

This is exactly the conclusion that Michel Foucault draws from his analysis of the place of psychoanalysis within the field of humanities in his *Les mots et les choses*.[4] Unlike other humanities that are part of modern knowledge, psychoanalysis represents such a mode of knowing which not only perceives the positivity of human being as based on its finitude, but actually gravitates toward that very finitude. As an analytic of finitude, psychoanalysis directly addresses that which other humanities can observe only indirectly. Its focus is the realm of the empirical, out of which emerge the empty figures of Death, Desire and Law, irreducible to any given system of representation. When human being exhausts itself in the infinite repetition of death, when desire becomes devoid of its object and language operates as an empty law, modern thought encounters the finitude which is the very basis of our existing, thinking and speaking. Since it is schizophrenia that reveals finitude in its crystal clear form, Foucault regards it as the ultimate vanishing point and simultaneously the ordeal proper to psychoanalytic inquiry. Although psychoanalysis can never by any means fathom the ground of schizophrenia, it must incessantly approach this peculiar form of experience, whose intentional structure collapses. What brings about this endless descent is not the fact that schizophrenic disturbance of existence is equivalent to a profound deficiency of the common sense. Rather, its necessity springs from the fact that schizophrenic inconsistency of experience reveals in non-sense and un-reason the bottomless depth of human facticity. Non-sense and un-reason are, strictly speaking, located outside of the sphere within which the categories of error, deceit and untruth are applicable, for what they unveil are the essential qualities of human existence: its contingency and finitude.

---

[4] Foucault, Michel. 1971. *Les mots et les choses*. Paris: Gallimard, 385–8.

It would be a mistake, however, to consider the idea of human finitude as some a-historical given. The issue of finitude as known to modern rationality emerges only with the epistemological rupture of discovering human being in the full positivity of its life. The change which, according to *Les mots et les choses*, takes place at the beginning of the nineteenth century consists not so much in the effort to improve our understanding human being as it is a new relation to human existence. While classical thought had perceived human being only through its incommensurability with the Infinite, the modern experience is grounded upon the finitude of its existence. The dusk of metaphysics is heralded when finitude is thought no longer against the background of the Infinite but in itself. The finitude of human existence thus refers not to the unattainable world beyond, but rather to man's factual position in the world.

It is by no means fortuitous that Heidegger's ontological description of being-in-the-world plays a principle role in the modern discourse of finitude, for it is here that the sublime relation between human existence and time is discovered. When Heidegger raises the issue concerning the basic evidence, conjoining the Cartesian "I think" with "I am" by means of questioning the peculiar nature of that "I am," not only does he extricate being (*das Sein*) from the captivity of representation, but also places in the forefront the question of its temporality. The phenomenological description of temporal existence then unfolds into the dwelling in the clearing of beings which is borne solely by its ecstatic temporality. The present, the past and the future, all manifest themselves to phenomenological seeing as three equally original ec-stases in which the temporary dwelling in the clearing of beings unfolds. This exposition also makes it possible to comprehend wherein the essentially inconstant and unanchored nature of human existence lies. Since the temporality of human existence is primarily future-oriented, human being is uncontrollably carried away from its origin. What follows from the inquiry into the modern episteme carried out in *Les mots et les choses* is that human being can never return to its own origin because it is constantly torn away from it by its own temporality. The descent toward the origin is always already a step into the future, and therefore human existence can never attain the pure presence that is given to things. Human existence can never encounter itself in the mode of full presence, but only in the transition from the empirical givens of the world to its own origin that keeps eluding its grasp. In contrast to the mute permanence of things, its individual character is determined by ecstatic temporality, which is the basis for existential historicity that stretches from birth to death. The individual integrity of human existence and the ensuing consistency of experience are preserved as the temporal unity of existence that temporalizes itself in the repeated search for the receding origin. The supremely modern way in which Heidegger tries to find human existence in its individuality leads him to the realm of sameness, maintained in the repeated experiencing of the irreducible difference. In his treatment of temporality, in which the idea of the Infinite and the hope of resting upon sheer self-presence are discarded, modern ontology achieves the cognition of the finitude of human existence.

Insofar as the individuality of human existence is inextricably connected with its temporality, one needs to ask what role, in this respect, is played by the possibility of a psychopathological disorder. If temporality is the only medium determining human existence in its individuality, how is it possible to relate to it that form of finitude which manifests itself in the inconsistency of human experience? As Foucault mentions in his *Naissance de la Clinique*, the experience of individuality in modern thought is born not out of relating to the Infinite, but out of experiencing death.[5] The relation to death cuts human being off from universality and bestows upon its existence a singular character. By virtue of its intimate experience with death, medicine obtains a privileged position among the other sciences about man, for it especially makes contact with the ontological status of human existence as such. In this respect psychiatry is no different from the rest of medical knowledge. Death which seizes human being in the disintegration of consistency of experience is by no means a mere event to be discerned among others, but it is first and foremost the foundational vanishing point of human existence. For schizophrenia or any other psychopathological disorder to develop, death must be there, already anonymously at work in the very heart of human existence. Accordingly, individual existence asserts itself in its resistance to this form of human finitude.

It is in any case clear from Foucault's picture of modern knowledge that the threat of the overall disintegration of individual existence provides the innermost potentiality, as well as the neuralgic point, of the phenomenological description of the temporal dwelling in the clearing of beings. A possible disintegration of the temporal unity of existence is adumbrated in Heidegger's ontological project from its very beginning, and yet it seems difficult to address the end of individual existence as such. The phenomenology of finitude finds itself in a deadlock when aiming to describe the demise of the individual existence. Pondering the schizophrenic disintegration of experience, Binswanger relies on the assumption of an integral being-in-the-world whose personal integrity is impaired by the influence of a pathological disorder, instead of taking the end of individual existence itself as the focus of his method. Such is the case in *Zollikoner Seminare* as well, where the essence of psychopathological disorders is determined on the basis of the integral unity of individual existence. The schizophrenic's alleged experience of being dead, the collapse of the world, and the disintegration of the self thus appear merely as expressions of a deficient dwelling in the clearing of beings and not as original, non-derived phenomena.

Hence, if we dare to enter the mine-field that is the realm of relations between psychopathology and Heidegger's conceptualization of the finitude of human existence, this is not done merely in order to follow in his footsteps. Although Boss's psychiatric erudition doubtlessly enriched the philosophical perspectives presented in *Zollikoner Seminare*, it is imperative that this work be treated at a critical distance, thereby allowing us to assess the tenability or untenability of the foundational principles of Heidegger's approach to the phenomenon of psychopathological disorder. A possible pitfall does not consist only in the clumsiness of a philosopher entering into the field of psychiatric inquiry without the basic knowledge that the specialist has. The very question of a psychopathologically

---

[5] Foucault, Michel. 1963. *Naissance de la Clinique*. Paris: PUF, 201–2.

conditioned end of individual existence reveals the limits of the modern episteme within whose framework human being is given the central place in the system of knowledge. This indicates the necessity of thinking that is devoid of any anthropological certainty. It is precisely this question that forces us to make a delicate and yet foundational semantic shift which, according to Foucault, consists in the transition from the finitude of man's being to the end of man as the vanishing point of all thought.[6]

In order not to set out in blindness to the border zone of the modern episteme, guidelines must be found which could serve us as a critical correlate of the results of Heidegger's inquiry. Apart from Foucault's archeology of knowledge, such guidelines should be sought mainly in the so-called schizoanalysis, created by the shared effort of Gilles Deleuze and Félix Guattari in opposition to the mainstream of modern psychiatry and its individualistic conception of psychopathological disorders. As the word itself suggests, the task of schizoanalysis is to comprehend schizophrenia as a crucial philosophical problem that casts light not only on the boundaries of the individual existence, but also on the limits of human existence as such. Insofar as Deleuze and Guattari object to Binswanger's approach to schizophrenia (and implicitly to the phenomenological project of the temporal dwelling in the clearing of beings) due to its methodical adherence to human individuality whose presupposition a priori precludes an adequate explication of clinical states of deep depersonalization or delirious states and the related hallucinations, their schizoanalysis is conducted with the intention of penetrating to the a-personal processes that repeatedly confirm the disintegration of individual existence.[7] Unlike the ontological description of the in-dividual being-in-the-world, schizoanalysis attempts at a terminological comprehension of the *dividual* nature of our experience. In this sense, it can be understood as a more radical conceptualization of the end of individual existence.

However, the sense of the confrontation outlined above is definitely not to merely substitute one philosophical conception with another. Since Heidegger's work, according to Foucault's claim in *Les mots et les choses*, surpasses the scope of the modern episteme in an intriguing way, the appropriate treatment consists not in quickly dismissing it, but rather in a detailed examination of those works by Heidegger that are, in one way or another, relevant to understanding psychopathological phenomena. Hence, apart from *Zollikoner Seminare* and *Sein und Zeit*, it is necessary to also to consider texts such as *Die Grundbegriffe der Metaphysik*, *Beiträge zur Philosophie*, or *Erläuterungen zu Hölderlins Dichtung*, the interpretation of which should not only point to some of the blind spots of the ontological project of the temporal dwelling in the clearing of beings, but also delineate the hitherto unrecognized possibilities of Heidegger's thought. This is the path that can lead us to the answer to the question concerning ontological conditions of insanity as such.

---

[6] Foucault. *Les mots et les choses*, 396.

[7] Deleuze, Gilles, and Guattari, Félix. 1975. *L'Anti-Œdipe. Capitalisme et schizophrénie*. Paris: Minuit, 30.

References

1. Binswanger, Ludwig. 1957. *Schizophrenie*. Pfullingen: Neske.
2. Deleuze, Gilles, and Félix Guattari. 1972. *L'Anti-Oedipe: Capitalisme et schizophrénie*. Paris: Minuit. English edition: Deleuze, Gilles, and Félix Guattari. 1983. *Anti-Oedipus: Capitalism and Schizophrenia*. Trans. Robert Hurley, Mark Seem, and Helen R. Lane. Minneapolis: University of Minnesota Press. Foucault, Michel. 1963. *Naissance de la Clinique*. Paris: PUF.
3. Foucault, Michel. 1963. *Naissance de la Clinique*. Paris: PUF. English edition: Foucault, Michel. 1973. *The Birth of the Clinic*. Trans. A.M. Sheridan. London: Tavistock Publications Limited.
4. Heidegger, Martin. 1987. *Zollikoner Seminare. Protokolle, Gespräche, Briefe*. ed. Medard Boss. Frankfurt am Main: Vittorio Klostermann. English edition: Heidegger, Martin. 2001. *Zollikon Seminars*. Trans. Franz Mayr and Richard Askay. Evanston: Northwestern University Press.
5. Heidegger, Martin. 1993. *Sein und Zeit*, 17th ed. Tübingen: Niemeyer. English edition: Heidegger, Martin. 1996. *Being and Time*. Trans. Stambaugh, Joan. Albany: SUNY Press.

Chapter 2
Methodological Pitfalls

2.1 Inhuman Science

Having situated Heidegger's thought in the epistemological scheme outlined by Foucault in his *Les mots et les choses*, we can discern not only its general contours, but also its limitations. We may even think of possible ways to transgress the limits of the ontological analysis of human existence and try to see mental disorders in a different light. It might be therefore effective to use the critical potential of *Les mots et les choses* to a maximum.

In the following chapter, Heidegger's critique of natural science and its domination in the area of psychiatry, as it is formulated in his *Zollikoner Seminare*, shall be confronted with Foucault's epistemological analysis of the classical thought that is conducted in *Les mots et les choses* and with the picture of classical medicine that Foucault presents in his *Naisannce de la clinique*. This confrontation brings to the fore the Cartesian idea of *mathesis universalis* which functions as a general matrix of scientific thought. The play of conceptual identities and differences based on the general matrix of *mathesis universalis*, however, leaves no place for the individuality of human existence. To grasp the individuality of human existence, both phenomenology and medicine must turn away from the conceptual scheme of *mathesis universalis* and from the classical notion of thought. Together with the individuality of human existence, phenomenology also uncovers the phenomenon of the lived body which reflects the psychosomatic nature of human existence. In his *Zollikoner Seminare* Heidegger then integrates the individuality of the human existence with the phenomenon of the lived body in the complex structure of being-in-the-world.

But before we reach the phenomenal structure of human existence, we must understand what prevents natural science from reaching the realm in which human existence finds itself. We need to examine methodological principles of natural science in order to discover the significance of the hegemony of natural science in the area of medicine. Despite an enormous progress in the effectiveness of medical treatment and the huge amount of information about the processes in human

© Springer International Publishing Switzerland 2015
P. Kouba, *The Phenomenon of Mental Disorder*, Contributions
to Phenomenology 75, DOI 10.1007/978-3-319-10323-5_2

organism, medicine formed by natural science is, according to Heidegger, deceived in its approach to human existence by its very understanding of reality. Only if one arrives at understanding of what is real for natural science, is it thus possible to declare that there are any phenomena beyond the reach of natural science.

The inquiry into the methodic principles of a specific discipline is usually understood as examining the methodology of a scientific work in the relevant field of study. In the case of physics, which in *Zollikoner Seminare* serves as a model of natural science, the key role is played by scientific experiments and theoretical hypotheses. These two aspects of scientific work are essentially interdependent. Inasmuch as the scientific experiment is derived from an underlying theory, its results can lead to a revision of the given theory. With the help of the scientific experiment, it is to be shown whether or not the theoretical hypothesis corresponds to reality. In their reciprocal correlation, experiment and theoretical construction contribute to the co-operative discovery of nature. The two research methods share their scientific exactitude which is manifested in the use of mathematical forms and relations. What physical science finds in application of mathematics is an undisputed confirmation of its general validity and effectuality. The undertaken experiments and formulated hypotheses obtain the hallmark of objective truthfulness as long as they correspond to the spirit of mathematical exactitude.

However, a given means of research, which (just as an experiment or a theoretical construction) is meant to result in scientific knowledge, represents a method only in the "instrumental"[1] sense. From the purely instrumental conception of method Heidegger distinguishes method in the more original sense of the word, substantially different from the methodology of scientific inquiry. As the sense of the Greek words μετά and ὁδός (the "way from here to there" or the "way toward") suggests, method in the original etymological sense denotes an approach by means of which the character of the examined area is revealed and delineated.[2] For the scientific theses and experiments to come into play at all, it is first and foremost necessary to gain access to the area under scrutiny. Only within the framework of an area open and determined by means of a certain method is it possible to invoke incontestable facts, while elaborating on theses and verifying experimentally their validity.

The question of method is therefore of outstanding significance within the realm of physics; the direction as well as the character of the inquiry is determined not by research practices, but primarily by the method that actually allows the implementation of these practices together with their mathematically exact treatment of facts. A similar conclusion is reached by Deleuze in his *Différence et répétition* when he considers the conditions enabling the repeatability of scientific experiments.[3] As long as science presupposes the repeatability of processes observed under the same conditions, this is done not so much by applying mathematics to natural phenomena as by operating within the framework of mathematizable relations. Compared to

---

[1] Heidegger. *Zollikoner Seminare*, 167.

[2] Heidegger. *Zollikoner Seminare*, p. 137.

[3] Deleuze, Gilles. 1968. *Différence et répétition*. Paris: PUF, 9–10.

preliminary access to the area under inquiry, the mathematical formality of the means of research is secondary, since the usage of mathematical forms can yield data only in the context of primary measurability. The realm of physical processes is thus always uncovered in advance with regard to their mathematical measurability.

Since the measurability of beings, as this is presupposed by exact science, entails comprehension of a purely quantitative character, physics must disregard the qualitative richness of life and focus exclusively on its mathematically apprehensible factors. Natural entities, stripped of their semantic potential, remain merely the sum of quantitatively recordable and mutually comparable data. However, the impact of the presupposed exact measurability of things is not restricted to their simple quantifiability. What lies in their measurability is also the preliminary calculability of all processes under observation. That is to say, the changes taking place are pre-adumbrated so that different eventualities of their course are predictable.[4]

Besides, Heidegger's exposition of the methodological principles of mathematical natural science shows that the prediction of changes is possible only under conditions that guarantee elementary regularity in nature. In order for such conditions to be met, there must take place idealization, which yields homogeneous space and homogeneous time. Without it the modern conception of physical science as realized by Galileo and Newton could never have been formulated. Galileo's principal point of departure that posits the conditions of empirical inquiry is the supposition in which the occurrence of change is regarded as a regular change of the position of mass-points in homogeneous space and time. What is postulated in this supposition is also causality without which exact predictability would remain inconceivable. The scientific rationalism proper to physics is based on the belief that every occurrence must be the effect of some cause.

However, Galileo's presupposition is something that cannot, unlike the theoretical hypothesis, be proven or refuted by means of undertaking an experiment, since it reaches the ultimate ontological foundations of mathematical physics. In order to comprehend the key principles of mathematical physics, it is necessary to explicate the ontological project that underlies its method.

Heidegger's clarification of the ontological sense of the method of exact sciences derives from the understanding that as soon as there is the continuous motion of mass-points discerned in the process of change, every single thing ceases to be an entity that is present in itself and instead becomes an object. Consequently, the field proper to physical science is created by nothing other than mathematically noticeable objects concatenated in causal relations. Everything that defies this framework is automatically considered as uncertain and as not truly real. Certain, i.e. true, is only what manifests itself in the sphere of objects of observation with a mathematical index to the eye of the observing subject. Nature, articulated as a set of observed objects, is placed in relation to the thinking subject. The dichotomy of the mathematically conceived *res extensa* and *res cogitans* corroborates the vast extent to which the method of mathematical natural science is informed by Cartesian dualism.

---

[4] Heidegger. *Zollikoner Seminare*, 135.

Even though the idea of mathematical natural science reflects not so much Descartes' own philosophical system as the whole legacy of his epoch, Descartes still continues to occupy an exceptional place, since it was he who pondered mathematical physics in its ultimate foundations.

Although the objective status of natural beings can seem, with hindsight, thoroughly natural, Heidegger connects it with the historical change of European thought occurring in the seventeenth century. According to him, neither Antiquity nor the Middle Ages were familiar with such a conception of beings: whereas ancient culture comprehended natural phenomena in the sense of the Greek φαίνεσθαι, i.e. as something manifested by means of disclosing itself out of concealment, medieval thought viewed all beings as created by the God. In comparison with these views of reality, objectiveness means a certain modification of the presence of beings. Natural science is made possible by a change due to which natural beings are no longer conceptualized as present in themselves; their presence can be manifested only by virtue of the ideas of the thinking subject. Although the reality of nature is not quite denied or condemned to the sphere of mere seeming or "semblance", the presence of natural beings is thus comprehended as re-presentation.[5] What in effect is at stake here is the radical reversal in the understanding of being of natural beings – their being is inextricably linked to their representation in the subjective mind.

The foundations of mathematical physics are revealed even further in the 1935/1936 lecture series published under the title *Die Frage nach dem Ding*, where Heidegger tries to explicate the character of the mathematical order (*das Mathematische*) underlying Galileo's and Newton's conception of nature. Here, just as in *Zollikoner Seminare*, it is demonstrated that Galileo's and Newton's natural laws make sense only within the realm that is projected from the outset in terms of measurability and computability of natural beings. For nature to be intelligible by means of mathematics, it needs to be axiomatically determined as equally distributed spatiotemporal nexus of mass-points; therefore, what can be projected into the scientific picture are only bodies integrated into this nexus.

In view of the fact that Descartes had indeed been the one who in an exemplary way pondered what Galileo and Newton achieved in science, a mere glance at his *Regulae* reveals that the mathematical order, out of which modern physical science is derived, must not be conceived of as *mathematica vulgaris*, but rather as *mathesis universalis*. What is at stake is not mathematics itself, but rather a project of the factual essence of beings that allows for a neat classification and gradual transition from the elementary toward the most complex of knowledge. The mathematical order as the principal standpoint of mathematical natural science creates the grounding that allows for the division of unclear and complex sentences into simple theses and, by drawing upon these in a rationally intelligible sequence, results in an understanding of the complex ones. In the overall arrangement and composition of everything within the order of *mathesis universalis* lies the broadest foundation on which mathematical physics is built.

---

[5] Heidegger. *Zollikoner Seminare*, 129.

This matrix, claims Heidegger, is not only the origin of mathematical natural science and modern mathematics (Leibnitz's discovery of differential calculus, etc.), but also Cartesian philosophy as such. Descartes' philosophical system is arguably the fruit of deep reflections upon the mathematical order; as if the mathematical tendency in thinking had awoken and grasped itself by considering itself the criterion of all thought and devising the rules it brings forth. It is only on the basis of the mathematical order that the need arises for the discovery of the first, altogether indubitable thesis that could serve as the ultimate axiom for all other sentences, irrespective of what they address. The statement "I think therefore I am" can be the absolute foundation for the certainty of cognition only because it relies on *mathesis universalis* as the basic matrix of the seventeenth century thought. The objectification of all beings present-at-hand would be meaningless without it, for these are put in relation to the subject of the axiom "I think – I am".

It is interesting to note here that the characteristics of mathematically organized knowledge mentioned above converges in many respects with Foucault's picture of the classical episteme. As the epistemological investigation undertaken in *Les mots et les choses* indicates, the arrival of classical science in the seventeenth century marks a rupture in the history of European thought. Not that science would have only at this point acquired a sense of measure and order; what occurred was that an altogether extraordinary importance was attributed to the values which had to some extent already been acknowledged. What is characteristic of the epistemological field of classical science is that measure and order serve as points of departure as well as the ultimate imperatives of thought.

The example of Descartes' *Regulae* clearly demonstrates that it is by virtue of the universal validity of measure and order that not only deductive derivation and clear, purely intellectual observation of a certain thing, but also the comparison between two or more things achieve a new formal status. Apart from comparing quantities for the sake of determining the arithmetical relations of equality and inequality among things, Descartes also acknowledges comparison by means of order, within whose framework the simplest term is found and from there also the progression from simpler to more complex elements. As the measurement of size or amount can be reduced to creating order (since arithmetic and physical quantities may be arranged into a continuous row), both of the types merely represent two different ways of determining the progression from the simple to the complex. Thus, Foucault concludes that it is the idea of *mathesis universalis*, of the overall, rationally observable order, that plays the key role in the classical episteme. No matter how prevalent mathematical formalism might be within certain scientific realms, the plane proper to classical knowledge is not the mathematization of all reality and the concomitant conversion of a qualitative difference into a quantitative one. The mathematization of the empirical asserts itself only in such realms of classical science as the Galilean and Newtonian physics, whereas the relation of understanding to the general order as proposed in *mathesis universalis* also concerns the non-quantifiable. Insofar as classical science as a whole shares some common characteristics, this lies, according to Foucault, in its preoccupation with what he terms "the calculable order" in the broadest sense of the word. The reference to *Regulae* also lays bare another consequence of general calculability: the possibility of an exhaustive inventory. Whether the issue under consideration is an exhaustive list of all elements of a given set, or a division of an observed field into specific categories, or an analysis of a sufficiently representative specimen, *mathesis universalis* always guarantees the possibility of an exhaustive inventory as well as a continual transition from basic levels of understanding to the most complex ones.

To remain within the field of natural scientific investigation: a good example of a science formed on the basis of classical episteme is so-called "natural history." According to Foucault, this science that deals with the order in the realm of living beings relies on the idea of a universal calculus, without necessarily resorting to mathematical reductionism. Unlike mathematical physics, natural history does not restrict itself only to quantitatively detectable values and relations, but also records other visible traits of natural beings. However, even here, a substantial reduction of the investigated area still does occur. Natural history does not inquire into the hidden qualities, forces and abilities that had determined the direction of natural scientific inquiry prior to the seventeenth century; nature is here relevant only insofar as it is accessible to the observing gaze.

Even the utilization of such an extraordinary means as the microscope is no exception to this rule. The exposition offered in *Les mots et les choses* proves the contrary: the implementation of the microscope is conditioned by a systematic reduction of the scientific perspective. Smells, tastes, and tactile sensations – all become excluded from the scientific observation. On the other hand, what is overtly privileged is sight, the sense of clarity and extension. Nevertheless, even sight is not accepted without certain limitation: especially the perception of colors is suppressed to the very minimum and what stands in the forefront are lines, areas, forms and surfaces. To observe is thus to determine natural beings with regard to their form, number, size and mode of their placement in space. However, this space is not the natural ambience of living beings, but an abstract space out of which all vital relations have been excluded. Whether concrete pieces of knowledge are ascertained quantitatively, or by means of geometrical forms, or through exact description, it is always within a visual field reduced to pure extension. The theme proper to natural history is therefore extension in which natural beings are manifested. In this respect, natural history is not by any means remote from mathematical physics that finds a guarantee for the quantifiability of natural beings in their position within the realm of *res extensa*.

The epistemological affinity of these two scientific disciplines, which emerges from their connection with *mathesis universalis*, does not, however, reach beyond the emphasis on perfect clarity and controllability of knowledge. Whereas the Galilean and Newtonian physics relies on nothing but mathematically formalized methods, natural history is content with an exhaustive inventory and a description of natural beings, thanks to which a certain specimen in various situations can be depicted in the exact same manner. The key to a reliable recognition of a certain animal or plant is their characteristic trait. Natural history focuses on determining the characteristic traits, thanks to which it states the differences among natural beings and classifies them, dividing them up into genera and species so that every creature finds its own place in the natural scheme of things. As every category must stand in relation to all others, what is peculiar to a certain specimen cannot be recognized except on the basis of a classification of natural beings. An animal or a plant has no identity of its own; it is that which others are not, as it is discernible only by means of differentiation. To identify a certain specimen is thus to ascertain what it is that sets it apart from other species. Any identification of natural beings encompasses a whole chain of differentiations. When natural history assesses the determination of genera and species of empirical specimens, it is not guided by vague similarities among natural beings. It persistently analyzes the relations of their affinity solely by means of the notions of identity and difference. These notions, however, don't only govern the natural scientific taxonomy; as arithmetical relations of equality and inequality, they are also to be found in mathematical measurement and comparison. Therefore, Foucault can indeed proclaim the classical episteme as a whole to be characterized not only by the universal science of order, but also by the search for identity and difference.

The structure of the classical episteme must have left its traces in many other disciplines, including medical thought – however, not only by means of the physicalization of the human body, as one might suspect, but in a manner much more subtle than that. The analysis of classical thought which is presented in *Les mots et les choses* shows that the idea of the body as a physical mechanism, as this is widespread thanks to the influence of Descartes', has dominated medicine only for a relatively brief time period. Natural scientific thought found its fulfillment in medical science, but it was natural history rather than mathematical physics that provided the model for scientific thought in this area. Its influence on medical thought is traceable on the pages of *Naissance de la clinique*, where Foucault addresses the so-called classificatory medicine. Similarly to natural history, classificatory medicine cannot do without a taxonomical system, within whose framework diseases are classified and hierarchized into various genera and species. What is important for its concerns is not so much the mechanical functioning of the corporeal apparatus or exact measurement of its blood pressure and temperature as the precise diagnosis of the type of disease and its ranking within the classifying system of diseases. The task of the classificatory medicine is to discern in the vast profusion of symptoms certain traits, to differentiate them from other pathological phenomena and to undertake their precise identification. In quest of the precise identification of pathological changes, the medical gaze functions as an instrument of scientific cognition that reveals, on the basis of the botanical model, the rational order of disease. The understanding of this "pathological garden," a reliable knowledge of specific types of diseases and their mutual differences, functions as the foundational guideline for the doctor and, at the same time, as the indispensable prerequisite of a successful treatment. Whether classical medicine conforms to natural scientific classification or to Cartesian mechanicism, it never loses its elemental relation to *mathesis* as the universal science of measure and order.

In the light of these observations, Heidegger's evaluation of the natural scientific mode of reasoning that is presented in *Zollikon Seminars* requires a certain adjustment. It is not problems of mathematical physics, but rather the foundational character of the mathematical project of beings as such that is to receive attention. In relation to the primary mathematical project, physics remains only one of the realms in which *mathesis universalis* has shaped itself as the cardinal standpoint to beings in general. Heidegger himself is very clearly aware of it in his *Die Frage nach dem Ding* where he stresses that the question of whether the utilization of mathematical procedures is indeed justified with regard to immediately present nature is not so important as the decision concerning the verification and limits of the mathematical order as such. It is not enough to confront the will to render nature quantifiable on the one hand, and nature essentially recalcitrant to it on the other. Behind the dilemma between mathematical formalism and the clarifying view of natural beings looms the question of limits beyond which the idea of *mathesis universalis* loses its justification.

From the perspective of the mathematical order itself the critical reflection on *mathesis universalis* may indeed seem to be a highly problematic undertaking. The mathematical order as the overall arrangement and distribution of observed beings has no limits, as it concerns both quantifiable and unquantifiable beings. Rather, *mathesis universalis* itself, from which not only mathematical natural science but also other scientific fields including philosophy evolve, is what determines the limits of scientifically exact reasoning. After all, any conceptual thought outside of the frame of measure and order is impossible, and so is any kind of science!

However, before accepting this presupposition, it is necessary to clarify what is understood by conceptual thought. In *Zollikoner Seminare*, the special position and function of scientific concepts receives careful scrutiny.[6] Scientific thought, derived from the mathematical project of beings, requires in the first place that the concepts should be thoroughly unambiguous. Any ambiguity is to be excluded by means of a clear definition of every single notion. A correct definition proceeds in such a way that characterizes an entity by means of primary generality and secondary specificity; a general definition of an entity is accompanied by a characteristic trait that differentiates a given entity from other entities of the same kind. Definition thus proceeds from a higher category to the delineation of a specific difference. By virtue of this procedure, it is possible to single out and delimit one entity as opposed to all others.

So far, a conceptual definition wouldn't be different from the way in which the Ancient thought used to differentiate various categories of beings. What is important, however, is to realize that conceptual thought as constituted on the basis of *mathesis universalis* is inextricably linked with representation. Heidegger claims a concept to be a re-presentation of something. The very word "concept" (*der Begriff*) inherently echoes "capture" or "concentration" which becomes, on the basis of the mathematical project, a representation of something. However, what is represented within the framework of conceptual representation is not a singular entity, but that which is common to all beings of a certain type. This representation is what remains identical in all individual cases.[7] Only with regard to identity that is contained

---

[6] Heidegger. *Zollikoner Seminare*, 169–73.

[7] Heidegger. *Zollikoner Seminare*, 171–2.

within every scientific concept is it possible to comprehend individual beings as representatives of relevant species. Although a concept is a representation of what is identically the same, it is still impossible to speak of this identity in positive terms. The identity represented in a concept has a sense only in relation to differences arranged within the overall system of understanding. Thus, the structure of *mathesis universalis* within the framework of conceptual thought is manifested as a complex order of identities and differences.

Nevertheless, conceptual thought grounded upon *mathesis universalis* runs against its limits once it is expected to comprehend the unique or the ambiguous. Since every notion must be absolutely unambiguous, it cannot grasp reality in its multitude of meanings. Faced with an ambiguous situation, the scientific notion becomes a hindrance in thinking. The same applies to every thing that needs to be shown in its irreducible singularity. To grasp what is peculiar to one single entity by means of concepts that assert themselves within the framework of *mathesis universalis* is altogether inconceivable, for their function is to highlight that remains identical in many beings. Even though abstraction as such does not quite explain what brings about the uncompromising unambiguousness of scientific notions, the necessity to disregard all singularities remains a side effect of conceptual thought. Any singularity gets lost by necessity in the interminable interplay of identities and differences.

It is this problem that Foucault alludes to while considering in his *Naissance de la clinique* the ambivalent attitude that classificatory medicine takes toward human suffering: as long as the view of medical science aims to penetrate through the plethora of pathological symptoms to their invariable foundation, it must suppress the uniqueness of every individual case and highlight what is common to all cases of the same kind. In order to pinpoint the basis of pathological disorder correctly, classificatory medicine must keep its distance from the individual experience of the patient and bracket all unclassifiable factors such as innate dispositions, temperament, or age. A qualified medical treatment cannot do without a perfected command of the classifying system of diseases that serves as a preliminary guideline of cognition, whereas the patient's individuality is merely a negative attribute of the illness. Rather than the personal uniqueness of the patient and the unmistakable nature of his individuality, what is really important is the precise identification of the disease and its differentiation from all other elements of the nosological system. The individual side of human ordeal, including the peculiar multivocal nature of the space in which the doctor meets the patient, is thus bound to stay in the background of theoretical interest. Although classificatory medicine does not remain altogether blind to these phenomena, this is not due to its methodical effort to identify and differentiate the various kinds of pathology, but rather in spite of this.

Since Cartesian medicine is no less dependent on the clearly structured schema of identities and differences, the same applies to it as well. One might object that Cartesian philosophy at least maintains a relation to individual experience that is echoed in the foundational tenet of "I think." However, as Heidegger observes in *Die Frage nach dem Ding*, the "I" as based on the mathematical order and promoted to the paramount status of the thinking subject contains nothing particular or unique.

The subjectivity of the "I" lies only in the sheer necessity of its presupposition. In every utterance or act of thinking there is always presupposed the *ego* that thinks. The *ego* is what is always already present prior to any representation. Thus, the basis of the Cartesian "I" is not the individuality of a specific human being, but the permanent presence of the thinking subject. The "I" means nothing more and nothing less than *res cogitans*, out of which all qualities except for the ability to think have been abstracted.

Of course, the ability to represent is not restricted only to conceptual determination. Another mode of representation is to be added to the conceptual utterance, and that is sensual perception. In both cases, something is rendered present for the conscious "I" by means of representation. Although this "I" does not have to be always explicitly aware of itself, it must necessarily retain its substantial identity. In relation to the "I" regarded as the subject of thinking, all other things appear as objects. The objective status of the observed beings is nothing given *per se*, since it follows from the turning point in the understanding of the being of beings as brought about by Descartes on the basis of the mathematical order. The so-called objective reality is an ontological construct arising from the quest for the absolute certainty of understanding. As soon as this certainty has been found in the constant presence of the substantial "I," all beings lacking the character of the "I" are regarded as objects.

It is nonetheless disputable whether such an ontology can in fact be adequately applied to human being. The exposition presented in *Zollikoner Seminare* most resolutely testifies against this possibility. Heidegger does not miss a single opportunity to point to the fact that an ontology that understands being from the viewpoint of representation does not do justice to human existence. In his opinion, the peculiar character of human existence cannot be understood as long as human being is rendered an object about which scientific thought obtains data by means of conceptual representations. The inadequacy of this approach is demonstrated by the fact that human experiences and moods are not objects within the sphere of *res extensa*, something which was already known to Descartes. It is insufficient to proclaim human existence to have, in addition to its somatic part, also a part pertaining to the realm of *res cogitans*, and go on to examine their mutual effects. The multivocal shades and minute nuances of mental life cannot be understood once converted into representations in the consciousness of an abstractly conceived subject. The same applies to the human body which can be imagined as a physical mechanism and whose components can be subjected to physiological inquiry, but only at the cost of losing all human uniqueness. What then remains of it is an object torn out of its relation to its environment, an object resisting inner development and changes that have to do with aging. At best, ageing can manifest itself as dilapidation or imperfection that science may manage to remedy one day, but not as a natural principle of life.

Although this reduction concerns every biological organism, it is most clearly conspicuous in relation to human being. Natural history and mathematical physics, which both rely on *mathesis universalis*, can perceive human being only as a natural species or as a mathematically intelligible object. However, once the question is raised as to who human being is and how it exists, both disciplines are faced with the limits of their possibilities. The way in which human being as the unique individual relates to things, to others, to itself and to its own end remains by necessity beyond the reach of their understanding.

In general, one can say that this limitation applies to all scientific fields based on mathematical project of being of beings. The mathematical order asserted itself within Western thought not because it enabled us to unveil the peculiar character of human existence, but because it guaranteed a lucid classification of all realms of knowledge, irrespective of the specific character of the beings under observation. The universal order based on the idea of *mathesis universalis* is not only a visible arrangement of things, not only a symmetrical configuration of their proportions and relations, but the modus of being attributed to them prior to every empirical inquiry. The question of the peculiar character of human existence is neither the central theme nor the guideline of scientific thought. It is therefore no wonder that human existence, recalcitrant both to classification by means of conceptual identification and differentiation, and to preliminary objectification, stakes out the limits beyond which the mathematical order can no longer guarantee an adequate understanding.

With regard to the central role played by the idea of *mathesis universalis* within the whole scope of classical knowledge, it is self-evident that to inquire into the boundaries of the validity of the mathematical project of beings is to contemplate the outer limits of the classical episteme. The universal science of measure and order acknowledges only its inner boundaries, beyond which all non-scientific opinions and confused utterances are brushed aside. Nevertheless, the mere fact that classical science has its historical beginning implies that one day it is bound to reach its end. The idea of universal calculability as born in the seventeenth century does not necessarily have to perish together with it, but it most definitely must be deprived of its claim to absolute validity. In that very moment, the question of the limits of the universal science of measure and order becomes topical.

It would therefore be inane to regard Heidegger's critical reference to the inadequacy of all attempts at thematisation of human existence by means of a method that is grounded upon preliminary objectification and conceptual identification of observed beings as an expression of ill-concealed enmity to science as such. Heidegger himself refuses such a suspicion when claiming: "By no means should our discussions be understood as hostile toward science. In no way is science as such rejected."[8]

However, what remains questionable is that the ideas grounded upon *mathesis universalis* assert themselves within a field where human existence is at stake. Pushing into forefront the question of human existence, Heidegger strives for nothing else but rendering human existence understandable and explicable out of itself. Judged by the prism of *Les mots et les choses*, an attempt at directing attention to what concerns man himself and what by necessity eludes him in the sieve of objectifying ideas reflects the rupture between classical and modern knowledge. On the epistemological plane, the philosophical critique of the mathematical

---

[8] Heidegger. *Zollikon Seminars*, 110. Heidegger. *Zollikoner Seminare*, 143.

project of beings, especially as far as its principal incompatibility with the human way of being is concerned, appears possible only by virtue of the rupture whereby the theme of human being breaks into the visual field of scientific inquiry. As long as classical discourse fuses the representation and the being of beings with the same certainty with which the *cogito* allies with the *sum* of the thinking subject, the question of human existence cannot be raised. The formulation of the question of human existence is thus accompanied with the retreat of thought from the space of representation and the breakup of the general project of *mathesis universalis*. With the arrival of modern episteme, a rearrangement occurs within whose framework the structure of the calculable order, and together with it the formal disciplines such as mathematics and physics, stands on one side, and in opposition to it is the realm within which interpretive disciplines such as hermeneutics and clinical diagnostics evolve.[9]

However, the very breakup and substantial narrowing of the sphere of *mathesis universalis* does not guarantee an adequate thematization of human existence. The mere discovery of the theme does not mean the final victory, but rather poses an interminable task. For the adequate approach to human existence to be safeguarded, it does not suffice to merely register details and personal peculiarities of individuals. Heidegger is well aware of the fact that attention to the human individual and its unique qualities alone cannot lead to anything quite yet. Insofar as human existence is to be thematized in an adequate manner, it is first of all necessary to find a method that would discover the way into the realm where human existence can be encountered as such.

This path cannot be procured by empirical observation, but only by philosophical inquiry. A real, and not merely illusory, approach to human being requires a philosophical method that would be fully appropriate to the specifically human way of existence. The demanded method must strictly adhere to the mode in which human existence shows itself, and leave it at that. A method that meets the given criterion and allows for the thematization of human existence without inadmissible distortion or confusion is found in phenomenological description. According to Heidegger, phenomenology provides us with the optimal approach to human existence whose reach qualitatively surpasses the mode of thematization based on *mathesis universalis*.

However, the peculiar mode of phenomenological description is to be strictly differentiated from a description used in, e.g., botanical classification. First of all, phenomenology is not a procedure for acquiring pieces of scientific knowledge, but a method in the original sense of the word, i.e. a way that opens a certain realm of beings. Moreover, human being from the phenomenological point of view does not manifest itself as a specimen of a certain species, be it a categorical determination of an entity traditionally defined as *animal rationale*. Unlike science shaped within the horizon of representational thought that reduces all phenomena to objects of conceptual comprehension, phenomenology strictly forbids such reductionism. Phenomenological description does not lie in the representation of facts stated in the

---

[9] Foucault. *Les mots et les choses*, 88–9, 358.

sphere of *res extensa*; its orientation is rather subjected to manifesting every phenomenon in terms of what is peculiar to it. Since they are not representations woven into any well established network of identities and differences, and their sense is drawn directly from what they speak of, phenomenological notions can reveal both the uniqueness and the ambiguity of concrete phenomena.[10] Although phenomenology is not devoid of the character of conceptual thought, its notions are not so much based on the uniform matrix of *mathesis universalis* as they are on the uniqueness and ambiguity of what manifests itself.

Inasmuch as phenomenology is led by the striving for thematization of pure phenomena, it remains to be clarified what is understood by the notion of "phenomenon." Heidegger's answer to this question is derived from the differentiation between the ontic and the ontological phenomenon. It is generally true that a phenomenon is what shows itself, but it can show itself to us in various ways. Therefore, phenomena shown to our senses are, according to *Zollikoner Seminare*, placed on the one side, and phenomena sensually imperceptible on the other.[11] Whereas the ontic phenomenon relates to sensually perceptible beings, the ontological phenomenon concerns the being of beings that can be observed only in its sense. The being of beings can be manifest only through thought that relates to it with understanding. Even though the being of beings does not show itself as such in the beginning, the preliminary evidence of its sense is a prerequisite for any ontic register. Compared to ontic phenomena, ontological phenomena therefore occupy the foundational position and are of primary philosophical importance. Since being as such often remains concealed behind beings that freely offer themselves to our attention, the task of phenomenology as Heidegger conceives of it is to bring being to its explicit manifestation.

The phenomenological effort to thematize the being of beings does not at all mean that beings are to be completely ignored. Heidegger is rather concerned with our relation to beings so that the being of these beings emerges thematically. This hermeneutic engagement in the relation with immediately manifest beings aims to overcome the obfuscation of ontological phenomena that remain hidden under a layer of philosophical tradition or merely filtered through it in the form of phenomenologically unclarified seeming. The need for penetrating to what remains unthought-of within the philosophical tradition necessarily leads to a revision of this tradition, and especially to a critical evaluation of the conceptual structures grounded upon the principle of *mathesis universalis*.

Heidegger's critique of ideas derived from the mathematical project of beings asserts itself most conspicuously in the destruction of Descartes' philosophical system. Against the unwavering certainty of *cogito – sum* that places being next to representation, *Zollikoner Seminare* focuses its scrutiny on the character of that *sum*. As Foucault in his *Les mots et le choses* claims that phenomenology is not so much a continuation of the tradition of Ancient thought as an expression of the rupture between the classical and modern episteme, the same applies to its Heideggerian

---

[10] Heidegger. *Zollikoner Seminare*, 184.
[11] Heidegger. *Zollikoner Seminare*, 7–8, 234, 281.

version.[12] Despite the proclaimed return to the Greek conception of phenomenon as that which shows itself from itself, what is corroborated here is the original connection of phenomenology with the question of the human way of being, and together with it occurs also a certain consummation of the analytics of the finitude of this being. Instead of the objective observation of a human being or a retreat to a predetermined, closed-off subject, the phenomenological approach to human existence entails a hermeneutical entry into an open relation with what encounters and addresses us. The starting point of the phenomenological approach to human existence is thus our unmediated sojourn (*der Aufenthalt*) with beings. The exceptional character of man's sojourn (*der Aufenthalt des Menschen*) is not given by occurring at some place, but rather follows from an openness toward the world that is peculiar to human existence. Our sojourn has an essentially worldly character, as it evolves within the significative whole of the world. Being-in-the-world must therefore be shown as the foundational ontological feature of human existence. In order to adumbrate the preliminary ontological structure of sojourning as formed by being-in-the-world, Heidegger uses a simple graphic schema[13]:

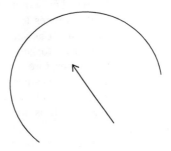

    This sketch makes the point of suggesting that human existence has nothing to do with an isolated, withdrawn subject which only secondarily relates to wordly beings. What is essential to sojourning is its openness to the possibility of addressing beings that manifest themselves in the horizon of the world. A verbatim translation of the German "sich aufhalten" (where "auf" refers to a certain openness, whereas "sich halten" means "to hold on to") suggests that the ontological character of sojourning lies in its maintaining an open horizon of the world, within whose framework significative and motivational connections present themselves in the shape of concrete beings. In the context of a disclosed and cleared sphere of the world, the sojourn always relates to that by which it is encountered and summoned to act. The sojourn finds itself always already in the world and only as being-in-the-world can it relate with understanding to specific beings as to its own possibilities.
    Since we relate to our possibilities not only spiritually, but unveil them mostly by its practical action, the question of the bodily character of human existence cannot be avoided. Should the human body be regarded as an entity occurring in a certain

---

[12] Foucault. *Les mots et les choses*, 336–7.

[13] Heidegger. *Zollikoner Seminare*, 3.

place in space, or is it to be comprehended from the viewpoint of the ontological structure of being-in-the-world? Heidegger resolutely opts for the second option when distinguishing the lived body (*der Leib*) from the corporeal thing (*der Körper*). The lived body is not a mere material given, but a factual expression of being-in-the-world. The facticity of our existence remains both in its openness to the world and in its bodiliness (*die Leiblichkeit*). The lived body is a natural center of gravity in our relating to possibilities around which the differences between near and far, up and down, right and left are organized. Corporeal things, on the contrary, have no relation to space at all, they merely occur in it.

The phenomenological description of the lived body can therefore not simply postulate it and go on to derive from this various directions and trajectories, but rather must persistently stick to the open spatiality of being-in-the-world. A dynamic transitional nature of the bodily existence can assert itself only on the basis of openness that characterises being-in-the-world. The peculiar character of this transitivity can be best illustrated by the fact that the boundaries of the lived body don't align themselves with the boundaries of the body in the sense of a mere corporeal thing. Whereas our corporeal frame ends with our skin, the lived body transcends this limit.[14] However, one can speak of a transcendence only in the phenomenal sense, since it reflects our ecstatic relatedness to surrounding beings. As hearing, speaking and seeing constitute an essential part of our lived body, its only limit is the horizon of our world. Unlike our corporeal frame whose content can change only by growing, gaining or losing weight, the horizon of our world is freely transmutable, and thus capable of vastly surpassing all tactile sensations, as well as receding in reverse into a single intensive feeling of physical pain. What then remains after our death is only *Körper*, whereas our lived body ends together with our existence.

If natural science derived from the mathematical project of beings neglects the lived body, it is because it mistakes it from the very beginning for a corporeal thing, ontologically interpreted as an object. With the help of measurements, causal-mechanical schemata and conceptual categorization, one can indeed track down many objective items of knowledge concerning the human body, but never understand the ontic aspects of the lived body. Pain, blushing with shame or weeping, all elude the view adjusted to facts represented within the realm of *res extensa*, and yet they remain inherent to the basic possibilities of our bodily existence. In order to find adequate access to these possibilities, it is not enough to consider them as traces of human psyche; it is rather necessary to understand them as various modes of being-in-the-world. After all, a sudden blush is not an expression of psychic processes, as it makes sense only in relation to some specific situation in the world. The same applies to all physical postures and gestures. All ontic phenomena that express our bodily existence have thus neither a psychic, nor a somatic, but a psychosomatic character. To split human existence into its psychic and somatic parts is for Heidegger to completely fail to regard their original whole as formed by being-in-the-world.

---

[14] Heidegger. *Zollikoner Seminare*, 112–3.

What is also bound with the overall unity of sojourning with beings is the fact that the lived body, unlike the anonymous corporeal thing, is endowed with a genuinely individual character. The lived body is always mine; or rather, I am my own body. It would be utterly absurd to contend that the eye sees, the mouth speaks, the hand works and the brain thinks, since it is always I myself who sees, speaks, works and thinks. Equally erroneous would be the assumption that the lived body presents a sort of substratum upon whose basis human individuality is sustained. This is evident from Heidegger's statement: "If the body as body is always my body, then this is my own way of being. Thus, bodying forth is co-determined by my being human in the sense of the ecstatic sojourn amidst the beings in the clearing [*gelichtet*]."[15]

That human being exists as an open being-in-the-world does not mean that its existence disintegrates into an incoherent welter of sensations, gestures and attitudes. In spite of remaining open to an address on the part of innerworldly beings, my relation to these beings is necessarily one and the same with the performance of my own existence. When coining in his *Sein und Zeit* for man's sojourn the notion of "being-there" (*das Dasein*), Heidegger says nothing of it except that it is myself, that being of being-there is in each case mine (*je meines*).[16] And the task of the ontological analysis of being-there is to reveal the locus of its peculiar individuality. Since being-there never has the character of an entity which is present-at-hand and whose qualities can be simply postulated, its individuality cannot be determined by marking out an essential substance. On the contrary, the ontological analysis must display the self in the various modes of its existence. That being-there exists as an individual follows only from the ecstatic nature of its relatedness to beings which it encounters. Heidegger's concept of the individuality is thus sharply different from the Cartesian conception of the "I" that remains identical throughout the incessant succession of its cognitive acts. While the subjective consciousness remains cut off from the world to which it is related, being-in-the-world ontologically belongs to our self. The "I" understood as individual being is not an isolated, abstract subject, but rather the specific "I am in the world."

Since individual existence does not remain detached from change, but actively engages in it, the difference between such existence and the Cartesian subject most conspicuously manifests itself on the temporal plane. The Cartesian "I" is posited as what is always already present-at-hand; that is to say, it is a substance that cannot be affected by time. The existential constancy of the self is, on the contrary, essentially connected with time. As Heidegger puts it, "[t]he constancy of the self is temporal in itself, that is, it temporalizes itself. This selfhood of [being-there] is only in the manner of temporalizing [*Zeitigung*]."[17] Ultimately the phenomenological description of the self thus extends to temporality which gives our existence its original sense. The ecstatic relatedness to beings in which our existence evolves is not

---

[15] Heidegger. *Zollikon Seminars*, 87. Heidegger. *Zollikoner Seminare,*, 113.

[16] The expressions *Aufenthalt* and *Dasein* (or *Da-sein*) are used by Heidegger basically as synonyms, and therefore we can use their English equivalents in the same way.

[17] Heidegger. *Zollikon Seminars*, 175. Heidegger. *Zollikoner Seminare*, 220.

"carried" by anything other than its own temporality. The ecstatic relatedness to beings that binds the future, the having-been and the present into one whole, ensures the essential coherence of existence, thereby endowing it with its individual constancy.[18] Much as this individual constancy remains open to change and existential rupture, it is also an expression of the fact that human existence always somehow understands its being, that it comprehends it as its own and, to some extent, as always the same.

The phenomenological description of the temporal unity of existence thus arrives at the idea of sameness which is irreconcilable with the epistemological character of classical rationality. Sameness, which encompasses in itself both constancy and change, which steps out of itself and becomes other, is according to Foucault's testimony one of the crucial components of modern episteme.

However, one must not forget that phenomenology is not the only mode of thought that on its quest for what is not identical with itself gains an understanding of individual life in its changes and duration. The revelation of human individuality is not a prerogative of only philosophical inquiry, but occurs in the much broader context of European thought, which has had its repercussions also within the field of clinical medicine, as it is documented in *Naissance de la clinique*. Ever since the eighteenth century, that is to say, with the arrival of modern episteme, medical thought has become increasingly appreciative of the importance of all unclassifiable factors that had thus far been supplanted by the classifying system of diseases. Individual dispositions, age or way of life have moved into the focal point of medical attention and, together with them, the specific human individual sees the light of day. Thanks to the reversal in the relation between the classifiable and the unclassifiable, the human individual becomes visible in its own singularity. Thus, according to Foucault, medicine is transformed into a science dealing with the ill and healthy individual. In spite of the fact that within the nosological system, the model of natural scientific classification is still utilized, there nonetheless occurs a shift that enables clinical medicine to penetrate into the inside of the human organism and reveal the dark depth of bodily existence. Only when pathological anatomy assumes the pivotal position within medical knowledge can medicine arrive at an understanding of a living organism, its development, aging and death. Rather than a classificatory table of diseases, what should henceforth be the focal point of medical interest is to be found in the various ways in which an ill organism resists or succumbs to pathological decomposition. The virtual boundaries between the disease and the patient are gradually wiped away to the point of vanishing, so that what remains is the patient and his pathologically transformed existence. Classical medicine of natural species is thereby changed into the medicine of pathological reactions.

The fact that empirical investigation of human health and disease, similar to phenomenological description of temporal sojourning, addresses the individual character of human existence does not imply that Heidegger's ontological analysis has nothing to offer to modern medicine. What gives phenomenology the hallmark of

[18] Heidegger. *Zollikoner Seminare*, 84–6.

exceptionality is both its understanding of the principal role of temporality and its sense of the integrity of the being-in-the-world that enables it to thematize complex psychosomatic phenomena without having to derive them from the functioning of the biological organism. The phenomenon of the lived body that obtains its sense against the backdrop of the overall structure of being-in-the-world is substantially different from the anatomical constitution of the human organism or the structure of the organic tissues. Even though modern medicine has marked a breakthrough in the understanding of inner development of organic structures, the lived body still remains inaccessible to it. The lived body, which forms an integral component of the ontological whole of being-in-the-world, is the key to the understanding of many psychosomatic disorders about which clinical medicine is still in the dark. Thus, the articulation of being-in-the-world can be regarded as the most important result of the phenomenological method for medicine.

The phenomenological approach to human existence is highlighted in *Zollikoner Seminare* especially in connection with psychiatry and psychotherapy which gradually free themselves from postulates determining mental disorder as a specific entity, situating it within the framework of the psychic totality of man instead. The phenomenological method can provide these disciplines with the needed philosophical foundation enabling them to adequately thematize not only the unity of psychic acts, but also the original unity of psychosomatic totality. With regard to the topic of the present study, we shall focus on the question of how, on the basis of ontological description of being-in-the-world, the nature of psychopathological disorders can be understood.

2.2 All-Too-Human Science

The focus of this chapter is Binswanger's psychiatric *Daseinsanalysis*, which represents the first attempt at the application of Heidegger's philosophy in psychiatry. The exhaustive study of Binswanger's concept of mental health and illness is followed by its criticism formulated by Heidegger in *Zollikoner Seminare*. Heidegger reproaches Binswanger for his anthropologism and for the complete misunderstanding of the ontological analysis of human existence. In order to avoid such misunderstanding, it is necessary to expound the ontological view on being-there to its full extent. While Binswanger understands human existence only as sojourn with beings, it is necessary to grasp it as sojourn in the openness of being. Sojourn is not only sojourn among beings, but – above all – sojourn in the openness of being. Only in this way can the individual character of our existence be understood properly. However, the question remains how to grasp the nature of mental disorders including the disintegration of the self that occurs in the most serious cases. This issue becomes even more crucial if we realize the limits of the ontological analysis of human existence that are highlighted by its confrontation with Foucalts' notion of Unreason and by Deleuze's critique of Heidegger formulated in *Différence et répétition*.

As regards the possibilities offered by the phenomenological description of our existence within the framework of psychiatric and psychological investigations Binswanger's work was indeed pioneering. Long before the Zollikon seminars took place, this philosophically educated psychiatrist attempted to work with the stimuli gained from Heidegger's *Sein und Zeit* and, based on these, to create a new conception of mental disorders. The result of his effort was the so-called psychiatric *Daseinsanalysis*, which drew upon the ontological analysis of being-there (*das Dasein*).

Even though no explicit mention of psychopathological phenomena is to be found in *Sein und Zeit*, Binswanger came to realize that the ontological analysis of being-there is of eminent importance for the realm of psychiatry. Psychiatry had already in his time achieved the understanding of mental disorders as having a reality and making sense only when treated as an inner disorder of the personality; however, it still lacked the means for thematizing the pathological aspects of the interaction between the human individual and his/her environment. In the given state of affairs, with medicine strictly distinguishing mental pathology from organic pathology, the overall position of the specific individual in the world, as well as his/her psychosomatic unity, remained an unsolved problem. In order to explicate pathological changes of personality without extracting it from its immediate standing in the world, Binswanger made use of the phenomenological interpretation of being-there, which highlights the individuality of our existence and considers being-in-the-world its inseparable component. It was against this background that the variegated forms of psychically disturbed behavior could be outlined and explained as various modes of being-in-the-world.

Before we embark on elucidating the various forms of psychically disturbed behavior, we must raise the question concerning the way one actually encounters that which common language describes as insanity. The reflections summed up in the collection of several casuistries, published under the title *Schizophrenia*, depart from the discovery that the primary encounter with insanity is an encounter not with mental illness but with otherness.[19] The lay view governed by the standard rules of social behavior regards certain comportment as crazed or deranged when inappropriate to the given situation. When, for example, Binswanger's patient Ilsa puts her hand inside a red-hot oven in order to show her father how far true love can go, her gesture is far-fetched to the point that none of her relatives can imagine themselves acting as she does. Others view her act not as a loving sacrifice but rather as senseless self-violence, which prevents them from identifying with it even hypothetically. The anxious fear of gaining weight felt by Ellen West, or the panic dread of being pursued sensed by Suzanne Urban – both seem equally foreign to "sane" reason. All of these patients of Binswanger's move away from their fellowmen in the same degree to which they alienate themselves from the stimuli and possibilities that spring from the framework of the everyday world of practical intentions and tasks. Thus, the inevitable lot of any individual whose action is not governed by the

---

[19] Binswanger. *Schizophrenie*, 44–6.

unwritten rules and requirements of everyday reality is to rupture the bonds that connect him/her to others.

Although behavior that defies the commonly shared semantic contexts is assumed to be deranged in a given situation, it could nevertheless seem perfectly normal in a different social situation or cultural context. What is accepted as a common or even desired way of behavior in one cultural environment is considered unacceptable in another. Whereas in the secular society, messianic visions, conversations with angels or deep dejection arising from the awareness of one's sinfulness are regarded as expressions of religious derangement, in a religious community these can be assigned the highest value. According to Binswanger, the significance attributed to insanity varies depending on the cultural environment: where modern rationality discovers symptoms of mental illness, the previous centuries had found signs of possession by the devil, fallenness and malediction. In the so-called primitive cultures, however, an individual can become a shaman only on the basis of his/her ability to confront others with something "beyond" their comprehension.

Irrespective of the system of social and cultural norms, insanity always first manifests itself in the form of a behavior devoid of sense. Since the deranged behavior does not correspond to the semantic context of everyday world, it must appear to others as unreasonable; its motives remain opaque and intentions inscrutable. As the madman's speech does not emerge from the context of the commonly shared world, it does not lay bare what it speaks about, but rather conceals it. Its nature is not apophantical but cryptic. The madman thus confronts others with the possibility of losing their mind and simultaneously lets them peer into the dark abyss that gapes beyond the boundaries of their understanding.

Only out of the primary encounter with the disturbing otherness of the insane could European culture have given birth to such sciences as psychology and psychiatry. The extent to which the encounter with un-reason had been constitutive of both disciplines was shown by Foucault in his early treatises *Maladie mentale et psychologie* and *L'histoire de la folie*. Binswanger is also aware that the primary point of departure of psychiatric inquiry is the arlarming otherness manifested in the madman's behavior. Just as the layman, the psychiatrist sets out from the original strangeness of this conduct (*die Fremdheit dieser Handlung*).[20] Unlike the lay public, the psychiatrist must not content himself with a mere statement of the nonsensicality of a certain behavior but must seek to understand it. His task is to penetrate into the welter of unclear motives and obscure intentions, trying to find his way around it and to discover the hidden sense of the pathological experience.

In order for that to be accomplished, psychiatry must resist the temptation to reduce the madman's otherness to the mere object of scientific inquiry. Scientific objectification would thereby only widen the gap between the doctor and the patient. Therefore, Binswanger refuses the naturalistic view of pathological phenomena derived from the legacy of classificatory medicine. It is by no means fortuitous that Foucault notes in his *Naissance de la clinique* that the tendency to conceive of a disease as a specific entity which can be integrated into a classifying system on the

---

[20] Binswanger. *Schizophrenie*, 46.

basis of its qualities does not come to an end even with the arrival of the nineteenth century. Psychiatry is also very slow to shake off the conviction that, thanks to the nosological system that makes it possible to divide illnesses just as natural entities into specific groups and subgroups, the culturally conditioned criteria of normality and abnormality can be surpassed and supplanted with relatively unequivocal benchmarks. If the psychiatrist should positively state the diagnosis, i.e. precisely discern the type of illness in each case, he/she needs a *Bezugssystem* different from that of the cultural norms, which he finds in the classifying system of the natural scientific sort. With the help of such a system, one can proceed from the original strangeness of the pathological behavior to the specific nosological unit with the same certainty with which the botanist regards a plant as belonging to the correct genus and species. Even though the psychiatrist does take into account the patient's individual dispositions, including various aspects of his personal history, and observes the deranged behavior in the subtlest of its shades and variations, he always betrays the original experience of un-reason from which he departs. Within the framework of the classificatory system of illnesses, the immediate evidence of un-reason is converted into a sort of foreign ingredient that impresses upon human existence a shape different from the one it has had so far. Instead of searching for the true sense of a deranged behavior, its meaning is predetermined as a pathologi-cal deficiency: contrary to health, mental illness is comprehended as a deficient state that jeopardizes the affected individual, while preventing him/her from carrying out certain life functions. In this respect, psychiatric medicine that relies on a given classificatory table of illnesses is no different from organic pathology.

Insofar as the medical gaze regards mental illness as a functional defect, it also implies that this dysfunction must be rooted in something that surpasses all observ-able symptoms, determining their pathological character. Pathological symptoms, such as stereotypical behavior, anxiety or hallucinations, are thus grasped as signs pointing to some hidden essence. To determine the right diagnosis is therefore sim-ply to judge the symptoms correctly and to decide the type, nature and anticipated course of the given illness.

However, such explicated symptoms have nothing to do with the phenomenon as understood by phenomenology. The incompatibility of the phenomenon and the pathological symptom is also noted by Heidegger, claiming in his *Sein und Zeit* that the phenomenon is what shows itself as such, whereas symptoms of a certain illness merely indicate that which lies concealed behind them.[21] Insofar as insanity is to manifest itself as a phenomenon, nonsensical behavior must not be regarded as a pathological symptom, but must be brought to light out of itself. Encountering the phenomenon of insanity requires that the empirical evidence of un-reason should not be evaded, but rather approached with the hope that it will show its meaning some day. More precisely, what is at stake is to explicate the phenomenon of un-reason, while thematically exposing that which, preliminarily and concurrently, remains evident only non-thematically.

---

[21] Heidegger, Martin. 1993. *Sein und Zeit*. Tübingen: Max Niemeyer, 29.

Part of this resolution is Binswanger's decision not to regard un-reason through the prism of clinical categories. Since his times the medical conceptualization of psychopathological disorders has changed significantly, and the jargon he uses is therefore obsolete, but we should not be too concerned about this, as he, instead of adopting purely functional criteria of the distinction between health and illness, prefers a different viewpoint – the ontological constitution of being-in-the-world. Nonsensical behavior, and, together with it, an entire set of personal, physiological and biographical data characteristic of a certain individual, must be, in his opinion, interpreted against the backdrop of the ontological structure of being-in-the-world and its temporal constitution. An integrated constitution of being-there functions as a unifying principle on whose basis all the seemingly disparate elements can be connected into a single whole, their meaning restored, and what eludes common understanding comprehended.

Taking the structural order of being-there (*die Gefügeordnung des Daseins*) as his point of departure, Binswanger is able to thematize specific traits that characterize the pathologically altered being-in-the-world as various modes of disturbance in this overall composition.[22] By virtue of paying heed to the ontological constitution of being-there, ontic features characteristic of an ill individual's being open themselves to his gaze as various forms of disarrangement and ruptures of the structural moments of sojourning amidst beings. However, this breach entails no disintegration into singular, mutually heterogeneous elements, but rather a change in the way the structural moments of sojourning combine, forming a united whole. Therefore, the original sense of psychopathological disorders manifests itself not in the loss of certain existential moments, but rather in the overall modification of existence is as such. As long as human being exists, none of the constitutive moments of its existence can be absent; being-in-the-world, the lived body and individual being form an inseparable whole that ontologically conditions all ontic changes as described in psychiatric *Daseinsanalysis*.

As long as phenomenological psychiatry is to thematize pathologically disturbed modes of existence reflected in the behavior of an individual, it must not content itself with a mere list of aspects due to which this behavior is labeled as deranged, exaggerated or eccentric. In this fashion, it would merely summarize the impression which the insane individual makes on others, without taking into account his/her own existence. Instead of the normative comparison of the "mentally ill" with the healthy, what is necessary is to explicate his/her behavior in the light of his/her own existence. To enter into an encounter with insanity in the way demanded by Binswanger is to cancel the distanced attitude, to cease to regard the ill merely "from the outside", and instead to try to view his/her situation from his/her own perspective. This is the only way to traverse the abyss of non-sense that divides the ill from other people, thus attaining the very center of pathological motives and intentions.

Nevertheless, the way in which the phenomenological view reaches beyond the framework of everyday reasonableness is, in the *daseinsanalytical* interpretation, by

---

[22] Binswanger. *Schizophrenie*, 12.

no means what the clinical psychiatry understands as empathy. In order to comprehend the situation of Binswanger's patients such as Ilsa, Ellen West or Suzanne Urban, it is definitely not enough to merely empathize with their minds. What is at stake in the search for the meaning of pathological experience is not to describe the mental states of certain individuals, but to discover the ways their worlds are structured. Binswanger emphasizes that phenomenological psychopathology explores not so much subjective experiences as pathologically modified modes of being-in-the-world, which makes it possible to overcome the difference between the mental states with which one can empathize and those with which one cannot. Insofar as the ability to empathize is conditioned "subjectively," as it varies in each of us, phenomenological description can render pathological experience understandable, even if the world of the mental illness is profoundly different from the commonly shared world, as is the case with various forms of schizophrenia. For the motives and intentions of pathological behavior to become understandable, there is a need to relinquish the semantic context of our everyday world, to find our way around in the significations of the pathological world, and to map the way this world is projected.

The notion of the world-project (*der Weltentwurf*), used by Binswanger in this respect, derives from Heidegger's text *Vom Wesen des Grundes*, where it denotes the fundamental act by which we project our own possibilities. However, there is nothing in the world-project itself that would derive from the tentative plan or outline; its "tentativeness" lies in its preliminary opening of the world as the horizon of significance, within whose framework the singular beings can become manifest as things with which one can set about doing something. Such a world-project is not given by some particular volitional act either, as it is only the world-project that makes possible our relation to beings. In this sense, the world-project is constitutive of all of our decision-making, thought and action.

Since the horizon of significance, which remains open through the world-project, confronts us with certain possibilities while excluding others, it reflects finitude as well as the individual diversity of being-in-the-world. As long as "individuality is that which is its world," as claims Binswanger, every individual can be understood on the basis of his/her world-project that determines the overall style of his/her existence.[23]

This discovery is important especially in the case of psychopathological disorders, in which the significative whole (*das Bedeutungsganze*) of the commonly shared world of everyday existence undergoes considerable changes. What is characteristic of manic excitations, for instance, is the feeling of boundless breadth, freedom and ease that shows everything in bright colors; a world of unlimited possibilities opens where "nothing is impossible", and therefore nothing is brought to a conclusion, since once one possibility has been seized upon, human being is lured to seize upon ten others that are even more tempting. An individual prone to depression, by contrast, experiences states of utmost dejection, in which all things and people are drowned in monotonous grayness and grime; his/her world is akin to a

---

[23] Binswanger. *Schizophrenie*, 149.

gutter, a wasteland, or an underground tomb, where all plans are stillborn and where nothing seems worth embarking on. Both the flamboyant world of celestial breadth and the underground world of dirt and decay are poles apart from the social and habitual bonds of the everyday world, in which action is governed by practical purposes and possibilities refer to one another without forming a vicious circle. With regard to the fact that the manic world of glamour and ease usually encompasses a reference to the dark depth of depression, it is of essence to grasp the individuality of existence thus structured on the basis of the alternation of two opposing, and yet innerly bound modes of being-in-the-world.

Other specific modifications of being-in-the-world and the correspondent individual dispositions, which determine the pathological form of existence, can be described in a similar way. In this respect, the phenomenological inquiry into world-projects goes even further than those branches of psychopathology that work with the notion of *personality*. This can be documented by Binswanger's confrontation with the clinical view of schizophrenic attack, which was common in his times.[24] The psychopathological concepts that focus on the investigation of personality disorders usually expound schizophrenia as the disintegration of personality, i.e. as a disturbance of psychic totality and an inner disorganization of its structures, with special emphasis on the feeling of lability that coerces a schizophrenic to seek support in some idea which could serve him as a point of reference, ridding him/her of his/her inner insecurity. Thus, schizophrenic delusions are conceived of as refuge and buttress of an innerly insecure personality, without raising the question of whence its essential insecurity actually springs. By what else could this insecurity be given if not by the insecure position of human being in the world? Therefore, psychiatric *Daseinsanalysis* addresses the schizophrenic experience in order to find in its gaps and discontinuities the expression of the fragility and unstableness of being-in-the-world. Explicating the inconsistency of experience observable in most schizophrenics, Binswanger inquires not about its causes, but about its structural conditions, which he finds in the world-project that is infiltrated by destructive intrusions of the Horrible, the Sudden and the Sinister.

The immensity of these destructive intrusions are far beyond whatever is usually an object of fear for human being. Therefore, the basic affective tuning of the schizophrenic world is not fear but anxiety, which unlike fear is not fixed upon a definite entity, but rather encompasses being-in-the-world as a whole. The correlate of the immediate presence of the Horrible, the Sudden and the Sinister, claims Binswanger, is anxiety, since nothing but anxiety can account for the fact that together with its intrusion there occurs the disintegration of the significative structure of the world, with which the individual is familiar. Anxiety carries the individual away from its familiarity with the world and casts it into uncanniness (*die Unheimlichkeit*), where all possibilities of action disappear and all beings fall into insignificance.

However, this frightful uncanniness must not be reduced to a common feeling of anxiety or anxious affect; its genuine character does not surface until the fundamental

---

[24] Binswanger. *Schizophrenie*, 452–4.

form of being-in-the-world is seen in the utter insignificance into which the world is submerged. Even though anxiety is a strange way of being-in-the-world, it is to be viewed as the fundamental disposition of being-there. The primary guideline in this direction is Heidegger's *Sein und Zeit*, in which anxiety is grasped as the fundamental phenomenon of being-there, whose source is not some external threat, but being-in-the-world as such. Anxiety confronts being-there with the bare fact of its own existence by means of unveiling it in its original uneasiness and precariousness.

The dark side of being-in-the-world announced in uncanniness is experienced by the schizophrenic in its worst form, that is to say, as exposure to the sheer horror of the loss of all possibilities and the rupture all significative connections. With the so-called normal individual, anxiety, if permitted at all, can always be overcome, whereas in the case of the schizophrenic, it becomes all-encompassing and inescapable. Instead of resolutely accepting the fact of his/her existence as his/her very own possibility, the schizophrenic is, over and over again, cast into a situation where his/her individuality becomes reduced to the pure capability of suffering. Out of the repeated confrontation with the traumatic experience of "the end of the world" evolves the overall mode of existing, marked by the persistent effort to piece together out of the shattered shreds of the significative whole of the world at least some sort of provisional space, within which one could freely move and breathe.

The need for establishing and maintaining a sort of refuge, and thus escaping the uncanniness of anxiety, can lead, among other things, to the tendency to objectify this uncanniness in the form of imminent jeopardy or the omnipresent enemy. Faced with a looming catastrophe or hostile machinations, one can at least do something, whereas the uncanniness of anxiety leaves no chance at all. No matter how perfect safety measures the schizophrenic may take, when turning his/her world into a fortress under strict surveillance, he/she can never escape out of his/her highly uncertain world-project, constantly at the risk of being exposed to disintegration and nothingness. That is why Binswanger likens the way one of his patients exists to walking on thin ice which can break any moment; in her world, to take one wrong step is to cause everything to tumble into an ice-cold dark depth.[25] Unlike the person that has, as it were, both feet firmly on the ground, the schizophrenic existence finds itself incessantly on the verge of a dismal abyss, in need to grasp at straws.

The schizophrenic therefore necessarily seems foreign and incomprehensible to a secured existence which confidently relies on the outer world. What comes into play then is condemnation, blaming the schizophrenic's behavior on his/her imbecility, mental defectiveness, or some other form of pathological deficiency. Understanding the meaning of the original anxiety of being-there (*die Daseinsangst*) within the schizophrenic experience, on the contrary, enables us to find the path to the world-project split between the desire for a safe haven where one can feel at home and the horror of falling into the abyss of uncanniness.

With reference to the sinister abyss of anxiety, psychiatric *Daseinsanalysis* can then unveil the essential insecurity also in the ideal of perfect safety, happiness and harmony to which the schizophrenic existence clings. The idealized world of beauty,

---

[25] Binswanger. *Schizophrenie*, 312–3 (the case of Lola Voss).

peace and order encompasses in its essence a reference to its opposite, to the dark world of uncanniness that is masked only imperfectly and provisionally. This receives its corroboration whenever the created ideal is doubted, which inevitably throws the person into the subjection to the very contrary of its ideal: the craving after leanness, delicacy and beauty, of which Ellen West keeps dreaming, can become reversed into bestial voracity; the desire for aristocratic nobleness and social recognition that permeates through the life of Jürgen Zünd turns into an uncontrollable downfall into the proletariat and social scorn; and finally the longing for total safety, which forces Lola Voss to make use of security rituals and superstitious practices, cannot ward off the arrival of "something horrible."

From this Binswanger concludes that the exaggerated ideal to which the schizophrenic clings offers no real way out of his/her situation, but merely conserves his/her state, preventing it from any possible development. The schizophrenic is incapable of stepping out into the future and seizing new possibilities, since he/she, bound by anxiety, is incessantly drawn down to what has already been. The paradoxical corroboration of this observation is also the suicide in which Ellen West, after 13 years of futile striving, found her last recourse.

Not only those pathological modes of being-in-the-world classified by psychiatry as "psychoses", but also those belonging to the sphere of "neuroses" can be expounded with regard to the basic anxiety of being-there. Anxious distress or panic appear in individuals suffering from such personality disorders as phobia, just as the various forms of compulsive or obsessive states.[26] In all of the aforementioned cases, anxious distress emerges as a clinically ascertainable symptom, influencing to a larger or lesser extent the pathological experience. Nevertheless, this crucial symptom could never surface without a much more original phenomenon that precedes, as well as retrospectively explains, all pathological structures. Anxiety, hidden in the foundations of being-in-the-world as the inner testimony of its unanchored and unsecured character, is the key prerequisite for even the usual fear to arrive; a phobia-stricken individual is then exposed to anxiety in an incomparably more radical way, as the extent of his/her "subjective" jeopardy is far beyond that of the real danger. What is at work here is not this or that threatening entity, but dread of something inexpressibly terrible, more precisely, horror of uncanniness, under whose onslaught the significative whole of the world collapses. Unlike the schizophrenic, whose existence is essentially marked by the collapse of the significative whole of the world and by the striving for a makeshift reconstruction, an individual suffering from phobia maintains a familiarity with the surrounding entities at least as long as he/she manages to evade encountering the object into which all of his/her anxiety has been incarnated. Insofar as the so-called psychosis manifests itself, from the *daseinsanalytical* perspective, as boundless exposure to uncanniness, neurosis must then be grasped as endangering anxiety and defense against this endangerment.[27] In the neurotic's world, anxiety plays a different role than in the psychotic's world: whereas in the first case, one seeks to displace and conceal it, or lives it in the form

---

[26] Binswanger. *Schizophrenie*, 272.

[27] Binswanger. *Schizophrenie*, 465.

of anxious expectation of frightful evil, punishment, incurable disease and inevitable death, in the other case it is directly exposed to the damaging effects of the awesome uncanniness that deprives his/her existence of all support. Hallucinations or the system of paranoid delusions, in which the whole world is laden with unclear threats and hostile schemes, have their place only within a world-project governed by anxiety. Nevertheless, both psychotic and neurotic disorders are connected by what Binswanger terms heightened susceptibility (*die Empfänglichkeit*) to the anxiety of being-there.

One must not forget, however, that anxiety is not only an expression of a pathological disorder, but also lies at the very heart of individual existence; it is that which lies hidden inside of being-in-the-world as its own otherness, endowing it simultaneously with its unique sense. Only in relation to it can we comprehend the facticity that differentiates the individual existence from others, lending it the character of *Jemeinigkeit*.

How can pathological proclivity to anxiety thus be discerned from determined confrontation with the uncanniness that is the prerequisite for discovering and developing one's very own possibilities of being-in-the-world? Is it merely a question of the extent of susceptibility and resistance, or are there two totally different modes of being-in-the-world at stake here?

This dilemma can be resolved only if we observe it from a temporal perspective. Speaking of "the weakness of existence" in connection with schizophrenic individuals, Binswanger has in mind the squeamishness of the temporal structure of their existence that prevents them from maintaining a genuinely open attitude toward the future.

For instance, the temporal continuity of Suzanne Urban's experience is so labile as to become incapable of integrating any new situation that would pertain to her familial environment.[28] Even though new experiences from other spheres present no serious problem for her, her family matters must remain the same; above all, no-one must ever fall ill, otherwise the temporal continuity of her existence is in jeopardy. Until her psychotic breakdown occurs, Suzanne Urban worries about the health and prosperity of her relatives, since any grave illness would entail a total catastrophe for herself. Characteristic of the pre-psychotic phase of her existence is her effort to take precautions against the breakdown of the temporal continuity of her existence that leads to the "self-denying" nursing of her ill relatives, especially her mother. Thus, what this family cult attests to is not so much a real mature love as it is the insecurity of her own existence. The news about her husband's incurable disease then necessarily comes as a devastating blow. As Suzanne Urban is incapable of processing this piece of information and integrating it within the order of her experience, she is inevitably cast into the abyss of sheer dread. The bottomless horror of the given situation, according to Binswanger, leads to an unprecedented torpor corresponding, on the temporal level, to time coming to a halt. Consequently to the extreme experience of total paralysis and loss of all security, paranoid delusions arise which enable temporal ecstasies to develop, but only at the cost of the overall

---

[28] Binswanger. *Schizophrenie*, 425–8.

order of experience being tied to the awesome uncanniness of anxiety. Every new experience that Suzanne Urban shall henceforth make is a mere confirmation of dark suspicions and unclear threats, all evolving from the primary theme of the persecution of her family. Her existence does not stand open to the new, does not project into the future, but is trapped in a vicious circle, which corresponds to the peculiar cyclicality of its temporality. No matter how unproblematic, consequential and inwardly sure this experience might seem, it always finally collapses under the onslaught of anxiety, which it itself brings to the surface by means of its cyclicality.

Binswanger notes a similar unreliability of experience with other schizophrenics, whose time is repeatedly shattered by the sinister proximity of the Sudden and the Horrible. The inconsistency of experience, which manifests itself in the multifarious forms of delusions and hallucinations, is merely another expression of the disruption of temporal continuity that occurs under the onslaught of anxiety. The peculiar form of temporalization, marked by intermittence, sudden leaps and irregularities, is described by Binswanger as urgency (*Dringlichkeit*), i.e. as a state of latent catastrophe, in which the individual existence is constantly jeopardized by destructive collisions and turbulences.[29] Instead of an unproblematic, fluent temporalization, the individual must exert all its strength to induce at least some semblance of continuity. The exhausting attempts at reinstating the temporal continuity of existence and piecing together the whole of experience keep casting the patient into increasingly emptier timelessness where nothing ever happens. The final stage of the futile effort to regain the temporal continuity of existence is thus the empty eternity, in which the exhausted individual wholly resigns from the active involvement in his/her own existence. "The schizophrenic process," claims Binswanger, "is in the first place a process of existential emptying and impoverishment in the sense of a gradual stiffening ('coagulating') of free self into an increasingly less free ('more dependent') object alienated from itself. From this perspective only can it be truly understood. The schizophrenic thinking, speech, and action are all merely partial expressions of this fundamental process." [30]

However, the reification and self-alienation in the empty timelessness where nothing happens any more does not by any means pertain to the ontological plane of being-there. The change in the overall way of existence that occurs in schizophrenia is of a purely ontic character; that is to say, it is an empirically evident modification, not a transformation in the ontological sense of the word. Binswanger outspokenly emphasizes that the ontological structure of being-there, and together with it the overall unity of temporality remains preserved, even if the schizophrenic existence is marked by a considerable degree of disturbance.[31] As being-there is primarily characterized by the ecstatic unity of its temporality, this unity can never be wholly absent; should that happen, the being-there would cease to be what it is, becoming *Nicht-mehr-Da-Sein*. Even the extreme self-alienation observable in many

---

[29] Binswanger. *Schizophrenie*, 255–6.

[30] Binswanger. *Schizophrenie*, 165.

[31] Binswanger, Ludwig. 1957. *Der Mensch in der Psychiatrie*, 11.

schizophrenics does not mean that the schizophrenic would cease to be a being with an interest in its own potentiality-of-being as described by Heidegger in *Sein und Zeit*.[32] Even though the incessant onslaughts of the awesome uncanniness shatter the schizophrenic's world to such an extent that he/she finds nothing by means of which he could understand himself/herself, what still remains with him/her is bare being as sheer horror of the emptied being-in-the-world. The disintegration of the self, of which Binswanger speaks in connection with the schizophrenic collapse of the significative whole of the world, does not invoke a total loss of interest in one's own being, but rather opens a whole series of defense mechanisms which aim for a reconstruction of the world and retrieval of one's self. All objective materializations of the awesome uncanniness that appear as foreign, hostile powers are to be understood primarily as attempts at self-determination and preservation of whatever remains out of its world-project and its own self. And even if the one becomes utterly incapable of an independent performance of one's own being, as is the case with the complete dissociation of personality, this does not mean that he/she has ceased to be being-there in the ontological sense of the term, but rather that he/she has distanced himself/herself from the possibility of a continuous existence open to the future, and of the correspondent individual being (*das Selbstsein*). The total collapse of individual existence, attested to by the catatonic torpor and mechanical movements repeated *ad infinitum*, is merely the extreme variation of weakness that prevents the individual from unraveling the autonomous existence, confident in his/her world and in himself/herself.[33] With regard to the possibility of a resolute existence oriented toward the future which does not shrink from even the potential threat of anxiety, it becomes evident to what extent the schizophrenic way of being lags behind the potential hidden within the ontological structure of being-there.

Since the psychiatric *Daseinsanalysis* departs from the united ontological composition of being-there, the schizophrenic's unstable being-in-the-world can appear only as a deficient mode of existence.[34] Against the backdrop of the temporal unity of existence, the intermittent and re-composed temporal continuity of experience looms as a deficient form of temporalization. The shakiness of the temporal structure interferes with the ability to maintain a truly open attitude toward new possibilities, which leads to a considerable narrowing of the openness to one's own possibilities. The sphere of possibilities that Ellen West is left with after she has clung to the ideal of leanness is so limited as to lead Binswanger to liken her life to the circling of a lioness that seeks in vain a way out of a latticed cage.[35] Instead of the primary orientation toward the future, what comes into view is anxiety related to the idea of obesity that binds her existence into an increasingly narrow range of possibilities. Urgency as a special form of temporalization rids the schizophrenic existence of its freedom, subjecting it to pathological compulsion;

---

[32] Binswanger, Ludwig. 1965. *Wahn, Beiträge zu seiner phaenomenologischen und daseinsanalytischen Erforschung*. Pfullingen: Neske, 24–6. Binswanger. *Schizophrenie*, 415.

[33] Binswanger. *Schizophrenie*, 261–2.

[34] Binswanger. *Schizophrenie*, 19.

[35] Binswanger. *Schizophrenie*, 104–5.

the repeated outbreak of temporal discontinuity supplants the freedom of one's continuous projecting oneself toward new possibilities with the unconditioned necessity to ward off the uncanniness that emerges from within the very basis of being-there. In Binswanger's opinion, the dependence and impotence of this mode of existence manifests itself all the more clearly, the more exposed to the pathological world the individual becomes, trying to save himself/herself from the destructive onslaught of anxiety. The extreme expression of the absorption in the world is the state, where the schizophrenic wholly succumbs to delusive images and sounds; "turning worldly" (*die Verweltlichung*) is here so radical that the schizophrenic perceives himself/herself merely as an object manipulated by the influence of external forces.

Regardless of the specific forms of the absorption in the world, all schizophrenic casuistries attest to the inability to accept one's existence as genuinely one's own and to live through it in a corresponding manner. Binswanger does not, however, forget to stress that the strange absorption in the world, observable in schizophrenic individuals, is incomparable with the everyday entanglement in the world where we are also prone to forgetting our own being, searching instead for the sense and support in what we are preoccupied with. The crucial difference lies in that the everyday existence always operates within the frame of an unproblematic familiarity with the world, whereas the pathological world to which the schizophrenic stands open is time and again subject to onslaughts of the awesome uncanniness. The individual settled in the familiarity with the world is thus always capable of overcoming his/her self-alienation and finding the way back to himself/herself, whereas the schizophrenic remains incapable of coming back to himself/herself, nor is he/she able to find reassurance and security in his/his world.

A different situation prevails in the case of pre-psychotic states and the so-called neurotic disorders, where the process of falling prey to the world still has a character of everyday being-together-with innerworldy beings. Since the familiarity with the world is not overtly disturbed and the consistency of experience does completely fail to disintegrate, the individual is able to find certain guarantees in his/her world, even though the shakiness of the temporal structure of his/her existence foists upon it a most rigid attitude toward all new experience, which brings the awesome uncanniness of anxiety to the surface. Just as the psychotic, the neurotic also remains incapable of fully taking over his/her own existence. From out of his/her heightened susceptibility to the anxiety of being-there springs the peculiar falling prey to the world, marked by compulsive actions or various phobias.

What is characteristic of all pathological modes of being-in-the-world is thus the greater or lesser extent of deficiency in the performance of the individual existence. Despite refusing the functionalist view on mental disorders, Binswanger does eventually arrive at addressing the phenomenon of existential deficiency which is common to all pathological modifications of being-in-the-world. However, as long as phenomenological psychiatry finds a certain deficiency in pathological modes of existence, this deficiency springs from neither the functional notions of health and illness, nor the basic application of the system of social norms, but from the overall ontological structure of being-there.

The primary prerequisite of such a way of thematization is Binswanger's assertion that the ontological structure of being-in-the-world has no invariant character, as every individual performs and experiences his/her own existence in slightly different way.[36] Insofar as all modes of being-in-the-world are never completely the same, it is then possible to demonstrate the individual differences in the arrangement, "consistency," "materiality," "tint" and temporality of existence arising from this or that world-project. Every mode of being-in-the-world that uncontrollably lags behind the possibility of an integrated, autonomous existence oriented toward the future appears, against the background of the formal ontological arrangement of being-there, as an example of "miscarried being-there" (*missglücktes Dasein*).

A deviation from the norm determined by the ontological composition of human existence is by no means always irreversible. Given that the patient's being-in-the-world has not deteriorated to the extent to which it would prevent him/her from entering an understanding relationship with the psychotherapist, the therapeutic conversation can endow him/her with the understanding for the fundamental character of his/her world-project and show him/her where and how he/she has confused, deranged or derailed himself/herself in the framework of its structure.[37] In this way the ill individual can step out of their pathologically distorted, insecure world, and find their way back to the integrated, autonomous being-in-the-world. The objective of the *daseinsanalytic* therapy is to rid the mentally ill of all pathological inhibitions by revealing to them those structural possibilities of being-in-the-world that are essentially their own. The point is to bring them, by means of a therapeutic conversation, to the determination to take over their own existence and to independently develop their very own possibilities, without necessarily entertaining the paranoid need to ward off the influence of others.

The psychotherapeutic effort to open for the mentally ill their very own possibilities of being-in-the-world is all the more important in that the notion of "miscarried being-there" – Binswanger's coinage for psychopathological states – denotes not only a deviation from the norm resulting from the ontological composition of being-there, but also carries within itself a reference to the eudaemonistic dimension of human existence. Opposed to the miscarried being-there is the "successful being-there," which uses being-in-the-world to the maximum of its ontological potential, leading to fulfillment of life. In psychiatric *Daseinsanalysis*, one can speak of a real fulfillment only when human existence is characterized not only by a bold orientation toward the future, but also by the possibility of love and friendship. Especially love as absolute openness to the other is considered here an existential moment that requires the ability to overcome one's own boundaries and rise to new possibilities. It is this ability that the "mentally ill" lack, expending most of their strength for protection against the awesome uncanniness of anxiety. If there is love in schizophrenic individuals, claims Binswanger, then it occurs merely in a deficient form, such as pathological jealousy and the ensuing need to possess the other.[38] When

---

[36] Binswanger. *Der Mensch in der Psychiatrie*, 11.

[37] Binswanger. *Der Mensch in der Psychiatrie*, 33–4.

[38] Binswanger. *Schizophrenie*, 19.

Suzanne Urban devotes all her life endeavor to struggle for the well-being of her loved ones, or when Ilsa shoves her hand into a red-hot oven in order to show her father the strength of real love, neither of these do so out of love, but rather out of the need to brace themselves against the onslaught of anxiety that coerces them to close themselves off from others, captivated by their outlandish ideal.[39] Their action is led not by love but rather by the care for themselves that leaves no room for openness to others.

A similar self-centeredness, resulting from the jeopardy of their own existence, is discernible also in other mentally ill individuals, who lack the ability of fully opening themselves to the other and create what the psychiatric *Daseinsanalysis* refers to as the "dual modus" of a common existence. The dual modus of being, manifested in the phenomenon of love, is according to Binswanger something more than purely singular mode of being-in-the-world that does also encompass coexistence with others, but the individual existence never surpasses in relation to them the primary interestedness in itself that springs from its original *Jemeinigkeit*.

By such a suggestion, however, Binswanger clearly leaves the line of Heidegger's thought, setting out in his own direction. His contemplation of the love phenomenon aims primarily to show where the phenomenological thematization of human existence, as sketched in *Sein und Zeit*, ends in an impasse. The crucial problem of the phenomenological description of being-there, in Binswanger's opinion, is the fact that it regards only the individual modus of being-in-the-world, while leaving aside the dual modus of being, consummated in loving relationships. The ontological project of being-there departs from the structure of *Jemeinigkeit* which reflects from the very beginning the finitude of one's own existence. If individual existence has a character of being-toward-death, it means that it always anticipates the possibility of its own end, which lays bare its essential loneliness. One can either accept this loneliness as one's own lot that is to be fulfilled by a determined and independent choice of one's own possibilities, or flee from it by falling prey to the possibilities of the everyday world that are offered to everyone. Whether being-there accepts its original loneliness, or rather in that it yields to the temptation of a convenient dependent existence, governed by how "they" live and by what "they" say, its existence always has an individual character. Only on the basis of the original *Jemeinigkeit* of existence is it possible to distinguish between both of the modes of being, the authentic and the inauthentic existence.

However, the *Grundformen und Erkenntnis menschlichen Daseins* states that love is incompatible with both the authentic and the inauthentic existence, as it exceeds the limits of individual existence as such.[40] The dual modus of being, at which the human being arrives in loving harmony with the other, is allegedly incompatible with being-there that primarily cares about its own existence, while relating, incidentally, as it were, to other beings. If Heidegger terms the structural whole of the individual existence interested in itself as "care," love must stay outside of the

---

[39]. Binswanger. *Schizophrenie*, 269–70.
[40] Binswanger, Ludwig. 1964. *Grundformen und Erkenntnis menschlichen Daseins*, 4th edition. München/Basel: Ernst Reinhardt Verlag, 58.

framework of existence thus determined. The very notion of care in the Heideggerian sense, which implies the idea of a cumbersome burden and personal effort, is for Binswanger a denial of the essential character of love.

Further inquiry also leads to the discovery that care does not remain in itself, but is borne by temporality. The structural whole of care, and so the individual character of being-there, is ultimately based on the ecstatic unity of temporality. But since one cannot proceed from individual existence to a single "us," love cannot be adequately thematized even on the basis of temporality that constitutes the ontological whole of care.

As long as love is to be comprehended as a certain mode of human existence, claims Binswanger, it is necessary to seek its uniqueness in that it surpasses the original loneliness of individual existence resulting from its being-toward-death. Despite failing to render it immortal, love enables human existence to cut the bonds of its own finitude and, merging with the other, to rise to the infinite. However, when touching the infinite in this way, human existence never reaches beyond time. Rather, what is conferred on the dual being of love is a peculiar temporality that temporalizes itself in the form of eternity. Unlike the empty eternity into which the schizophrenic descends, what is at work here is not the ontic modification of the original ontological unity of temporality, but rather a completely new type of temporality that has the character of the eternal moment. This is the reason why Binswanger considers love the ontological contrary of anxiety, which exposes the individual existence to uncanniness, giving it the feeling of its own loneliness, insecurity and finitude.[41] Anxiety appears, especially when the individual has fallen into despair, incessantly having to tackle uncanniness of being-in-the-world, as is corroborated by the casuistry of Ellen West and Jürgen Zünd.[42] Love, on the contrary, extricates us from the snares of uncanniness, as the encounter of two lovers creates the open space of trust and secureness that cannot be shattered even by the inexorable certainty of death. This encounter oscillates as the eternal moment of love, in whose intimacy the lovers find their real home.

What is typical of the dual mode of being, whose temporal basis is formed by the eternal moment of love, is the fact that one no longer exists solely for one's own sake, but for the sake of "both of us." In love, we care about "our common" being, which is in *Grundformen und Erkenntnis menschlichen Daseins* attributed the character of *Unsrigkeit*. Just as the *Jemeinigkeit* characterises the individual existence, *Unsrigkeit* belongs to the loving co-existence[43] In Binswanger's opinion, it is only on the basis of *Unsrigkeit* that it is possible to comprehend the integrity of one's own existence that gives itself to the other in a loving relationship, while accepting it at the same time.[44] The integrity of the loving co-existence is corroborated not in the determined acceptance of one's own loneliness that springs from the finitude of human existence, but in the faithful sharing of common *Unsrigkeit*.

---

[41] Binswanger. *Grundformen und Erkenntnis menschlichen Daseins*, 54.

[42] Binswanger. *Schizophrenie*, 135–6, 230–2.

[43] Binswanger. *Grundformen und Erkenntnis menschlichen Daseins*, 59.

[44] Binswanger. *Grundformen und Erkenntnis menschlichen Daseins*, 126.

Depicting the eternal moment of love and the associated space of trust and secureness, Binswanger goes so far as to speak not of being-in-the-world, but of being-beyond-the-world (*Über-die-Welt-hinaus-Sein*). This expression means that the loving existence rises above the purely utilitarian sphere of practical possibilities, offered by the everyday world. Being-beyond-the-world is different from practical action, within whose framework things manifest themselves as what they are used for, others as those who handle them, and the individual as the one who can concern himself/herself with one thing or another. Unlike the everyday being-in-the-world, in which a certain possibility is understood only insofar as the individual existence finds in it a concretization of its own potentiality-of-being, being-beyond-the-world is governed not by what we can do but by what we are allowed to do.

By claiming this, Binswanger occupies himself not so much with wordplay as with a much more substantial revision of Heidegger's ontological project of being-there that allegedly adheres too strictly to the logic of power for it to open the pathway to the ontological character of love.[45] As long as being-in-the-world in its whole is imbued with the idea of power, manifested both in the consummate sovereignty with which one takes care of one's own existence, and the fatalism with which one embraces his/her own finitude, being-beyond-the-world, necessarily stands beyond all power and powerlessness. The crucial moment of being-beyond-the-world is not the individual determination to take over the burden of one's own existence or the effort to shun it, but a gift that renders individual existence richer and more complete than it could ever become on its own. This gift is not given by our loving counterpart either, as it is given to both of us. The act of giving, occurring in love, happens as a revelation, as self-manifestation of the infinite and eternal intimacy. Those to whom the gift is given are not required to do anything but to remain gratefully in the openness that is revealed in the loving encounter.

As regards Heidegger's ontological analysis of being-there, Binswanger claims that "the beginning with the *Jemeinigkeit* of being-there cannot be overcome by prudency or reason, but by something quite different, namely by imagination".[46] If phenomenology is to arrive at a dual mode of being, then imagination, whose scintillation binds together the loving "I" and "you", must stand in its focus. Opposed to the understanding of one's own existence that involves the understanding of other beings one is dealing with, it is the shared being-beyond-the-world that is imbued with imagination, by whose virtue the we dwell in the sphere of loving trust, safe intimacy and eternity.

Imagination, however, must not by any means be mistaken for mere phantasy, let alone illusion. Binswanger repeatedly emphasizes that love is not a passionate affection or some other psychic process, but rather the fundamental feature of human existence that has its own "reality." More precisely, love requires for itself a special ontological status, one that springs from the dual mode of existence. In view of the fact that the ontological nature of the dual mode of existence is exhaustively described on the 700 pages of *Grundformen und Erkenntnis menschlichen Daseins*,

---

[45] Binswanger. *Grundformen und Erkenntnis menschlichen Daseins*, 147.

[46] Binswanger. *Grundformen und Erkenntnis menschlichen Daseins*, 14.

it is no exaggeration to call this work the phenomenological book of love. As opposed to Heidegger's phenomenological description of being-there, which primarily emphasizes the moment of practical understanding, the erotic *Daseinsanalysis* explicates the dual modus of existence as the cardinal phenomenon.

Binswanger's phenomenology of love is tangible also in the works such as *Schizophrenie* where the notions of eternity, safe trust or being-beyond-the-world refer to that which the pathologically disturbed existence painfully lacks. It would therefore be mistaken to surmise that Binswanger highlights love as an isolated phenomenon. The crucial motif that directs his intellectual work is the effort to obtain the overall picture of human existence. While Heidegger's thought is governed by a purely ontological interest, as its primary focus is nothing but the question of being and accordingly omits many aspects of human existence, Binswanger situates his conception within the anthropological realm. As he points out, his aim is to supplement the ontological description of being-there so that it captures the whole of human existence in its completeness.[47]

This prompts the need to broaden the ontological picture of human existence by including therein not only loving imagination, but also the ability of imagination that gives rise to the work of art. One can mention in this connection that both types of imagination stand quite near each other within Binswanger's anthropological conception, as they both surpass the pragmatic context of being-in-the-world in a similar way. Both the artistic and loving imagination accomplishes the full scope of its dimension when it ascends from being-in-the-world to being-beyond-the-world.[48] Despite their consubstantiality, the two types of imagination are to some extent different from each other, which is given by the fact that loving imagination, unlike the artistic imagination, functions as a linking element within the loving harmony between "I" and "you."[49] That is not, however, to say that the creative imagination should close itself off in an ivory tower of its own images. The creative genius opens through the imagination to the totality of beings, without becoming fixed upon a specific entity as something to be utilized practically. In the light of this inspiring encounter, the genius appears as one who traverses from the intimate closeness to the world into the "height above the world," into a genuine eternity of loving harmony with nature, mankind and God. Dealing in his *Schizophrenie* with the question of genius, Binswanger notes that his exceptionality consists in the ability to bring beings in general into a completely new connection and revelation.[50]

In an absolutely different situation is the madman, who lives in the world as an emergency asylum or banishment from which there is no escape. Incapable of ascending to being-beyond-the-world, the madman is doomed to a barren, lonesome being-in-the-world, which stands in the way of both the loving encounter with the other and the act of creation. Whether a schizophrenic, depressively or neuroticaly structured individual, the madman is incapable of opening to a real encounter,

[47] Binswanger. *Grundformen und Erkenntnis menschlichen Daseins*, 640.

[48] Binswanger. *Grundformen und Erkenntnis menschlichen Daseins*, 14, 158.

[49] Binswanger. *Grundformen und Erkenntnis menschlichen Daseins*, 505–6.

[50] Binswanger. *Schizophrenie*, 252–3.

clinging instead to ideas or things at hand in order to seek in them the support for being-in-the-world jeopardized by anxiety. The incessant tension between the understanding being-in-the-world and the imaginative being-beyond-the-world that stands in the primary focus of Binswanger's anthropological conception is thus translated into his interpretation of the "diametrical opposition" between the madman and the genius.

Unfortunately, however heavily the psychiatric *Daseinsanalysis* and the resulting concept of love and artistic genius draw upon a vast wealth of experience, this approach cannot stand the test of strict philosophical criteria. Leaving aside the psychopathological dimension of human existence for the moment, one can start by mentioning the critical notes of Paul De Man, who occupied himself with Binswanger's work in the context of literary theory. His observations summed up in the essay "Ludwig Binswanger and the Sublimation of the Self" concern especially the doubtful role played within Binswanger's conception by the phenomenon of the self, but what does not pass unnoticed either is the problematic status of imagination, asserted in artistic or loving enthusiasm.[51] Both of these difficult questions, according to De Man, have to do with the overall humanistic orientation of phenomenological description of the creative and the loving mode of being. Cognate with this is the normative tendency manifested in the emphasis on the ideal of a balanced, fully harmonious existence.

De Man arrives at this discovery against the background of Foucault's archeology of the Western thought which puts phenomenology into the context of the modern episteme. Insofar as the epistemological inquiry undertaken in *Les mots et les choses* reveals the bond that ties phenomenology to the fate of modern knowledge, what it implies is that even phenomenology is not safe from the fundamental jeopardy designated by Foucault as "anthropological sleep." What the modern episteme brings into focus of all knowledge is human being, perceived as the empirical object on the one hand and as the transcendental precondition of all knowledge on the other. Therefore, phenomenology must continuously combat the temptation of anthropologism that springs from this empirical-transcendental bifurcation. The basis of anthropologism, according to Foucault, consists in the fact that "[a]ll empirical knowledge, provided it concerns man, can serve as a possible philosophical field in which the foundation of knowledge, the definition of its limits, and, in the end, the truth of all truth must be discovered."[52] Once we relate the mentioned criterion to Binswanger's conception, it becomes crystal clear that what we are dealing with here is a model case of falling into the trap of anthropologism.

If phenomenology cannot completely evade its fateful proclivity for anthropologism, this does not mean that it must fall prey to it. This is clearly attested to by *Les mots et les choses* itself, where phenomenology is grasped as not only an attempt to bridge the empirical and the transcendental regions, but also the place of birth of a

[51] De Man, Paul. 1983. *Blindness and Insight. Essays in the Rhetoric of Contemporary Criticism.* Minneapolis: University of Minnesota Press, 36–50.

[52] Foucault. *Les mots et les choses*, 352. English edition: Foucault, Michel. 1970. *The Order of Things*, ed. Ronald. David Laing. London: Tavistock Publications Ltd., 341.

new ontology. Despite its rootedness within the transcendental realm of thought, phenomenology falls apart from within and becomes the description of experience, which is still empirical, and ontological inquiry, focusing on the question of being as such.[53] The lion's share in this split within the phenomenological project belongs to Heidegger, who decidedly rejects the Husserlian theme of transcendental consciousness, replacing it with the question of being. In his case, what is at stake is no longer the search for the transcendental foundation of the empirical contents of knowledge, but rather the fundamental ontology accessible through the ontological description of individual being. Although Heidegger's fundamental ontology does depart from the *Jemeinigkeit* of being-there, its main aim is not so much the empirical inquiry into the human individuality, but rather the ontologically purified description of being-there that pays heed only to those existential moments that are tied to the openness of being. Insofar as individual existence relates to its own being with understanding, this relation cannot be mistaken for the egoistic preoccupation with oneself, as it always already encompasses the understanding of being as such.

On the other hand, the effort to supplement the ontologically strict description of individual being with the phenomenological description of a creative genius and a loving encounter rests on purely empirical foundations, which De Man condemns as an inadmissible blending of the empirical with the ontological subject matter. In spite of relying on the ontological analysis of being-there, Binswanger cannot resist the "tendency to forsake the barren world of ontological reduction for the wealth of experience."[54] As a consequence, his phenomenological project lapses into the very anthropologism Heidegger seeks to avoid.

It is therefore not surprising that Heidegger resolutely distances himself from Binswanger's psychiatric-erotic orientation. Even though it is Binswanger's merit that the phenomenological way of thinking had been introduced into the psychiatric realm, his work is assessed in *Zollikoner Seminare* with extreme severity. The very attempt at supplementing the ontological insights demonstrated in *Sein und Zeit* with a phenomenological treatment of love is subjected to harsh criticism. The reason for declining the effort to complement the individual with the dual mode of existence lies not in the very fact that Binswanger supplements the ontological description of being-there, but rather in the fact that being-there is rendered in a way that is full of distortions.

To see how Heidegger rectifies Binswanger's anthropological conception, it is important to remind ourselves that in *Zollikoner Seminare* the concepts of being-there (*Dasein*) and sojourn (*Aufenthalt*) are used as synonyms. As being-there relates not only to its own being, but to being as such, its basic structure lies in the understanding of being. The understanding of being is not only a side, abstract addendum to sojourning with beings, but rather the key to comprehending our sojourn as such, notes Heidegger with an emphasis on the important role played by this fundamental determination in the overall clarification of being-there and its

---

[53] Foucault. *Les mots et les choses*, 336–7.
[54] De Man. *Blindness and Insight*, 49.

existentials.[55] The description of existential structures, whether of being-in-the-world, care or being-toward-death, is carried out in *Sein und Zeit* solely with regard to the understanding of being.

In opposition to that, Binswanger completely disregards the understanding of being and contents himself with the general designation of human existence as being-in-the-world, care and being-toward-death. Nevertheless, all these formal classifications obtain their true sense only against the background of the principal delineation of being-there, i.e. the understanding of being. Therefore, Heidegger observes that "'[p]sychiatric *Daseinsanalysis*' operates with a mutilated being-there from which its basic characteristic has been cut out and cut off."[56] Approaching being-there without paying respect to its original relatedness to being, the psychiatric *Daseinsanalysis* changes all its ontological features into purely anthropological classifications. When being-in-the-world, care and being-toward-death have become parts of the mosaic out of which the overall picture of human being is to be composed, it seems only logical that the irresistible need arises to supplement them with love and its corresponding being-beyond-the-world that rises even above the certainty of death.

Once, however, being-in-the-world, care and being-toward-death have been comprehended on the basis of the understanding of being, such supplementation would immediately turn out to be redundant, as the understanding relation to being already encompasses all empirically differentiated modes of behavior, including – among others – love. We can even concur with Heidegger in that through the understanding of being, one can arrive at a much deeper and richer grasp of the phenomenon of love than the one offered in the picture of the loving being-beyond-the-world.[57] Due to the fact that the sojourn relates to being, it can see the other also in a non-expedient and non-pragmatic way. For such a change of perspective to be thematized, it is imperative to stick consistently to the restrictive character of the ontological description of being-there and set out only from those structures revealed by fundamental ontology.

Ignoring the understanding of being leads also to the incorrect interpretation of the role played by the moment of transcendence. As the fundamental moment of our existence, transcendence is established by our relation to being that remains different from all beings, and yet essentially concerns every single one of them. Insofar as transcendence in the common sense of the word denotes proceeding from one level to another, Heidegger specifies it further as proceeding from beings to being. Our existence is in the process of transcending only inasmuch as it advances beyond the framework given by beings and relates to the *being of beings* that radically differs from all beings. Transcendence occurs as advancing from beings in their discoveredness toward being, which guarantees their discoveredness; it can be, in other words, characterized as ecstatic dwelling in the difference between beings and being. Without transcending in precisely this way, without having secured in

---

[55] Heidegger. *Zollikoner Seminare*, 236.

[56] Heidegger. *Zollikoner Seminare*, 237. English edition: Heidegger. *Zollikon Seminars*, 190.

[57] Heidegger. *Zollikoner Seminare*, 237–8, 287.

advance access to being in its utter difference from all beings, we could discover no beings at all. In order to arrive at beings, we must always already advance from beings toward the being of beings.

As beings in their unmediated discoveredness are not that "toward which" our existence advances, but that "from which" our existence advances, a transcendence of this delineation can have nothing to do with the relation of the subjective consciousness to reality. Insofar as the subject-object division is surpassed solely by means of the structure of being-in-the-world in which the understanding of being is omitted, as is the case within psychiatric *Daseinsanalysis*, the temptation cannot be resisted to consider being-in-the-world only as a new determination of the subjectivity of the subject and regard transcendence only as an act by which the consciousness reaches reality. Both being-in-the-world and transcendence are thus extracted out of the context of fundamental ontology, playing once again the roles of transcendental structures of consciousness, where they serve as a foundation for the empirical investigation of human being.

Failing to think the movement of transcendence through to being itself, Binswanger also misses the phenomenon of disclosedness (*die Erschlossenheit*), characteristic of being-there. The fact that being-there is essentially open for the encounter with beings, is understandable only on the basis of its primary disclosedness. In order to encounter some beings, being as such must stand open to us. The disclosedness of being is tied to our existence as that which makes possible the discoveredness of beings. Insofar as the transcending existence always advances from beings to being, insofar as it moves on the edge of the ontic-ontological difference, it simply advances from the discoveredness of beings to disclosedness of being.

The meaning of the disclosedness of being is manifest with special prominence in the phenomenon of anxiety, whose uncanniness removes individual existence from its familiarity with beings, thus allowing it to experience the fearful emptiness of its openness. The disclosedness of being-there remains misunderstood within psychiatric *Daseinsanalysis*, despite the numerous passages analyzing the pathological aspects of uncanniness that deprives the individual existence of all common certainties and confronts it with the bare fact that "it is." Even though the disclosedness is briefly dealt with in *Grundformen und Erkenntnis menschlichen Daseins*, Binswanger does so only to point out its purely individual character.[58] In order to grasp the phenomenon of a loving being with the other, it is, according to him, necessary to rid the disclosedness of the limitation springing from the focus of the individual existence purely on itself, substituting it with an openness pertaining not only to "myself," but to "both of us." However, precisely this statement testifies to a total misunderstanding of the ontological disclosedness and of how it is bound with the overall structure of being-there. The possibility of its most radical individuation might well lie in the act of transcendence, but what is made accessible to individual existence in its relation to disclosedness is not only its own being, but being as such. Disclosedness is also not so much an attribute of the individual existence as an open dimension in which it belongs. Being-there is not a proprietor of

---

[58] Binswanger. *Grundformen und Erkenntnis menschlichen Daseins*, 34.

this open dimension; it is merely allowed to dwell in it. Being-there is someone who remains in the openness of being, and only as such can it encounter that which is; its sojourning with beings is possible only as dwelling in an open dimension in which beings can at all be present.

In order to see being-there in the right light, one must not view it only as sojourn with beings, but rather grasp it as a sojourn in the openness of being.[59] Insofar as Heidegger terms our existence as being-there, this "there" denotes precisely the open dimension of being. The determination "there" refers to no locality within space, but to the openness of being in which being-there dwells.

Only when human existence is explicated as a dwelling in the openness of being is it possible to explain how its *Jemeinigkeit* belongs to it. One's own self is maintained as self-collected dwelling in the clearing of being.[60] Only individual being thus explained allows one to shun his/her individual role, to get enmeshed in beings and lost in the possibilities offered by the world. Nothing but such being can also give it the opportunity to meet the other as partner and together go beyond what has hitherto been considered given and possible. Falling in love, one departs not from an isolated subject, but from the world in which we find our possibilities and where we play our social and sexual roles. Nevertheless, a possible step beyond the framework of the given and certain presupposes the preliminary disclosedness of being, without which the question of how one can abandon one's world and build a new one amidst the ruins would be unanswerable. For love and other crucial moments of human life to be adequately thematized, we need to see that the phenomenon of disclosedness vouches our existence not only for its "being-open" (*das Offen-sein*), but also for its "being-free" (*das Frei-sein*), thanks to which one can break free from all the habitual roles, adopted possibilities and accepted interpretations of one's own existence.

It is this phenomenon that gets lost in Binswanger's concept of the world-project, which forms the cornerstone of his empirical inquiries in the field of psychopathology. When psychiatric *Daseinsanalysis* describes the pathologically structured world-projects determining the character of this or that individual existence, it remains therefore unclear how one can abandon the pathologically distorted world and advance toward new, hitherto inaccessible, possibilities, which is a necessary prerequisite of an effective therapy. Binswanger contents himself with the statement that the psychotherapeutic treatment can be successful once the patient realizes the deficient structure of his/her own world-project, which is a realization that the psychotherapist can facilitate.[61] This, however, gives the impression as if the world-project were the working of some transcendental consciousness which can merely be confronted with its own creation in order to evoke the revision of its relation to the world.

Despite referring to *Vom Wesen des Grundes*, where the world-project is conceived of as the fundamental act by which being-there confronts its own possibilities, Binswanger still neglects the very understanding of being, which in the first place

---

[59] Heidegger. *Zollikoner Seminare*, 188–9.

[60] Heidegger. *Zollikoner Seminare*, 240.

[61] Binswanger, Ludwig. 1955. *Ausgewählte Vorträge und Aufsätze*, Bd. II: *Zur Problematik der psychiatrischen Forschung und zum Problem der Psychiatrie*. Bern: Francke, 293, 306.

allows anything to be understood. "[O]nly in the illumination granted by our understanding of being can beings become manifest in themselves, (i.e., *as* the beings they are and in the way they are)," claims Heidegger.[62] However, in psychiatric *Daseinsanalysis*, the world-project is considered only with regard to the discoveredness of beings that manifest themselves within its framework, not as regards the disclosedness of being that makes it possible for beings to appear as something that is. This leads to an incomplete picture of the phenomenon of being-in-the-world, in which its ontologically constitutive dimension is omitted, and thus the overall image of being-there distorted.

The misunderstanding of the overall structure of being-in-the-world occurring in psychiatric *Daseinsanalysis* affects not only the general exposition of being-there, but also the phenomenological interpretation of the specific forms of the pathological being-in-the-world. Inasmuch as the world-project determines the way in which beings manifest themselves, what this means according to Binswanger is that it determines the configuration, consistency, materiality and tenor of the concrete being-in-the-world. However, Heidegger objects to this, claiming that materiality, consistency or tenor are not determinations of the world as such, but mere designations of beings that appear therein. To consider these qualities moments of the world-project is therefore to mistake that is discovered within the world for the structural alignment of the world as such.[63]

A similar confusion of being-in-the-world with the innerworldly beings occurs when Binswanger describes the temporal continuity of existence which is in jeopardy once being-in-the-world has been pathologically disturbed. The weakening of the temporal continuity can for him be manifested in the forms of phobic fear, compulsive behavior, or eventually the schizophrenic inconsistency of experience, where the fluent temporalization of existence is disturbed by the irresistible onslaughts of the Sudden and the Fearful. However, the key problem of this exposition is the fact that the expression "continuity" does not correspond to the phenomenological structures of the sojourning in the openness of being. The notion of continuity corresponds rather to one's own self-understanding that gets lost in the innerworldly beings, grasping one's own existence according to their criteria. By no means does the idea of continuity, or the possibility of "time coming to a halt" as a consequence of a shock, belong to the phenomenological description of being-in-the-world. "To speak about a break in continuity here, or to characterize the [existential] projection of the word by the category of continuity, as Binswanger does, is a formalization of [being-there's] existing emptying it of any factical [existential] content," says Heidegger.[64]

Nevertheless, this critique of psychiatric *Daseinsanalysis* does not imply in the least the necessity of relinquishing the possibility of grasping pathologically

[62] Heidegger, Martin. 1949. *Vom Wesen des Grundes*. Frankfurt am Main: Vittorio Klostermann, 169. English edition: Heidegger, Martin. 1998. On the Essence of Ground. In *Pathmarks* (trans: McNeill, William). Cambridge: Cambridge University Press, 130.

[63] Heidegger. *Zollikoner Seminare*, 253.

[64] Heidegger. *Zollikoner Seminare*, 257. English version: Heidegger. *Zollikon Seminars*, 206.

disturbed being-in-the-world in its empirical evidence. According to Heidegger, the fundamental presupposition of such a thematization of psychopathological disorders which, unlike psychiatric *Daseinsanalysis*, does not lapse into the anthropological picture of human existence is to pay heed to the overall ontological composition of sojourning in the openness of being. In order to prevent the structures that characterize the sojourning in the openness of being from appearing as merely isolated elements, but rather to allow them to emerge in their original interconnectedness, what one must reveal is their temporal constitution. The temporality proper to being-there has nothing to do with the uninterrupted, homogeneous sequence of moments following one another; its character is given only by the fact that being-there is always already somewhere and somehow situated, that it relates to its own being and being as such, and still is together with beings to which its proclivity is to fall prey. In spite of the fact that the situatedness amidst the understanding of and being together with beings do not as such form temporality, they refer to the dimensions of the having-been, the future, and the present, in which our existence temporalizes itself. It temporalizes itself in that it encompasses the having-been, the future and the present that form together the integral unity of temporality.

Only when the sojourning in the openness of being is considered on the basis of the inseparable unity of the three temporal ecstasies can it be shown where its primordial unity and integrity lie. The existential *Jemeinigkeit*, which encompasses not only the possibility of an integrated individual existence, but also the possibility of self-oblivion and self-evasion, is thus grasped as the ecstatic unity of temporality, in which the overall dwelling in the disclosedness of being becomes constituted. What is also corroborated by this observation is that the threat of the breakdown of the temporal continuity Binswanger speaks about when dealing with psychopathological disorders does not correspond to the phenomenal contents of being-there, since its temporal unity is bound to remain intact during the whole existence. As long as the ontological unity of temporality is preserved, one cannot speak of a factual disintegration of temporality, not even on the ontic level of experience.

It becomes thus evident that the thematization of psychopathological phenomena which is meant to be adequate to being-there cannot do without clarifying the relation between the ontological analytic of being-there and the empirical inquiry into mental disorders. Whereas the ontic investigation adheres to empirically ascertainable phenomena, in which the experiences and attitudes of a certain individual manifest themselves, the ontological inquiry pertains to the being of beings; that is to say, in the relation to human existence, it deals with the phenomenal structures that are accessible not sensorially, but only by means of hermeneutic exposition. The hermeneutic interpretation of being-there must not be confused with the understanding of a specific individual, since what occurs in the first case is the ontological interpretation of basic structures of sojourning in disclosedness, whereas what is at stake in the second case is the understanding of a situational context in which the given individual exists.

Insofar as they strive to understand the patient's situation, a psychiatrist or psychotherapist can unveil the ontic phenomena and their interconnections, but the ontological phenomena as such are accessible only to philosophical inquiry. Therefore, Heidegger stresses that one can, in connection with the psychopathological and psychotherapeutic problematic, speak of "phenomenology" only in the sense of an ontic examination that focuses on the specific possibilities and modes of behavior in the world, not in the sense of the ontological inquiry into being-there.[65] The investigation of pathological symptoms of a certain individual, however, can be guided by the ontological phenomena as unveiled by the hermeneutic exposition of being-there, though it has no right whatsoever to be their master and corrector. This right pertains only to philosophy that reveals the very ontological composition of being-there.[66] Psychiatry and psychotherapy with a *daseinsanalytical* orientation should never lose sight of the fact that their relation to ontological analytic of being-there is that of dependence. As long as the empirical investigation of psychopathological disorders should correspond to the basic character of being-there, it is on Heidegger's view necessary for all the diagnostic and therapeutic action to operate in the light of human existence projected as dwelling in the openness of being. Otherwise, one is in danger of going astray as Binswanger did, seeking on the basis of empirical data to arrange and supplement the ontological structures obtained within the frame of the analytic of being-there.

However, to do him justice, one should note that Binswanger later became aware of his "productive misunderstanding" of the hermeneutic exposition of being-there and tried to make amends. Especially his lecture titled *Der Mensch in der Psychiatrie* testifies to his effort to rectify the relation between the ontic and the ontological level of inquiry, and thus to prevent the ontological description of being-there from becoming contaminated by items of medical knowledge and observations. Apart from confusing the ontological structure of being-in-the-world with ontic phenomena treated by psychiatry or psychotherapy, what is refused here is the anthropological picture of human existence which Heidegger surpasses by determining being-there purely on the basis of the understanding of being.[67]

No matter how steadfastly phenomenological psychiatry may cling to the overall ontological composition of sojourning in the openness of being, the question remains how it can on the basis of the understanding of being explicate the phenomenon of un-reason to which Binswanger alludes in his treatise on schizophrenia. Thematizing that which originally appears as un-reason and non-sense, the psychiatric *Daseinsanalysis* relies on the ontological structure of being-there that remains invariable in its nature; all changes occurring in the course of pathological disorders pertain merely to the ontic plane of experience. Nevertheless, the emphasis lain on the ontological unity of being-there ultimately leads to a normative view of psychopathological phenomena, as the pathologically altered being-in-the-world is perceived as a deficient mode of being. Despite rejecting the normative approach to psychopathological disorders as used in the framework of clinical medicine and turning instead to the primary encounter with un-reason, Binswanger brings his

[65] Heidegger. *Zollikoner Seminare*, 279–81.

[66] Heidegger. *Zollikoner Seminare*, 255.

[67] Binswanger. *Der Mensch in der Psychiatrie*, 21–2.

psychiatric conception again to the notion of deficiency, this time deficiency in the ontic structure of being-in-the-world that is reflected against the background of the integral structural whole of being-there.

The way in which the primary experience with un-reason is depicted in Foucault's *Histoire de la folie* or *Maladie mentale et psychologie*, however, is totally different. The prefix "un" in the word un-reason is understood here not in the negative sense, but rather as an expression of a positive difference. It is no privative negation, by means of which someone is labeled as "devoid of reason," but rather a primary otherness that looms at the limits of our experience. Un-reason and non-sense show themselves no longer as mere shortcomings of sane reason, but as original, non-derived phenomena. It can be concluded from this that the normative view of psychopathological disorders is unnecessary and non-self-evident, and corresponds not so much to un-reason itself as to Binswanger's own psychiatric orientation.

Is it, however, possible to evade the normative view of psychopathological phenomena if at the same time one is to adhere strictly to the ontological description of sojourning in the openness of being? Is it possible at all on the basis of the dynamic structure of existence, created by the understanding of being, to reach a thematization of insanity that would reveal un-reason as its initial and ultimate truth? Inasmuch as every relation with beings is grounded upon the understanding of being, insanity can appear as a certain form of entanglement and absorption in beings, not as un-reason in the strong sense of the word. Insofar as Heidegger derives the ontological character of being-there from the understanding of being, it is possible that this understanding remains concealed, but it can never turn into total non-understanding. Being-there always somehow understands its own being and being as such.

Moreover, what is also reflected in the understanding of being is the exceptionality of human existence, since there is nothing else but this existence that could relate to the disclosedness of being. Animal, unlike the material nature, relates to its environment, but still is not exposed to the openness of being. The uniqueness of human existence manifests itself even where it forgets its innermost character, which is the dwelling in the openness of being, losing itself in its absorption in beings.

In spite of evading the temptation of anthropologism, Heidegger still ensures for the human existence a prominent position in the whole of knowledge, which corresponds to the rootedness of his philosophy within the modern episteme, as described by Foucault in *Les mots et les choses*. From this also springs the emphasis on the constancy of the individual existence that is maintained in the advancing from the discoveredness of beings to disclosedness of being. As the analytic of being-there attributes to it the character of *Jemeinigkeit*, it also secures its individuality in the ecstatic unity of temporality. In the light of *Jemeinigkeit* thus conceived, it is perhaps possible adequately to thematize the neurotic shunning of one's own existence; but once we are faced with the stark reality of un-reason that is manifested in the form of schizophrenic depersonalization, the phenomenological description of sojourning in discloseness has little to offer. The only remaining possibility is to grasp the schizophrenic disintegration of personality as a deficient form of the self-collected individual existence that implicitly refers to the unity of the integrated and autonomous existence. On this point Heidegger's view of the pathologically structured individual existence is no different from Binswanger's psychiatric *Daseinsanalysis*.

If we are to attain the taciturn and disquieting truth of un-reason, we have no option but to turn to a source of inspiration other than fundamental ontology and the ontological project of sojourning in disclosedness. In order to view even so extreme a form of un-reason that manifests itself in the schizophrenic breakdown, where the occurring "end of the world" is accompanied by the disintegration of the individual existence, as an original phenomenon, we need to bring to our aid a conception capable of problematizing the idea of the temporal unity of existence, with which the phenomenological conception of individual existence stands or falls.

The example of Binswanger warns us that, rather than psychological or psychiatric literature, we should prefer the philosophical work which alone can serve for a possible revision of the pillars of Heidegger's ontological project of being-there. In order to avoid the trap of anthropologism, in which one can get stuck by deducing the transcendental structures of human experience from the specific empirical data, we must seek a work that examines and thus already surpasses the boundaries of modern episteme. With regard to a selection thus narrowed, what appears as the most suitable besides Foucault's examination of the relation of Western culture to un-reason is Deleuze's thematization of the extreme forms of thought, not the least of which is insanity. Already in Deleuze's first great oeuvre – *Différence et répétition* – insanity is characterized in such a way that is far from the normative approach to psychopathological disorders. Instead of the clinical view of the mental disorder that reduces it to a mere empirical fact, what comes to the forefront is the effort to grasp schizophrenic, compulsive behavior and dementia as well not only as something observable in human being, but as an outstanding possibility of thought. As the very extremes and limits of thought, all these phenomena fall into the region in whose foundations Deleuze discovers non-sense. Within the framework of thought, non-sense is not a deficit. It does not stand in the same relation to thought as error to true cognition. Both error and truth belong to the region of sense, where they refer to each other. Non-sense, on the contrary, defies all categories of error, deception and non-truth, as it can be neither true nor false. As non-sense stands in the relation to sense as its extreme otherness, what it thus reflects is the finitude of thought as such.[68]

In order for this peculiar finitude to be explicable, it is necessary to reinterpret the traditional picture of thought and of the thinking individual. The first step is to dismantle the idea that thought is a performance of the subject that preserves its constant identity. The thinking subject, whose own identity is the guarantee of the identity of all objects, which creates the prerequisite for their reliable recognition, allows for only one form of cognitive failure – error; other lapses of thought are then understood as mere consequences of outer circumstances. Insofar as the manifold forms of non-sense are to be taken seriously, it is imperative that the question of the condition of their possibility be raised, which Deleuze deems hidden in the link between the process of thinking and the process of individuation. This link has

---

[68] Deleuze. *Différence et répétition*, 199–201.

nothing to do with the structure of *ego cogito*, as it occurs on a plane where no "I" exists. Through individuation, the individual only becomes instituted, but even that is still far away from the constant identity of the thinking subject, as this is open to breaks, changes or encounters that are irreducible to mere recognition of a certain object. In all these situations where the other appears as other and not as representing the identical, what comes into play is a-subjective individuation, and it is its unquiet relation to thought that renders the act of thought a risky venture that can at any moment fall in the bottomless abyss of non-sense.

However, it is not only the constant identity of the thinking subject, but also the phenomenologically projected individuality of human existence that renders unfathomable the dimension proper to non-sense. No matter how resolutely fundamental ontology diverges from the Cartesian picture of thought, it still fails to comply with the requirements of philosophical inquiry into the conditions enabling insanity, which can be documented by the example of *Sein und Zeit*, where the transcending relation to being is connected with the possibility and necessity of "the most radical individuation."[69] Individuation in this context occurs within the framework of the advancing from the discoveredness of beings to the disclosedness of being. Being-there individuates itself in the instance of abandoning its settled-ness amidst things and its social bonds with others which incessantly tempts it to lose itself in them and forget its very own character that consists in dwelling amidst the openness of being. Advancing from the familiarity with beings condemns being-there to solitariness, throwing it into to uncanniness where nothing addresses it in terms of what it has thus far understood. It is only this total solitariness that gives being-there the experience of that in which the foundation of its personal uniqueness lies. In this way it is enabled to re-discover and re-assume itself. Individuation in *Sein und Zeit* is thus conceived of as lonesomeness that opens up a path from self-oblivion back toward individual being-there and its irreplaceable position in the openness of being.

As regards uncanniness Heidegger also adumbrates the dimension of the abyssal depth, but Deleuze ventures even further when he links individuation to the loss of ground (*effondement*) that reveals beneath all grounding the bottomless, formless chaos, where relatedness to oneself is no longer possible. The process of individuation as expounded in *Différence et répétition* presupposes a much more radical getting "outside-itself" than is the case in the ecstatic advancement toward openness of being. What is at stake there is not only the turning away from worldly matters. Nor is it only the loneliness in the depth of uncanniness, but the uncertain search for coherence and stability that may, and then again may not, turn out successful. What is at play here, instead of the polarity of self-oblivion and self-discovery, is the much more radical vacillation between disintegration and reintegration that form the two opposing moments in the process of individuation.

The specificity of an individuation conceived in this manner lies in its impersonal character, as the processes of disintegration and reintegration occur already at a pre-personal stage. The individual, constituted in the field of individuation, is not indivisible, but on the contrary keeps constantly going through moments of

---

[69] Heidegger. *Sein und Zeit*, 38.

decentralization and disorganization, after which there must come the phase of re-consolidation.[70] The ceaseless alteration of disintegration and reintegration attests to the fact that individuality as such is not a lifelong permanence, but only temporary and provisional.

Thus, the conception of individuality as delineated in *Différence et répétition* is substantially different from the phenomenological project of individual being that guarantees beforehand its unity and constancy. Despite the possibility of forgetting its own existence and losing itself in the innerworldly beings it encounters, being-there always retains the character of *Jemeinigkeit* that enables it to re-discover itself at any instant. This unflagging possibility essentially springs from the temporal unity of sojourning in the openness of being. The individuation that occurs in the advancement from the familiarity with beings does not actually run any real risk, as it merely reveals what being-there always already is. Not even the uncanniness into which the solitary existence lapses can explicate the possibility of non-sense unless the temporal unity of existence, and together with it the individual structure of existence, becomes jeopardized. Moreover, as long as the process of individuation is united with the understanding of being that foregrounds sojourning in disclosedness, the mystery remains how something like non-sense and un-reason could appear there.

It may seem that the ontological project of being-there that binds the understanding of being with the ecstatic unity of temporality has its justification insofar as it enables the unveiling of the ontic-ontological difference that occurs in the advancement from the discoveredness of beings to the disclosedness of being. However, one may object to this that even the ontic-ontological difference cannot be adequately comprehended unless the ecstatic unity of temporality that bears the whole structure of the understanding of being is challenged.

As much as he appreciates that Heidegger liberates the ontological difference from the entrapment of representation reducing it to the negative aspect of identity, Deleuze adds in one breath that this step as such is not enough. The first step, which is the realization that being is characterized not by any sort of negativity, but only by its difference from all beings, must be followed by the second step which shall show the ontological difference without any reference to a given unifying principle, be it the unified ontological composition of sojourning in the openness of being.[71] The individual, according to Deleuze, can stand in relation to the total otherness of being only insofar as it is a disintegrated individual, whose moments disassemble and re-assemble themselves on the basis of temporal structures.

What it means in the context of the analytic of being-there is that the advancing from the discoveredness of beings to the disclosedness of being corresponds to the self which is not unified, but rather shattered, by its temporality. But as long as he persistently clings to the temporal unity of individual existence, Heidegger remains incapable of seeing the ontological difference in its purity, as he subjects it to the principle of the Same; in spite of abandoning the notion of identity, to which

---

[70] Deleuze. *Différence et répétition*, 331.
[71] Deleuze. *Différence et répétition*, 89–91.

difference is bound merely as its additional complement, and inquiring instead after the Same which encompasses difference as such, Heidegger does not go far enough, for he still explicates difference on the basis of sameness.[72]

This view leads Deleuze to the necessity of surpassing the Heideggerian philosophy of ontological difference, which serves in *Différence et répétition* as one of the landmarks, and substitute it with a new conception of a pure difference that can do without reference to any *a priori* unity or sameness whatsoever.[73] From this point there thus evolves his philosophical collaboration with Guattari, within whose framework the model of individuality falling apart and a-personal individuation is further worked out.

As this brief and global evaluation necessarily evokes a certain mistrust, our next task will be to show the extent of the validity of the above-mentioned assertions and the extent to which there are exceptions to the given "rule" in Heidegger's philosophy. It may as well be that fundamental ontology already encompasses a certain awareness of the problems that Deleuze points out, and the following stages of Heidegger's thought exhibit various attempts at their solution. Before coming back to the problem of psychopathological disorders, we shall therefore have to explicate in detail the ontological structure of sojourning in disclosedness, especially with regard to the phenomenological project of being-there as adumbrated in *Sein und Zeit*.

References

1. Binswanger, Ludwig. 1955. *Ausgewählte Vorträge und Aufsätze, Bd. II: Zur Problematik der psychiatrischen Forschung und zum Problem der Psychiatrie*. Bern: Francke.
2. Binswanger, Ludwig. 1957. *Schizophrenie*. Pfullingen: Neske.
3. Binswanger, Ludwig. 1957. *Der Mensch in der Psychiatrie*. Pfullingen: Neske.
4. Binswanger, Ludwig. 1964. *Grundformen und Erkenntnis menschlichen Daseins*, 4th ed. München/Basel: Ernst Reinhardt Verlag.
5. Binswanger, Ludwig. 1965. *Wahn. Beiträge zu seiner phaenomenologischen und daseinsanalytischen Erforschung*. Pfullingen: Neske.
6. De Man, Paul. 1983. *Blindness and insight. Essays in the rhetoric of contemporary criticism*. Minneapolis: University of Minnesota Press.
7. Deleuze, Gilles. 1968. *Différence et répétition*. Paris: PUF. English edition: Deleuze, Gilles. 1995. *Difference and Repetition*. Trans. Paul Patton. New York: Columbia University Press.
8. Foucault, Michel. 1963. *Naissance de la Clinique*. Paris: PUF. English edition: Foucault, Michel. 1973. *The Birth of the Clinic*. Trans. A.M. Sheridan. London: Tavistock Publications Limited.
9. Foucault, Michel. 1964. *L'histoire de la folie à l'âge classique*. Paris: Gallimard.
10. Foucault, Michel. 1966. *Maladie mentale et psychologie*. Paris: PUF.
11. Foucault, Michel. 1970. *The order of things*, ed. Ronald D. Laing. London: Tavistock Publications Ltd.
12. Heidegger, Martin. 1949. *Vom Wesen des Grundes*. Frankfurt am Main: Vittorio Klostermann.

---

[72] Deleuze. *Différence et répétition*, 188, 384.

[73] Deleuze. *Différence et répétition*, 1–2.

13. Heidegger, Martin. 1962. *Die Frage nach dem Ding*. Tübingen: Niemeyer.
14. Heidegger, Martin. 1987. *Zollikoner Seminare. Protokolle, Gespräche, Briefe*. ed. Medard Boss. Frankfurt am Main: Vittorio Klostermann. English edition: Heidegger, Martin. 2001. *Zollikon Seminars*. Trans. Franz Mayr and Richard Askay. Evanston: Northwestern University Press.
15. Heidegger, Martin. 1993. *Sein und Zeit*, 17th ed. Tübingen: Niemeyer. English edition: Heidegger, Martin. 1996. *Being and Time*. Trans. Joan Stambaugh. Albany: SUNY Press.

Chapter 3
The Strategy of *Sein und Zeit*

3.1 Ontological Analysis of Being-There

In order to see whether there is validity in the Deleuzian critique of Heidegger, a detailed examination of the ontological structure of human existence as depicted in *Sein und Zeit* is necessary. The examination of all basic components of being-there initially brings to light surprising similarities with Deleuze's philosophical conception, but finally uncovers the fundamental divergence between the two philosophical positions. It is the divergence between the autonomy and unity of thought on the one side, and the heteronomy and multiplicity on the other. This divergence is evident especially in the existential analysis of anxiety where Heidegger finds not a possible disruption of the integrity of the self, but an affirmation of the individual unity of its existence. Such an interpretation of anxiety bears all the signs of what one may call the "romantic strategy" of thought. Supposing that this is the strategy Heidegger applies in *Sein und Zeit*, it becomes comprehensible why he cannot articulate the pathological disintegration of the self as an original phenomenon.

Insofar as reading *Différence et répétition* brings us to contemplating the basic principles of fundamental ontology, it is worth mentioning that this is not the only text in which Deleuze explicitly comes to terms with Heidegger's philosophy. In the last work he wrote together with Guattari, *Qu'est-ce que la philosophie?*, he comes back to it. The pivotal point of their meditations on the character and object of philosophy is the statement that the categories of subject and object are insufficient in grasping the true character of thought. Thought is for Heidegger not a connecting line between subject and object or one of them revolving around the other, for he situates it instead in the difference between beings and being. More precisely, what is at work within the framework of thought is the difference between the discoveredness of beings and disclosedness of being. The question of the onto-logical difference that resonates in the tension between the discoveredness of beings and disclosedness of being, according to Deleuze and Guattari, refers also

© Springer International Publishing Switzerland 2015
P. Kouba, *The Phenomenon of Mental Disorder*, Contributions
to Phenomenology 75, DOI 10.1007/978-3-319-10323-5_3

to the themes of territory and of deterritorialization that play an important role within their own philosophical project.[1]

However incompatible with Heidegger's inquiry into being the notions of territory and deterritorialization may seem, their adequacy becomes apparent if we realize that territory is, in *Qu'est-ce que la philosophie?*, tied together with home, with what is familiar, whereas deterritorialization belongs to what is *unheimlich*.[2] Territory is a region in which we feel at home. As such it presents the frame within which we know our way about, where we can thus act effectively. Deterritorialization, on the contrary, entails a process of abandoning territory and exposing oneself to uncanniness. This occurs once the frame of territory has been shattered and thought has set out for a journey into the unknown. In relation to the homelessness of deterritorialization, territory is not only the lost home; from the outset, territory and the deterritorialization are inextricably linked, which finds its corroboration in the fact that territory always includes possible paths of escape.

The topic of dwelling, which belongs to the character of territory, appears also in *Sein und Zeit* as part of the discussion of being-in-the-world. According to Heidegger, the world is primarily a region in which we dwell and around which we find our way.[3] Our being-there is initially and for the most part situated in the world as the familiar. Nevertheless, being-in-the-world can at any moment show itself also in the mode of uncanniness that reminds us of the true character of our being-there, i.e. sojourning in the openness of being.[4]

Insofar as the notions of territory and deterritorialization are projected onto the context of the ontological analytic of being-there, one can say that the former corresponds to the region where the familiarity with beings prevails, whereas the latter refers to the moment in which the open dimension of being uncovers itself. As long as territory is characterized by the discoveredness of beings, what emerges in deterritorialization is disclosedness of being. The ontological project of being-there, as adumbrated in *Sein und Zeit*, is then marked by the deterritorialization being unified with transcendence, within whose frame we advance from the discoveredness of beings to disclosedness of being.

Even though the basic motives of territory and deterritorialization can be found within the frame of fundamental ontology, it is by no means something which makes Deleuze and Guattari accept Heidegger's position. According to them, Heidegger approaches but cannot fully come to grips with the deterritorialization, for he constantly links it to the understanding of being anchored in the ontological unity of human existence. The uncanniness of being-in-the-world,

---

[1] Deleuze, Gilles, and Guattari, Félix. 1991. *Qu'est-ce que la philosophie?*. Paris: Minuit, 90–1.

[2] Deleuze and Guattari. *Qu'est-ce que la philosophie?*, 176.

[3] Heidegger. *Sein und Zeit*, 54. English edition: Heidegger, Martin. 1996. *Being and Time* (trans: Stambaugh, Joan). Albany: SUNY Press, 50–1.

[4] Note: Although the notion of "*Aufenthalt*" is practically nowhere to be found in *Sein und Zeit*, we shall still make use of it in our discussion, especially for stylistic reasons. As has been already said, the notions of "sojourn" and "being-there" operate in Heidegger as synonyms, and we will keep using them in this way.

through which disclosedness as such appears, is therefore not nearly as radical as the deterritorialization exposited in *Qu'est-ce que la philosophie?*.

The key prerequisite for depicting the revolutionary dynamism of thought, which invalidates all opinions and habitual viewpoints, is the differentiation of relative and absolute deterritorialization. These are not to be differentiated by placing relative deterritorialization occurring within the scope of psychic, social, geographical and political coordinates, and ascribing absolute deterritorialization only to pure thinking. Their difference is rather given by absolute deterritorialization occurring not by means of unification but by the breaking down of all unity, whereas relative deterritorialization always maintains a certain unity in one way or another. It is absolute deterritorialization that exposes thought to chaos which dissolves all coherence. Thought in this case appears an utterly perilous business, since chaos affects it as an endless variability and disorganization that provides no support whatsoever. Dissatisfied with the relative certainty of the opinion, thought necessarily runs the risk that brings it closer to rapture, intoxication or pathologically altered experience. The primary need of thought is thus the search for consistency that would enable it to resist chaos. Thought must undergo consolidation that would give chaos at least some coherence.

The need for finding an anchor, clinging to it and finding one's way, however, already lays the foundations for the establishment of new territory. Absolute deterritorialization must therefore go together with correlative reterritorialization, or at least with the effort to establish new territory. The same applies to relative deterritorialization, which is always secondary in relation to absolute deterritorialization. In this sense, it is therefore possible to comprehend the movement of thought as an interplay of deterritorialization and reterritorialization, which is exactly what Deleuze and Guattari have in mind when they claim that "to think is to voyage" in *Mille plateaux* [5]

But does not Heidegger claim something similar in the 1929–1930 Freiburg lecture series published under the title *Die Grundbegriffe der Metaphysik*, when he describes the mood belonging to philosophical thought as homesickness?[6] Unlike science, philosophical inquiry does not allow itself to be restricted to a predetermined domain of investigation. It creates its own domain only by means of its activity and keeps it open through inquiry. According to Heidegger, philosophical thought is characterized by Novalis's dictum that ascribes to it the unquenchable desire for being home everywhere. However, this desire can arise in philosophy only because the one who philosophizes is nowhere at home. He/she is continuously on the way home, but home always lies beyond.

Yet, homesickness is not a peculiarity of a few eccentrics, for philosophical inquiry essentially springs from human existence as such. Not only the philosopher, but we all are homeless. Considering that being-there is on the way, or indeed its

---

[5] Deleuze, Gilles, and Guattari, Félix. 1987. *Thousand Plateaus* (trans: Massumi, Brian). Minneapolis: Minnesota University Press, 482.

[6] Heidegger, Martin. 1983. *Die Grundbegriffe der Metaphysik*, Gesamtausgabe Bd. 29/30. Frankfurt am Main: Vittorio Klostermann, 7–8.

very being *is* the way, Heidegger attributes to it the character of transition (*der Übergang*). He sees in this transitoriness not only transitivity that enables it to advance from the ontic to the ontological level, but also its finitude. Determining the very basis of our being-in-the-world, finitude distinguishes us from animals, which can indeed perish, and yet are not transitory in the proper sense, for they remain instinctively attentive to their immediate environment. As finite, our existence necessarily remains incomplete and unclosed, from which springs also its openness to what is yet to come. As long as we do not evade our finitude, but rather accept it as our essential lot, we exist transitorily. The decision to come to grips with one's own transitoriness brings one back upon itself, throwing it into radical solitariness. The possibility of accepting and bearing the finitude of its existence thus makes individuation possible for being-there.

Insofar as the acceptance of the finite character of one's own existence, its "becoming finite" (*die Verendlichung*) in Heidegger's terms, remains bound with the act of individuation without the disruption of overall integrity of existence, it cannot be confused with the finitude of thought as suggested by Deleuze and Guattari. The conception of finitude as indicated in *Qu'est-ce que la philosophie?* is much more radical than Heidegger's conception of existential transitoriness. Finitude understood as exposure to chaos leads not to mere revelation of the unique individuality of existence, but to an unstoppable disintegration of individuality as such. Its main challenge is the consolidation of life which loses all its certainty in deterritorialization.

As the processes of deterritorialization and reterritorialization occur not only in the case of human beings, it seems also that the conception of finitude as presented in *Mille plateaux* or *Qu'est-ce que la philosophie?* pertains to all living, i.e. self-forming organisms that actively resist the destructive forces of chaos. Insofar as human being is distinguished from animals, this is a distinction only in the degree of factual and potential deterritorialization.

The mere statement of the disproportion between these two divergent views of deterritorialization, however, is still dissatisfactory. If we want to grasp the strategic reasons compelling Heidegger for "betraying" the deterritorialization, we must map out exactly the points in *Sein und Zeit* that indicate its direction and scope. This requires that we initially focus on those parts of the ontological analytic of being-there that exposit the secured dwelling in the world and also on passages where uncanniness comes into play. Another theme which must be brought into focus is the finitude of the individual existence.

Inquiring into the ontological structure of being-there, Heidegger departs from the conviction that this structure should be discerned by how we exist initially and for the most part, and not by some exceptional or ideal state. Therefore, the phenomenological description of sojourning in the disclosedness focuses primarily on our common, everyday mode of existence. What is reflected in this way is not only some sociological average of the manifold lifestyles. Regardless of the ontic differences among the various individuals and their lifestyles, one can state that we are always in one way or another familiar with the world and with beings therein. All common modes of behavior by which we relate to beings are based on a familiarity with the world we inhabit. Heidegger terms the world with which we are familiar "the surrounding world" (*die Umwelt*).[7] This world is not only a mere set of things, but rather an open horizon in which we orientate ourselves and understand beings and the possibilities they offer. As such, the surrounding world is that "in which" the everyday existence is situated. Insofar as the phenomenon of the everyday being-in-the-world is to be comprehended, we must grasp thematically the open horizon of the surrounding world and to describe its ontological structure.

Familiarity with the surrounding world is primarily reflected in the certainty with which we treat the beings shown in the horizon of this world. In our everyday being-in-the-world, we are concerned and occupied with beings. According to Heidegger, we take heed of beings, even while doing nothing in particular. All possible forms of behavior in which we treat or disregard beings are thus already certain modes of "concern" (*das Besorgen*).

Insofar as we deal with beings practically, we encounter them as useful things. Beings, which we treat within the frame of our everyday being-in-the-world, don't manifest themselves in their presence-at-hand, but as that which serves some purpose. The useful thing, however, is never given in isolation, for it always has its place within a certain context of useful things. Every useful thing can show itself as what it is only in the referential totality of useful things (the hammer referring to the nail, etc.). Considering their utility and availability, Heidegger attributes to useful things the character of handiness, or literally: readiness-to-hand (*die Zuhandenheit*). This readiness-to-hand, revealed by practical sight, is ontologically dependent on the referential whole of their mutual relations with which we are always already familiar. The bond connecting the specific thing with the referential context of useful things becomes apparent especially when the thing in question is broken and no longer serves its purpose. As a result, this thing shows itself as something merely present-at-hand. The referential whole of useful things thereby becomes conspicuous, contrary to its original nonthematic evidence.

In the everyday concern this nonthematic evidence retains yet another characteristic of beings that are ready-to-hand – their "relevance" (*die Bewandtnis*). Relevance is not an isolated quality either, for it always functions in the framework of the previously disclosed totality of relevance. We can understand what this or that thing is relevant for, only as long as we disclose particular beings as parts of the overall context of relevance. As long as we remain familiar with the surrounding world, we always have the totality of relevance already disclosed, understanding thereby not only the things that are ready-to-hand, but also our own possibilities.

The whole context of relations and references through which we understand beings ready-to-hand as well as ourselves and our own possibilities is referred to in *Sein und Zeit* as "significance" (*die Bedeutsamkeit*). Significance is the ontological structure of the surrounding world with which we are familiar. It is by virtue of this structure that we can uncover specific beings as ready-to-hand. This structure is the prerequisite for the signification of some entity to manifest itself. In this sense, signification can be regarded as the condition for the practical uncovering of beings.

---

[7] Heidegger. *Sein und Zeit*, 66. English edition: Heidegger. *Being and Time*, 62.

On the ontological level, the structure of signification thus proves that the surrounding world is not what we simply exist in but what forms the inseparable part of the whole constitution of our sojourning in disclosedness.

Moreover, what also finds its foundation in the ontological structure of the surrounding world is the existential spatiality that demarcates space for our everyday encounter with beings ready-to-hand. Within the framework of practical treatment of things, the useful thing is always situated in an environment where it has its place. Heidegger calls this environment, where all useful things have their appropriate place, "region" (*die Gegend*). Region is the segmented diversity of places that is disclosed together with the totality of relevance and significance and as such provides room for singular beings ready-to-hand. In its open vastness, region is delimited by the horizon that preserves the familiarity of its places and the inconspicuous certainty of its directions for endeavors. Familiar with region in our everyday treatment of things ready-to-hand, we always somehow know our way around. By the same token, our existence has always already taken a direction, i.e. it discerns right from left, near from far. The existential spatiality therefore always concerns our lived body (*der Leib*) that is not to be mistaken for a corporeal thing present somewhere in space. Unlike the corporeal thing, the lived body takes active part in the overall context of region, in which it traverses distances and retains its directionality. The prerequisite for factical directionality and traversing distances thus lies in the previous disclosedness of the totality of relevance and significance that provides room for practical dealing with beings ready-to-hand.

A further inquiry into the everyday being-in-the-world departs from the fact that one is never totally alone within the surrounding world. Since the practical dealing with beings that are ready-to-hand always refers to other users, these others are virtually present, even though no one is close by. Their existence is encoded in the ontological structure of the surrounding world as primordially as the relevance of beings ready-to-hand. Everyday existence is therefore being-with others and the space of region is a socialized space. Others appear in the world not as strange subjects, but in their practical dealing with things ready-to-hand. As long as we understand them, it is not due to some self-projection or empathy, but on the basis of the overall structure of the surrounding world with which we are familiar. *Socius* is primarily understandable for us as one who shares with us the same context of relevance and significance.

Inasmuch as we immediately grasp the sense and aim of what our neighbors do and strive for, we cannot be outright apathetic to them; we always, in one way or another, attend to them. This "solicitude" (*die Fürsorge*), which expresses the essential interest in the others even in the moment of turning away from them, is contrasted with concern in that it relates to the existents that have the character of being-in-the-world themselves. Yet, similarly to the concern with things, solicitude itself is no random momentary state, but rather the existential determinant of sojourning in disclosedness as such.

Paying heed to others in our everyday existence, we always compare ourselves to them in one way or another. The dependence on others necessarily entailed in this comparing leads us to conformity. This tendency to conform to others results in the impersonal anonymity of the everyday being-in-the-world. Instead of bearing responsibility for one's own opinions and deeds, the individual submits to the rule of "the they" (*das Man*) that decides what is reasonable, appropriate, and valid. Prescribing the possibilities of everyday existence, the public anonymity establishes the rule of mediocrity that excludes everything original, exceptional and unique. Its medium is superficiality of opinion that understands and judges everything. By allowing it to shun the responsibility for its own existence, the public anonymity provides individual existence with a relief from the burden of its own being. As long as the individual shuns the weight of its own existence, preferring rather the relief offered by public anonymity, its way of being is necessarily dependent and non-autonomous.

In *Sein und Zeit*, the way of existence in which the individual turns away from itself and succumbs to the impersonal anonymity is characterized as "falling prey" (*das Verfallen*). As an everyday mode of being-in-the-world, falling prey presents the existential movement in which the individual existence falls away from its being in disclosedness, falling prey to the surrounding world with the familiar. By falling prey, being-there becomes wholly absorbed in the possibilities and matters offered by the surrounding world. Thus, the movement of falling prey creates a sort of "whirlpool" in which the existence ceaselessly revolves.[8]

Paradoxically, absorption in the surrounding world provides us with peace consisting not so much in slothful idleness as in the feeling that the given mode of being is in order, i.e. in accord with how everybody lives, speaks and thinks. However, it is this accord that alienates the individual existence from itself, concealing from it its very own possibilities. Instead of searching for and projecting such possibilities, being-there strays into the surrounding world, which leads it to the point where it understands itself on the basis of the things it finds in this world.

However hard the individual existence may try to relieve itself of the burden of its own existence and rest in public anonymity, this wish can never completely be fulfilled. It is mood rather than knowledge that discloses the existential burden. The individual existence can turn away from itself only because it is led ontologically to itself through the basic disposition of anxiety. It is precisely this disposition that gives rise to the burden which will never just go away, however hard one tries to be rid of it.

Unlike fear, which is necessarily connected with some innerworldly entity, anxiety is not about some entity that endangers us. It is rather concerned with being-in-the-world as such. This indefinite threat, which is by no means external, presents itself as uncanniness. As such it is the very opposite of the familiarity with the surrounding world that determines the character of the common everydayness. In anxiety one realizes what it is "not to be at home," torn out of the referential and relational context of the surrounding world and banished into exile where there is nothing for it to hold on to. No innerworldly thing is relevant here any longer. When the ontological structure of the surrounding world collapses, one experiences the utter loss of significance. Since the significative structure of the surrounding world

---

[8] Heidegger. *Sein und Zeit*, 179–80. English edition: Heidegger. *Being and Time*, 167–8.

provides a diversity of places, what is also paralyzed by anxiety is the practical orientation in space.

Moreover, in uncanniness the bonds are torn that connect us with others. In this state the rule of public anonymity comes to an end. The individual existence thus becomes de-socialized and left in utter solitariness. In anxiety, the individual existence is deprived of the possibility of understanding itself from the standpoint of the public anonymity, left only with its own being.[9] By no means, however, does this mean that the individual existence thereby finds itself completely outside of the world. Anxiety "individuates being-there to its ownmost being-in-the-world," claims Heidegger, "being-there is individuated, but *as* being-in-the-world."[10] Anxiety is an outstanding existential disposition because it tears being-there out of its familiarity with the surrounding world only in order to reveal to it the empty openness of the world and its thrownness therein. In the disposition of anxiety, the individual existence is faced with the brute fact that it is nothing other than "thrown being" in disclosedness and that this is what it must remain, despite its preoccupation with innerworldly things and public anonymity that endow it with the feelings of security, sureness and fullness of life.

In its disclosedness, however, the individual existence also finds its "being-free" (*das Freisein*) that enables it to abandon all social roles, all adopted possibilities and to grasp itself as it truly is. In the *solitariness* brought by anxiety, individual existence in disclosedness shows itself in its difference from all habitual roles and easily accessible possibilities, offered in the surrounding world. This difference is eventually nothing but difference from all beings, both with and without the character of being-there. Therefore, it is only in anxiety that there can appear both the uniqueness of one's position in disclosedness and a fundamental difference of this disclosedness from all beings, which *Sein und Zeit* terms the ontological difference.

Mention should also be made here of the phenomenon of the lived body, especially because it never shows itself in the connection with the original disclosedness as revealed in anxiety. When Heidegger leaves the question of the lived body aside in his interpretation of anxiety, this is not an oversight. Nor is it done because fundamental ontology is not supposed to serve an exhaustive description of human existence. What is at work here is the philosophical decision that is explicitly formulated in *Zollikoner Seminare*: the phenomenon of the lived body is linked to sensuality and as such codetermines the character of being-in-the-world, but this does not pertain to the fundamental structure of existence, which is the understanding of being.[11] Insofar as being-there understands being as such, the lived body has no share therein. As the openness of being can manifest itself only in pure thought, and not in a sensual perception, the understanding of being reaches beyond the limits of the lived body that is always delineated by the horizon of the surrounding world. It is therefore understandable that the lived body can play no role in the phenomenological exposition of anxiety either.

---

[9] Heidegger. *Sein und Zeit*, 188. English edition: Heidegger. *Being and Time*, 176.

[10] Heidegger. *Sein und Zeit*, 187–9. English edition: Heidegger. *Being and Time*, 176.

[11] Heidegger. *Zollikoner Seminare*, 244–5, 254.

The exclusion of the lived body from the movement of transcendence does not change anything about the fact that the phenomenon of anxiety has its physiological correlates and preconditions. These, however, pertain only to the body as a corporeal thing or biological organism, and not to the body as integral part of the ontological constitution of being in disclosedness. Physiological processes thus remain secondary in the relation to anxiety. In spite of conceding that anxiety can also be evoked physiologically, Heidegger stresses that this is only because our existence is "anxious in the very ground of its being."[12]

This does not mean that uncanniness always shows itself in its truly ontological sense. Rather, the point is that uncanniness is the original mode of being-in-the-world. Uncanniness in this respect is a more primordial mode of sojourning in disclosedness than the everyday secured being-at-home in the surrounding world. Although we initially and for the most part remain familiar with the surrounding world, this being-at-home is a mode of the original not-being-at-home, and not vice versa.[13] In comparison with the groundless depth of anxiety, the everyday solicitude for others or concern with things ready-to-hand is merely a superficial mode of being. This also explains the attractiveness of the shallowness and unoriginality of public anonymity that enables us to veil the abyss of anxiety. Since uncanniness reveals being in disclosedness as uneasy and precarious, we seek refuge from it in the familiar surrounding world and in the possibilities it offers. But since being-in-the-world is essentially permeated by uncanniness, being-at-home in the surrounding world can at any time and for no obvious reason change into desolate not-being-at-home.

Another "intrusive" factor that disrupts the peaceful being-at-home in the surrounding world is conscience, whose voice claims our attention. Conscience as explicated in *Sein und Zeit* is not what is commonly understood by this word, i.e. a phenomenon operating in relation to a certain performed or intended deed in the polarity of "good" and "bad" conscience. The ontological interpretation treats conscience as a purely "formal" structure of being-there, i.e. as an existential phenomenon belonging to being in disclosedness. The existential role of conscience lies in its appeal to being-there that has become lost in public anonymity, rousing it from its absorption in the surrounding world. Insofar as conscience deprives being-there of its everyday refuge, it is only because its call comes from uncanniness in which the original homelessness of sojourning in disclosedness is unveiled. The primary tuning of the conscience's voice is the uncanniness of anxiety.

What conscience gives to individual existence is its own guilt. To be guilty, "*schuldig sein*" in German, generally means "to owe," or "to bring about a lack." With reference to the formal conception of guilt articulated as a certain cause of negativeness, Heidegger finds the original being-guilty of individual existence in its thrownness, i.e. in that it is thrown being in disclosedness. The reason for the negativeness is the fact that individual existence has not given its disclosedness to itself, and yet it can exist only on its ground.

---

[12] Heidegger. *Sein und Zeit*, 190. Heidegger. *Being and Time*, 177.

[13] Heidegger. *Sein und Zeit*, 189. English edition: Heidegger. *Being and Time*, 176.

Disclosedness is the enabling ground for being-there because, as Heidegger claims, "[t]hrough disclosedness, the being that we call being-there is in the possibility of *being* its there."[14] Although being-there has not laid the ground of its own existence, it is bound by its weight that shows itself most primordially in the uncanniness of anxiety. That being-there is guilty in the very foundation of its being appears most clearly in uncanniness, where all it is left with is the sheer fact that it is "there" as being in openness. In uncanniness, the negativeness of one's own existence has its essential source.

However, it is not only the ground of sojourning in disclosedness that is imbued with negativeness – it is also its existential performance. We can always choose only one of our possibilities, whereas others elude us by the mere consequence of the act of choice. Our existence is thus permeated by negativeness throughout. This negativeness, claims Heidegger, does not have the character of *privation*, i.e. of lack relative with regard to the unachieved ideal, since it determines sojourning in disclosedness as such.[15]

When it is said that the voice of conscience gives us to understand our existential guilt, this does not mean that conscience coerces us to somehow fill in the negativeness of our own existence; it rather summons us to accept it and keep it as such. The voice of conscience, stemming from uncanniness, calls us to return from the impersonal anonymity of everyday existence back to the ground one's own existence; at the same time, conscience also invites individual existence to accept the limitedness of its possibilities, from which one possibility is to be chosen and other ones foregone.

As long as it wants to have a conscience, individual existence corroborates the authenticity of its being in disclosedness. Conversely, as long as it silences the voice of conscience and wants to hear nothing of its essential being-guilty, the individual exists only in an inauthentic way. In the first case, what is characteristic is the readiness to bear one's own solitariness amidst uncanniness, while in the other case individual existence falls prey to the surrounding world and to public anonymity.

In order to describe the authentic way of existence Heidegger uses the term "resoluteness" (*die Entschlossenheit*). This represents a prominent way of sojourning in disclosedness whose uniqueness lies in that it, unlike inauthentic irresoluteness, reveals "the most primordial truth of being-there."[16] The uniqueness of resoluteness does not lie in bringing the individual automatically into uncanniness, leaving it there to itself. Even the resolute existence cannot do without being-with others and without the surrounding world, since it must, as being-in-the-world, project itself into certain possibilities, which does not however mean that it should fall prey to them in the way of inauthentic existence. In these possibilities, the authentic existence opens its own way in which it allows itself be led by its ownmost potentiality of being. In this sense, the resolute existence transcends the horizon of the surrounding world, grounding its understanding of specific possibilities in the understanding

14 Heidegger. *Sein und Zeit*, 270. English edition: Heidegger. *Being and Time*, 250.
15 Heidegger. *Sein und Zeit*, 285–6. English edition: Heidegger. *Being and Time*, 262–4.
16 Heidegger. *Sein und Zeit*, 297. English edition: Heidegger. *Being and Time*, 273–4.

of singularity and the contingency of its being in disclosedness. The understanding of its insecure and yet irreplaceable position in disclosedness shows being-there the innerwordly beings, as well as being-with others, in a light entirely different from the one of inauthentic existence that perceives them as the be-all and end-all of its being. In its inauthenticity, existence is absorbed by the surrounding world and its public anonymity to such an extent that it is "lived" by them, rather than assigning them their value and sense. On the contrary, the authentic existence breaks free from its subjugation to them, and even if it never fully abandons them, it still discloses them in an entirely original fashion, understanding them out of itself and out of its own being in disclosedness.

In this manner, the authentic existence is stretched between the commonly shared surrounding world and the empty disclosedness of the world, in which it stands absolutely alone. The tension of these two extremes determines the authentic existence in its unique individuality, simultaneously referring to what might be called the "heroic pathos" of *Sein und Zeit*. Authentic is the existence which resolutely advances from impersonal anonymity in order to take on its solitary being in disclosedness. "He who is resolute knows no fear, but understands the possibility of anxiety," from whose uncanniness the inauthentic existence hides in the familiar and habitual surrounding world.[17] If we speak, however, of the difference between the resolute and the irresolute existence, all moral judgments are to be left aside. When the ontological inquiry juxtaposes the gregarious, dependent and fallen existence with the essentially resolute and individualized existence, its aim is not to establish any criterion for estimating specific deeds. This differentiation is meant to be purely descriptive.

Since resoluteness, unlike everyday irresoluteness, reveals the most original truth of being-there, it is possible to use it as the ground for grasping the overall ontological constitution of being-there. What belongs to the ontological structure of being-there is both the disclosedness of the world and the surrounding world, and thus being-there can show itself in its integrity only in the moment when it stands resolutely in between these two. This standing entails also the manifestation of the difference between discoveredness of beings and disclosedness of being.

As long as we relate to our individual being in disclosedness, and together with it to being as such, it means that we essentially care about them. Only when caring about one's own being can one be interested in something else, be it innerworldly things or others with whom one shares the surrounding world. Both concern with things and solicitude for others are grounded upon this relation to oneself called "care" (*die Sorge*) in *Sein und Zeit*. Care in the ontological sense has nothing to do with a temporary state of mind such as everyday worry, since it expresses the whole structure of sojourning in disclosedness that encompasses the possibilities of both the authentic and the inauthentic existence.

If we take the schema of being-in-the-world as drafted in *Zollikoner Seminare* and complete it with moments of authentic standing in disclosedness and inauthentic

---

[17] Heidegger. *Sein und Zeit*, 344. English edition: Heidegger. *Being and Time*, 316.

entanglement in the surrounding world, we can imagine the ontological structure of care in the following fashion[18]:

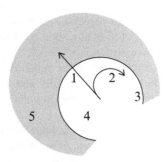

What should be evident from the draft is not only the ecstatic-horizontal structure of sojourning in disclosedness, but also the difference between the surface level of everyday being in the surrounding world and depth, that is the original dimension of the openness of being.

Since the ontological constitution of care is not a static structure, but rather determines the individual existence in its dynamism, Heidegger articulates it by means of the moments of thrownness, projecting and falling prey. These three moments together form one whole whose unity corresponds to the ontological phenomenon of care. Thrownness, projecting and falling prey conjoin not as isolated elements from which one of them may be missing at times, but rather as integral components of one ontological whole. This counts for both the authentic existence that operates in the same surrounding world as falling prey and the inauthentic existence that also cares about its being, thus projecting itself in its own "inauthentic" manner toward its own ground. Both of these two modes of being in disclosedness represent two different ways of thrownness, projecting and falling prey conjoining in one structural whole. In order for the whole ontological structure of care to show itself in detail, it is necessary to further delineate the character of each of its three constitutive moments.

The first of the three fundamental moments of sojourning in disclosedness is thrownness, also termed "facticity", since it is by its means that the individual existence is brought to face the fact of its being in disclosedness. Facticity lies in individual existence being confronted with the fact "that it is … and has to be" as an open being-in-the-world. The manner in which the individual existence always finds itself in the open region of the world is ontologically grounded in "disposition" (*die Befindlichkeit*), i.e. in what we commonly know as mood. Disposition decides how individual existence finds itself in the openness of its world. In disposition, being-there "is always already brought before itself, it has always already found itself, not as perceiving oneself to be there, but as one finds one's self", claims Heidegger.[19]

---

[18] 1. authentic existence and the ensuing movement of transcendence, 2. inauthentic existence and movement of falling prey taking the form of a whirl, 3. the horizon of the surrounding world, 4. discoveredness of beings, 5. disclosedness of being.

[19] Heidegger. *Sein und Zeit*, 135. English edition: Heidegger. *Being and Time*, 128.

In this respect, individual existence is brought face to face with its disclosedness most primordially by the fundamental mood of anxiety. Of all possible moods, anxiety is exceptional in that it reveals one's own being as a burden. As such, anxiety is the ground for all other moods, both depressed and elevated. Unlike anxiety that renders being-there radically solitary by expelling it from the context of the surrounding world, all other emotions determine not only how the individual existence finds itself, but also how the innerworldly beings or other people manifest themselves to it. Nevertheless, individual existence cannot uncover beings in their entirety unless it is exposed to the surrounding world by means of disposition.

In this way, a certain set of possibilities becomes accessible to individual existence. Finding itself in some disposition, it becomes situated in possibilities in which its potentiality of being is made clear. In order for a possibility to be its own possibility, individual existence must understand it in relation to its own potentiality of being. Thus, we get to the second moment constitutive of sojourning in disclosedness – the project that characterizes understanding. This existential project pertains to being in disclosedness as primordially as thrownness of disposition. Insofar as disposition determines individual existence in its facticity, projecting characterizes it in its existentiality, testifying to how one performs and manages one's own being in disclosedness.[20] Hence, individual existence exists in the mode of a "thrown project."[21]

What individual existence understands in its self-projecting is its being in disclosedness which it essentially cares about. Together with it individual existence understands also the referential relations of the surrounding world with which it is familiar. That is to say, understanding itself in its very own potentiality of being, individual existence projects the significative structure of the surrounding world that determines its own possibilities.[22]

The difference between authentic and inauthentic existence thus results from the question whether individual existence itself, on the basis of its potentiality of being, really projects its own possibilities, or whether it settles for possibilities already given and accessible within the frame of everyday being-in-the-world. Insofar as it understands its own possibilities out of its very own potentiality of being, it exists authentically; conversely, if it exposes itself to possibilities revealed in the surrounding world in which it loses itself, it exists inauthentically.

The third existential moment that fits in the overall ontological constitution of care is falling prey. More suitable than "falling prey", however, is the term "being-together-with" (*das Sein bei*), also used by Heidegger in this connection. Being-together-with, as Friedrich-Wilhelm von Herrmann explains in his *Subjekt und Dasein*, is more suitable since it encompasses not only the inauthentic mode of existence, but overall being together with innerworldly beings.[23] Being-together-with

---

[20] Heidegger. *Sein und Zeit*, 143. English edition: Heidegger. *Being and Time*, 134–5.

[21] Heidegger. *Sein und Zeit*, 148. English edition: Heidegger. *Being and Time*, 147–8.

[22] Heidegger. *Sein und Zeit*, 143–5. English edition: Heidegger. *Being and Time*, 134–6.

[23] Herrmann, Friedrich-Wilhelm, von. 1985. *Subjekt und Dasein*. Frankfurt am Main: Vittorio Klostermann, 198–224.

beings does not necessarily have to express only the entanglement in the surrounding world and the escape from the uncanniness of anxiety, as it can also take the form of resolute existence ready for anxiety, which understands itself, in its concern with innerworldy beings, out of its potentiality of being.

Only with this in mind can we understand that the phenomenon of being-together-with comes into play in the formal description of the ontological structure of care that encompasses both the authentic and the inauthentic existence in all their essential aspects. In *Sein und Zeit*, the ontological structure of sojourning in disclosedness is described as an original whole including the moments of being-ahead-of-itself, being-already-in and being-together-with.[24] As has been implied, being-together-with corresponds in this respect to concern with the innerwordly beings, whereas being-ahead-of-itself is characteristic of the project-ing, and being-already-in refers to the thrownness and situatedness of being-in-the-world. All the three moments constitutive of care can be separated from each other only for the sake of philosophical exposition, but none of them can be missing within the factual being in disclosedness.

Only on the ground of the structural whole of care described above is it possible to comprehend the peculiar structure of individual existence that characterizes being-there. Insofar as being-there is "always mine", it is not because it appears as a substantial subject or that it exists as the "I" that retains its invariable identity in the alternation of its experiences and attitudes. The individual character of sojourn-ing in disclosedness can be preserved only as the ontological unity of thrownness, projecting and being-together-with innerworldly beings. The unity of individual existence is the unity of the ontological constitution of care, whose whole is most primordially revealed in the authentic existence.[25] It is from there that we should depart if we are to comprehend the original constancy of individual being that has nothing to do with the permanent occurrence of the identical subject.

The authentic constancy of individual existence also sheds light upon the incon-stancy of the self characterizing the inauthentic existence.[26] Whereas the authentic existence retains its individual self-subsistence by resolutely projecting itself toward its solitary potentiality of being, the inauthentic existence becomes deprived thereof when scattered in the surrounding world, losing itself in the impersonal anonymity of common everydayness. Even though we exist, initially and for the most part, in the mode of public anonymity, it is necessary to expound the volatile unsteadiness of existence that falls prey to the surrounding world and public anonymity on the ground of the authentic existence, and not vice versa. "It is true that existentially the authenticity of being a self is closed off and repressed in entanglement, but this clos-ing off is only the *privation* of a disclosedness which reveals itself phenomenally in the fact that the flight of [being-there] is flight *from* itself," claims Heidegger.[27]

---

[24] Heidegger. *Sein und Zeit*, 192. English edition: Heidegger. *Being and Time*, 179–80.

[25] Heidegger. *Sein und Zeit*, 322–3. English edition: Heidegger. *Being and Time*, 296–7.

[26] Heidegger. *Sein und Zeit*, 322–3. English edition: Heidegger. *Being and Time*, 296–7.

[27] Heidegger. *Sein und Zeit*, 184–5. English edition: Heidegger. *Being and Time*, 172–3.

The inauthentic individual being that loses itself in the surrounding world and succumbs to the dictate of public anonymity is thus the privation of authentic individual being, in whose endurance the real character of sojourning in disclosedness manifests itself. Every privation expresses the missing of something and therefore derives its sense from what is its positive correlate. In the case of inauthentic existence, this means that its dependence and inconsistency must be understood on the ground of the autonomy and self-consistency of the authentic existence. The inauthentic existence still remains being in disclosedness, but by closing itself off from its own potentiality of being it forgets its own disclosedness and dwells only on the public surface of the common everydayness. It is this difference between surface and depth, non-originality and originality that forms one of the strategically important motifs of *Sein und Zeit*.

Insofar as public anonymity, governed by ambiguity, curiosity and idle talk, seduces us to superficiality and unoriginality, the uncanniness of anxiety opens the dimension of depth in which individual existence discovers its very own origin. Uncanniness provides individual existence with the possibility of returning back to itself by accepting this origin as what eludes its power. Insofar as we can indeed talk here of a "heroic pathos" it is only in connection with resolution and ability to bear the bottomless depth of sojourning in disclosedness. Whereas the authentic existence resolutely faces the groundless depth of its own being in disclosedness, the inauthentic existence tries to shun it, seeking support in the familiar surrounding world and its public anonymity. Authentic existence is thus the primordial mode of being in disclosedness not only because it reveals the original steadfastness of our individuality, but also because, unlike the inauthentic existence, it abandons the familiar surface of the surrounding world, revealing the proper depth of our existence.

If we sum up what has so far been said of the ontological picture of being-there, we see the extent to which it is marked by the contrast between familiarity with the surrounding world and uncanniness in which the groundless openness of being-in-the-world is unveiled. Whether our existence be authentic or inauthentic, it is affected by the tension between the surrounding world and primary disclosedness in which it dwells. Both the surrounding world and the phenomenon of disclosedness form the fundamental component of the overall ontological constitution of being-there. All this, together with the existential conception of individual existence that can do without the notions of substance and identity, is to be considered while enquiring after the methodical principles that create the ontological picture of being in disclosedness. The above-mentioned inquiry can be narrowed down to the question as to why one and the same existence can be both sojourning with beings and sojourning in disclosedness.

The answer to this question lies concealed in the ontological structure of care that encompasses the familiarity with the surrounding world, as well as the uncanniness of being-in-the-world. The way Heidegger depicts the whole ontological structure of care bears the basic features of one of the three specific arrangements (*agencement*) discerned by Deleuze and Guattari in their *Mille plateaux*. The themes of familiarity and uncanniness as sketched in *Sein und Zeit* attest to the fact that the ontological picture of the structural whole of care corresponds to the so-called romantic orientation that is expounded, together with the classical and modern ones, in chapter "*De la ritournelle*." Just like the other two arrangements, romanticism is not conceived of here as part of some evolutionary process or epistemological structure delineated by impermeable boundaries. All the three arrangements, claim Deleuze and Guattari, are not so much in the relation of succession as of mutual over-layering.[28] Thus, every arrangement creates certain perceptive and cognitive conditions that modulate the event of thought in different ways.

Whereas classicism lays particular emphasis on the question of form and the gradually formed matter, which is observable in e.g. Kant's first two critiques, romanticism brings into play the problems of territory and deterritorialization, confronting the themes of home and homelessness.[29] Against the being-at-home in territory stands the disquieting not-being-at-home that appears in the deterritorialization.

The fact that Heidegger's ontological picture of being-there corresponds to the romantic orientation is corroborated not only by the themes of familiarity with the surrounding world and of uncanniness, in which individual existence finds its unsecured being-in-the-world, but also by the heroic resolution of authentic existence that is confronted with the groundless depth of sojourning in disclosedness. The ontological picture of being-there as exposited in *Sein und Zeit* makes clear that being-there, provided it does heed the call of its conscience that issues from the very depth of its own being-in-the-world, sets out on the path leading out of the being-at-home in the surrounding world and its public anonymity. The path following the call of one's conscience requires the readiness to endure the exile and the uncanniness that is heralded therein. The individual existence that hears and wants to hear the summon of its conscience returns back to itself as to solitary being in disclosedness; its lot is to be on the way from out of the familiar surrounding world toward uncanniness which heralds the empty disclosedness of being-in-the-world. All this fits in the overall framework of the romantic orientation as described in *Mille plateaux*.

With the help of this concept, we can also understand the peculiar tension between the disclosedness of being and the surrounding world in which being-there dwells initially and for the most part. Insofar as individual existence is stretched between the familiar surrounding world and the uncanniness of its primordial disclosedness, it is not only because these two modes of being-in-the-world essentially belong to it, but also because they refer to each other. Insofar as the surrounding world operates within the framework of the ontological structure of being-there

---

[28] This means, among other things, that the description of the three arrangement discerned by Deleuze and Guattari cannot be confused with Foucault's epistemological inquiry, where the ruptures between the classical, modern and the coming "post-modern" thought are stated with positivistic severity. Insofar as some overlap of these opposing perspectives does take place, it is definitely not that the classical and modern episteme as sketched in *Les mots et les choses* would correspond to classical and modern arrangement as described in *Mille plateaux*. The names themselves are inevitably misleading, which should also be taken into account in any generalizing comparison.

[29] As concerns the issue of Kant's philosophy cf. Deleuze, Gilles. 1963. *La Philosophie critique de Kant*. Paris: PUF.

as *ratio cognoscendi*, the phenomenon of disclosedness can be termed as *ratio essendi*. In other words, inasmuch as the surrounding world is the reason enabling the cognition of disclosedness, disclosedness is the reason enabling the being of the surrounding world. By the same token, the surrounding world is more familiar and intimate, whereas disclosedness itself seems to be quite strange. Despite this strangeness, however, disclosedness is primary from the viewpoint of its ontological constitution. In describing the ontological constitution of being-there it is therefore necessary to depart from our familiarity with the surrounding world and to arrive at the phenomenon of disclosedness itself only by means of a increasingly deeper exposition.

By situating thought within the framework of territory and deterritorialization, the romantic orientation, according to Deleuze and Guattari, also brings a new view on boundaries, danger and insanity.[30] The romantic hero who abandons the being-at-home in the territory and confronts the groundless abyss is in a constant danger of becoming immersed too deeply in it. That is the danger Heidegger alludes to when he terms the uncanniness of anxiety as a threat that does not come from the outside, but rather "comes from [being-there] itself."[31] The existential disposition of anxiety casts being-there into the empty abyss of its being in openness. In uncanniness individual existence has nothing to hold on to, losing all its support in beings. It is left to itself.

The possibility of failing to find a way out of uncanniness is not explicitly thematized in *Sein und Zeit*, and still it is suggested by the statement that anxiety itself does not correspond to either inauthentic or authentic existence, as it reveals being-free (*das Freisein*) for the possibility of a resolute being in disclosedness. *Vereinzelung* into which one is thrown in anxiety is a state of undecidedness in which one is only offered the possibility of opting for authentic existence. But even if one is incapable of seizing this possibility, the imperilment arising from anxiety has a limited impact. One can get hopelessly stuck in uncanniness or keep constantly falling into it. This, however, would only doom individual existence to loneliness and isolation, not to losing itself. Even if it did give in under the weight of its own being that gets manifested in uncanniness, it can never be shattered so much as to cease being itself.

Deleuze and Guattari explain it by the fact that the romantic orientation in principle goes no further than classicism in that it retains the a priori primacy of the unity of thought, no matter how much duration, development and variation it brings to the formal synthetic identity. As far as *Sein und Zeit* is concerned, this becomes conspicuous in that the "I" conceived of as the transcendental subject of thought is substituted with the ontological unity of the structural whole of care, enabling individuality of existence. Although it is no invariable identity and shows itself not as a pre-existing substratum, this unity is an incontestable guarantee of the self-subsistence of individual existence. By virtue thereof being-there never loses its individual character – least of all when it exposes itself to the uncanniness of anxiety

---

[30] Deleuze, and Guattari. *Mille plateaux*, 418–9.

[31] Heidegger. *Sein und Zeit*, 189. English edition: Heidegger. *Being and Time*, 177.

in which it finds itself in its very own potentiality of being. Even when it loses itself in the impersonal anonymity of being-with others and falls prey to the surrounding world, being-there does not lose its *Jemeinigkeit*, since it still cares about its own being in disclosedness. The self-forgetfulness and self-in-consistency to which the inauthentic existence resorts are always relative to selfhood and self-consistency of the authentic existence. The absolute demise of individual existence is not possible in the framework of the everydayness, since the inauthentic existence is merely a privative modification of the authentic being in disclosedness and as such never loses the possibility of returning to what being-there always is.

Contrary to that, Deleuze and Guattari show in their philosophical conception that the self is not constant and self-contained, since it more or less disintegrates in the process of deterritorialization. Insofar as Heidegger really betrays the deterritorialization, as we learn in *Qu'est-ce que la philosophie?*, it therefore seems that the causes are to be sought in the romantic orientation of the ontological picture of the structural whole of care. The stress laid on the inseparable unity of the ontological whole of care which assures the individuality of existence brings *Sein und Zeit* to the conclusion that the uncanniness of anxiety does not subvert the integrity of individual existence, but rather confirms it. Since anxiety renders being-there solitary without interfering with its integrity, this reverberates also in the understanding of the overall insecurity and precariousness of the individual sojourning in disclosedness. Insofar as *Sein und Zeit* contains no mention of a truly radical disintegration of individual existence that would inherently belong to the existential act of transcendence, it is because the integral unity of ontological constitution of care excludes in advance the disintegration of one's own individuality. As long as one exists, the ontological unity of facticity, existentiality and being-together-with the innerworldly beings remains incontestable. Nevertheless, the overall ontological constitution of care does not lie simply in itself, as it has a primordially temporal sense. Thus, if we are to decide about the solidity and stableness of the structural whole of care, we cannot but unveil its temporal constitution.

3.2   Being-There and Temporality

Investigations summarized in this chapter give evidence that one must be careful with any schematic criticism. The detailed examination of Heidegger's notion of temporality makes it evident that there are certain hidden possibilities in *Sein und Zeit* that Heidegger himself overlooked or neglected. Even though he mentions only two basic modes of temporality – one connected with the authentic existence, the other with the inauthentic existence – it seems that besides the temporality oriented toward the future and the temporality oriented toward the present, there might be a temporality oriented toward the past as well. This realization would have very important consequences for psychopathology, as it is precisely in anxiety where the temporal dimension of the past plays a decisive role. But even more important is the discovery that what occurs in anxiety is the temporally conditioned disintegration of the self. Although Heidegger does not admit such possibility, a careful reading of his temporal analysis of anxiety implies that anxiety opens a temporal gap in which the existential integrity of the self falls apart. To acknowledge the possibility of the temporally conditioned disintegration of the self, however, would require a complete revision of the ontological structure of being-there, which is something Heidegger is not willing or able to do in *Sein und Zeit*.

If being-there has primarily a temporal character, it means that temporality is the sense of sojourning in disclosedness. Sense, generally speaking, is what makes it possible to understand something in its being. However, Heidegger determines the sense of being-there with even more precision by grasping it as that which makes possible the unity of the ontological constitution of care. Insofar as the sense of being-there lies in temporality, this establishes the unity of the structured whole of care and consequently the existential structure of *Jemeinigkeit*.

Still, temporality does not precede being-there, nor is it situated somewhere "beyond" it, since it is one with the performance of sojourning in disclosedness. As long as the ontological structure of care encompasses the moments of thrownness, of projecting and of being-together-with innerwordly beings, there must be some temporal sense pertaining to these as well. As three constitutive moments of the ontological whole of care, thrownness, projecting and being-together-with innerwordly beings are three different modes of temporality. This is evident already from their existential determination, where thrownness corresponds to being-already-in, projecting to being-ahead-of-itself, whereas concern with innerworldly beings becomes being-together-with. From the temporal perspective, the sense of facticity consists in the having-been, the sense of understanding in the future, and the sense of being-together-with innerworldy beings in the present.[32] The temporality of sojourning in disclosedness is thus perceived in the ecstatic unity of the having-been, the future and the present. It is this unity of the three temporal ecstasies that constitutes the integral whole of the ontological structure of care. As such, temporality does not arise by piecing together separate ecstasies, but temporalizes itself in their primordial interdependence. However, the integral unity of the having-been, the future and the present requires further elaboration, especially with regard to the existential moments of thrownness, of projecting and of being-together-with beings.

The having-been appears primarily in disposition which brings one back to what one already is. Disposition elucidates how being-there always already is and gives it to understand its being-in-the-world. Inasmuch as disposition brings being-there back to its own thrown being in disclosedness, it is due to the fact that the having-been essentially determines the character of sojourning. "Having-been does not first bring one face to face with the thrown being that one is oneself, but the ecstasy of having-been first makes possible finding oneself in the mode of how-I-find-myself."[33] In other words, disposition is anchored in having-been, and not vice versa. This applies not only to fear or anxiety, but also to elevated moods such as hope, joy or

---

[32] Heidegger. *Sein und Zeit*, 327–8. English edition: Heidegger. *Being and Time*, 300–1.
[33] Heidegger. *Sein und Zeit*, 340. English edition: Heidegger. *Being and Time*, 312–3.

euphoria that are in their own way also anchored in the facticity of sojourning in disclosedness, and thus also in its having-been.

What enables being-there to understand its own being is the ecstasy of the future. It is by virtue thereof that being-there can relate to its potentiality-of-being.[34] "The future," says Heidegger, "makes ontologically possible a being that is in such a way that it exists understandingly in its potentiality-of-being."[35] Together with it, the understanding becomes concretized in the possibilities into which we project ourselves.

The possibilities manifested to us don't show themselves primarily as purely logical potentialities, but rather follow from our encounter with innerworldly discovered beings. Thus, we get to the third existential moment of sojourning in disclosedness that is being-together-with beings. Inasmuch as disposition is ontologically made possible by having-been and projecting by the future, concerned being-together-with beings derives its temporal sense from the present. The ecstasy of the present provides the ontological horizon in which beings ready-to-hand or present-at-hand can be encountered as what we are concerned with.

Therefore, the present creates the conditions for one's own falling prey to things of concern and getting lost in them. Being-there devoured by the present holds on to only what is closest, roving from one possibility to another. What ensues is the circulative movement of falling prey, which is governed by the inflated present. However, not even in the falling prey that becomes entirely absorbed in the present does being-there cut itself off from its thrown being in disclosedness; even here, being-there still somehow understands its ownmost potentiality-of-being, albeit only in that it outwardly alienates itself from it.[36] Even in uttermost subjection to the present our existence remains temporal, preserving its having-been and its future.

Still, the interdependence of the three temporal ecstasies is not to be doubted in the cases of thrownness and projecting either. The fact that each of the constitutive moments of sojourning in disclosedness is endowed with its own primordial ecstasy does not, in any case, mean that the other two remaining temporal structures should be absent. The ecstatic unity of the having-been, the future and the present always preserves its integrity regardless of which temporal ecstasy plays the key role. Only because it temporalizes itself in every ecstasy as a whole can temporality carry the overall ontological structure of sojourning in disclosedness.[37]

As the carrying foundation of sojourning in disclosedness, temporality is necessarily of an ecstatic character. Temporality is the primordial "outside-of-itself" that does not depart from any interior, but is always already carried away into the open dimension of being. The phenomenon of the ecstatic advancing outside-of-itself, however, does on no account destroy the individual structure of existence that consists in its *Jemeinigkeit*, but rather preserves it in the indivisible unity of the having-been, the future and the present. That the ecstatic being outside-of-itself

---

[34] Heidegger. *Sein und Zeit*, 327. English edition: Heidegger. *Being and Time*, 300.

[35] Heidegger. *Sein und Zeit*, 336. English edition: Heidegger. *Being and Time*, 309.

[36] Heidegger. *Sein und Zeit*, 348. English edition: Heidegger. *Being and Time*, 319–20.

[37] Heidegger. *Sein und Zeit*, 350. English edition: Heidegger. *Being and Time*, 321.

does not hinder the permanent maintenance of the individual unity of existence cannot be changed even by the fact that the temporality of being in disclosedness is, according to Heidegger, essentially finite.[38] The finitude of the ecstatic temporality in fact innerly conditions and enables the individual unity of existence. As long as being-there is of an individual character, as long as it is interested in its own being, it is ultimately because its temporality is finite.

The reason why the temporality of sojourning in disclosedness manifests itself as finite ensues from the analysis of the phenomenon of being-toward-death as rendered in *Sein und Zeit*. In the ontological description of being-there, being-toward-death is addressed as the fundamental existential. As being-toward-death, human existence is always in a certain relation to its own end, which distinguishes it from the animal that can perish, and yet, remaining throughout its life instinctively bound to its surrounding, it never relates to death as such. Unlike the living organism, our existence is finite not only because death awaits it, but also because it always in some way understands death. Even when reluctant to know about the possibility of its death and thus trying to forget about it, we can never entirely cover up the indistinct certainty of our end. Death is the ultimate and extreme possibility of our existence. In this basic possibility of our existence, every one is utterly irreplaceable, as it is each one who must die his/her own death.

Whereas every possibility of being-in-the-world relates to other possibilities with which it is connected by the invisible web of referential relations, death is absolutely non-relational. Death makes the individual existence face the utter impossibility of being-in-the-world. When one dies, one ceases to be being-there (*das Da-sein*), becoming no-longer-being-there (*das Nicht-mehr-da-sein*). As long as being-there is characterized as being in disclosedness, death is nothing else but radical closure. Death is not a privative form of being in disclosedness such as the inauthentic existence, but non-being in disclosedness. But as long as one exists, this closure remains the last possibility of one's own existence.

Insofar as death is grasped as the unique possibility of being-in-the-world, it means that death is, in *Sein und Zeit*, addressed as an existential phenomenon. Thus, within the frame of the ontological analysis of being-there, "the existential analytic of death is subordinate to the fundamental constitution of [being-there]."[39] Dying is conceived of not as a sudden or gradual disintegration of the united ontological constitution of being in disclosedness but as a way of being by which individual existence relates to the possibility of its end. Consequently, the phenomenon of dying must be interpreted as being-toward-death on the basis of the integral ontological structure of being in disclosedness, that is, on the basis of care.

Therefore, the crucial constitutive moments of care must be projected in being-toward-death. Having it ahead of itself, individual existence understands its death as its own possibility. Relating to it as to its very own, non-relational possibility, individual existence understands its death necessarily with regard to its own being-in-the-world it cares about in its being. For individual existence, death is the

---

[38] Heidegger. *Sein und Zeit*, 331, 425. English edition: Heidegger. *Being and Time*, 304, 398–90.

[39] Heidegger. *Sein und Zeit*, 247. English edition: Heidegger. *Being and Time*, 229.

possibility of its impossibility-to-be and, as such, brings it back to its very own potentiality-of-being. Face to face with the possibility of death, individual existence is extricated from the relational network connecting it with the surrounding world and brought back to its solitary potentiality-of-being. The existential relation to death therefore appears to fall into one with relation to one's own being.

But even before being capable of realizing the sheer fact that everyone sooner or later must die, individual existence senses its own vulnerability to death by means of disposition. The existential certainty of death announces itself most primordially and urgently in the fundamental disposition of anxiety. This disposition manifests to being-there the jeopardy springing from its own "there" – in it, being-there is brought back to its own solitary existence to which also the possibility of the impossibility of its existence belongs.[40] In anxiety, individual existence is exposed to the possibility of death as to the all-pervading nothingness that constitutes the very foundation of its being.

Since the *possibility* of death is primordially uncovered in anxiety, individual existence strives to cover up this disposition and the ensuing perspective of its own end. Turning away from its ultimate and very own possibility, however, individual existence turns away from its ownmost potentiality of being as well. This happens by the self-exposure to the surrounding world and to public anonymity where one seeks shelter from the uncanniness of anxiety. Individual existence then does not cease to be being-toward-death, but its mode of being-toward-death is merely inauthentic.

Though individual existence may initially and for the most part shun the possibility of its death, it can take a contrary attitude to it. This attitude lies neither in suicide nor in gloomy ruminations about death that sooner or later end in suicide but in accepting death as a unique possibility of one's own being. As being-toward-death is anchored in the ontological structure of care, the change in the way individual existence addresses its very own and ultimate possibility must bring also a total change in the performance of being in disclosedness.

What changes in authentic existence is, above all, being ahead-of-itself that constitutes the existential moment of understanding. Being-toward-death that is not led by the common sense of the public anonymity is characterized in *Sein und Zeit* as the anticipation of possibility (*das Vorlaufen in die Möglichkeit*). This mode of existential being-toward-possibility relates to death as to the absolute impossibility of sojourning in disclosedness, without diminishing the indefiniteness and inscrutability that spring from its character of possibility. Death means the impossibility of any relating to anything; it is the possibility of the definitive end of all further possibilities. As long as individual existence understands the possibility of its death in this way, individual existence projects itself also toward its very own potentiality of being-in-the-world. In the anticipation of its ownmost, non-relational and most ultimate possibility, individual existence understands its potentiality-of-being-in-the-world in that it extricates itself from the subjection to the public anonymity that exercises control over it. Individual existence finds itself in solitariness facing the extreme possibility of its end.[41]

---

[40] Heidegger. *Sein und Zeit*, 265–6. English edition: Heidegger. *Being and Time*, 244–6.
[41] Heidegger. *Sein und Zeit*, 263. English edition: Heidegger. *Being and Time*, 242–3.

As long as the solitary existence understands itself from its very own potentiality of being, what belongs to this understanding is the fundamental disposition of anxiety, in which individual existence uncovers the hidden jeopardy springing from its own disclosedness.[42] Anxiety brings individual existence to face the possible impossibility of its being in disclosedness. Despite not necessarily falling to uncanniness, the existential anticipation of one's very own and ultimate possibility requires the readiness to anxiety. As long as it is to accept the possibility of its death, individual existence does not have to factually abandon the surrounding world or the co-existence with others, but must understand them from its solitary and anxious being in disclosedness. This suffices for individual existence to see both its lostness in the public anonymity and its entanglement in the possibilities of the familiar surrounding world, and thus to take the opportunity to exist on its own.

The individual existence that anticipates its ultimate and very own possibility thus exists not only independently, but also integrally. The existential integrity of sojourning in disclosedness lies in opening all possibilities from the perspective of one's very own and ultimate possibility. This happens when individual existence chooses one out of all the possibilities that precede death and invests its whole being in this possibility, despite being aware of the fact it thus necessarily loses all others. In this way, individual existence extricates itself from the entanglement in random possibilities offered by the surrounding world, surpassing inconsistency and carelessness that spring from the supremacy of the public anonymity. This, however, is merely the ontic side of one's own integrity.

It is of essence to mention also the ontological side of existential integrity that pertains to the existential structure of being in disclosedness. The anticipating resoluteness with regard to death is exceptional in that it brings to light the overall structure of the individual being that understands itself from its very own potentiality-of-being-in-the-world. The individual existence that anticipates the possibility of its own end exists integrally, as it advances from the surrounding world and the public anonymity toward its unique and irreplaceable position in the disclosedness of being. In the anticipation of its very own, non-relational and ultimate possibility, it exists transitorily. Its being-toward-death thus loses the character of evading its finitude and becomes genuinely transitory. This transitoriness marks not only the finitude of individual existence, but also its primordial transitivity characterizing the existential act of transcendence.

As the advancing from the discoveredness of beings to the disclosedness of being, transcendence is the fundamental act of existence; all specific deeds and attitudes by which the existing individual relates to beings rely on this act. Transcendence is the primary act by which individual existence incessantly goes beyond the immediate context of the surrounding world. By doing so, individual existence transcends itself in its familiarity with the surrounding world and in its subjection to the public anonymity without losing its own integrity. On the contrary, going beyond the familiar surrounding world and its public anonymity opens for individual existence a way to self-discovery in the sense of grasping its primordial

---

[42] Heidegger. *Sein und Zeit*, 266. English edition: Heidegger. *Being and Time*, 245–6.

being in disclosedness. Thus, the existential self-transcendence manifests itself as self-gaining and self-fulfillment.

We must not forget, however, that the transitory being in disclosedness has a primordially temporal sense. Existential transitoriness is therefore most primordially anchored in the ecstatic nature of temporality. The very fact that the individual existence is self-transcending, adumbrates the ecstatic character of temporality in which there lies the primordial "outside-itself" of being-there. Existential self-transcendence would be inconceivable without the ecstatic unity of the future, the having-been and the present, by virtue of which the existential moments determined as being-ahead-of-itself, being-already-in, and being-together-with innerworldly beings are tied together. It is the ecstatic unity of temporality that allows being-there to advance out of its dwelling in the surrounding world and to attain its ownmost being in disclosedness. Since being-there sustains itself in the ecstatic unity of the future, the having-been and the present, the disintegration of this unity means the definitive end of being in disclosedness. But as long as one exists, the possibility of such disintegration remains the ultimate possibility of individual existence.

The transitory existence always somehow relates to the possibility of its end. Since the primordial constancy and integrity of individual existence appears in the anticipation of one's ultimate and very own possibility of its being, Heidegger can designate the future as the primary dimension that endows the ecstatic unity of the three temporal ecstasies with its meaning. When the future proves itself to be the key phenomenon of time, what comes to the fore is the anticipatory structure of understanding, out of which being-there approaches its thrownness and discloses its present.[43] This applies, however, only to such an existence which resolutely accepts the extreme possibility of its end. As long as it shuns its finitude, seeking to cover up or objectively explain its ultimate possibility, being-there exists out of its present. In that case, the ecstatic unity of the three temporal ecstasies temporalizes itself not out of the future but out of the present. The transitory existence then uncontrollably entangles itself in the surrounding world and in the innerworldly beings it encounters therein; its self-understanding evolves not from its very own being in disclosedness but from the public anonymity of the world with which it is concerned.

Even though none of the three temporal ecstasies can be missing in the ecstatic unity of temporality, one of them always dominates. The fact that temporality temporalizes itself in two different ways, out of which one derives its sense primarily from the future, whereas the other from the present, allows us to grasp the difference between the authentic and the inauthentic existence on the temporal level. By anticipating its very own and ultimate possibility, and thus accepting being-toward-death as its essential determination, the authentic existence is primarily aimed toward the future. The inauthentic existence that strives to shun its own finitude while seeking support in the public anonymity of the surrounding world is, on the contrary, fully exposed to the present.

Insofar as it anticipates the possibility of its death, the authentic existence relates to its ownmost potentiality of being and to its thrown being in disclosedness. Thus,

---

[43] Heidegger. *Sein und Zeit*, 326–9. English edition: Heidegger. *Being and Time*, 299–303.

authentic existence fulfils the transitory character of being in disclosedness, whereas the inauthentic existence seeks rest in the familiar surrounding world where it dwells.

However much it refuses to accept the transitoriness of its being and closes itself off in the surrounding world, inauthentic existence cannot extricate itself from its transitory character, as long as it is being in disclosedness, i.e. as long as it exists. Inauthentic existence also projects itself toward its very own potentiality-of-being-in-the-world, but it lags behind its very own potential while clinging to beings offered by the surrounding world and falling prey to the public anonymity. Even the inauthentic existence understands its being in a certain way, albeit in that it increasingly alienates itself from its ownmost potentiality-of-being-in-the-world.

It follows that the temporality of inauthentic existence is not devoid of the ecstatic character, but only effectuates its modification. Since the three temporal ecstasies that carry away the transitory being in disclosedness are absolutely inseparable, it is only the form of this temporal unity that can change. In the case of the authentic temporality, the ecstatic unity of the future, the having-been, and the present appear as *anticipation, retrieve*, and *moment* (*das Vorlaufen, die Wiederholung, der Augenblick*). Insofar as the future ontologically enables the existential projecting, the having-been establishes the factual thrownness and the present discloses concerned being-together-with beings, the authentic existence comes in its anticipation of death back to itself as to its ownmost potentiality-of-being-in-the-world, retrieving repeatedly its thrown and solitary being in disclosedness, and disclosing in the ecstatic moment its own situation. Conversely, the inauthentic existence is marked by the awaiting itself out of what the surrounding world and the public anonymity have to offer, forgetting about the solitariness of its thrown being in disclosedness, and thus making present its possibilities. The ecstatic unity of the future, the having-been and the present is therefore temporalized in inauthentic temporality as *awaiting, forgottenness*, and *making present* (*das Gewärtigen, die Vergessenheit, das Gegenwärtigen*).[44]

Nevertheless, the two different modes of temporalizing represented by authentic and inauthentic temporality are not equally primordial. Enabling ontologically the mode of being in which being-there shuns its own transitoriness, the inauthentic temporality is grasped in *Sein und Zeit* as a modification of the authentic temporality that allows individual existence to take over and fulfil its transitory being in disclosedness. With regard to the fact that authentic temporality expresses the primordial ecstatic unity in which the whole ontological structure of the transitory being in disclosedness is established, inauthentic temporality must be derived from this temporal origin, and not vice versa.

Despite moving away from its origin, the inauthentic temporality can never completely fall off from it, for it always has the authentic temporality behind itself as its possibility. Inauthentic being in disclosedness that temporalizes itself in awaiting, forgottenness and making present never loses the possibility of returning back

---

[44] Heidegger. *Sein und Zeit*, 336–9. English edition: Heidegger. *Being and Time*, 309–12.

to the authentic way of existence whose temporal structure has the character of anticipation, retrieve and moment.

Individual existence is situated between its beginning and its end, i.e. between birth and death, and it is in this situation that individual existence maintains its constancy by virtue of ecstatic temporality that reveals its true character in authentic temporalizing. To put it more precisely, individual existence does not stand between birth and death as between two points that are present-at-hand, but stretches itself along by opening itself into the three temporal ecstasies.[45] The authentic manner of this ecstatic rapture establishes the primordial self-subsistence and constancy of individual being. Their opposites are the dependence and inconstancy of individual being that arise from the awaiting, forgetting and making-present mode of temporality. Hence, neither the dependence nor the inconstancy of individual existence spring from a disintegration of the ecstatic unity of temporality, but only from its inauthentic temporalizing.

Everything may be clear so far. But the question remains, how psychopathological phenomena are to be conceived of in such a framework. Are we to regard them through the prism of authentic existence that embraces in anticipation the possibility of its own death while setting out into the uncanniness of anxiety, or are we to perceive them in the light of inauthentic existence that closes itself off in the familiar surrounding world, falling prey to the innerworldly beings and to the constraints of possibilities imposed by the impersonal anonymity of being-with others? The first option is absurd already at first glance, as the self-subsistence and consistency of authentic existence can hardly correspond to the shakiness and uncertainty of a pathologically disturbed self. The other option does not seem plausible either. To expound the self shaken by a pathological disorder as a certain form of dependent and inconsistent individual being that is characteristic of the inauthentic existence is possible only provided that no regard is paid to the serenity and ease which, according to Heidegger, spring from the familiarity with the surrounding world in which inauthentic existence dwells. However, a pathologically disturbed individual is anything but serene and at ease. It therefore seems that psychopathological disorders can be addressed neither on the basis of authentic temporality, whose sense is determined by the future, nor on the basis of inauthentic temporality, which temporalizes itself out of the temporal dimension of the present.

Departing from the presupposition that temporality temporalizes itself always as the ecstatic unity of the having-been, the future and the present while one of the temporal dimensions always dominates the other two, we still have one more possibility of grasping the temporal, and thus also the ontological sense of psychopathological disorders. Even though *Sein und Zeit* does not explicitly address this possibility, we can surmise that in the case of psychopathological disorders, the ecstatic unity of temporality temporalizes itself neither out of the future, nor out of the present, but out of the having-been. Once the having-been has become the fundamental dimension of temporality, the primary position is occupied by thrownness, from which both projecting and being-together-with beings derive their sense.

---

[45] Heidegger. *Sein und Zeit*, 374–5. English edition: Heidegger. *Being and Time*, 343–4.

The key moment of thrownness is nothing else but the fundamental disposition of anxiety, by means of which individual existence is cast into the uncanniness of its being-in-the-world. The pathologically structured being-in-the-world is repeatedly thrown into uncanniness, in which the significative context of the surrounding world collapses, or at least, it must, time and again, face the devastating onslaught of anxiety. Anxiety is the fundamental factor of pathological being-in-the-world, which can be best documented by the casuistries of schizophrenics, who are exposed to the uncanniness to the highest possible degree. What corresponds to this is the overall change of their existence and the implicit change in the way their temporality temporalizes itself.

In one of his casuistries, Binswanger describes the temporality of the schizophrenic existence as a special modification of temporality in whose frame experience turns into a vicious cycle.[46] The schizophrenic who suffers from paranoid delusions finds in everything he encounters a confirmation of his old suspicions; everywhere he finds traces of conspiracy and persecution he has long suspected. All fearful suspicions, nevertheless, essentially refer to anxiety, concealed behind them as their dark truth. Tied to that which has been, the schizophrenic can neither project himself freely to the future, nor dwell at ease with what is offered in the present. The temporality of his existence is governed by the having-been so much as to allow the future and the present to manifest themselves merely as its derivates. It is a temporality of a world where everything remains as it has been, where everything must remain as it has been unless anxiety should hold the stage once again. Every single hint of the genuine future or the disclosed present is perceived here as extreme peril that once again exposes the schizophrenic to the uncanniness.

In any case, it is not only the psychotic who shuns the challenge of the future and the claim of the present, but also the neurotic, repetitively reliving the old drama, endlessly repeating one obsessive gesture or fearing the object whose power is to cast him/her into the abyss of uncanniness.

Generally speaking, the pathological mode of temporalizing is marked by both the impossibility of authentic future, in which being-there keeps itself ahead of itself, as well as of all that with which it is familiar, and the impossibility to meet the claims of the present, albeit only to the extent to which they are met by the inauthentic dwelling in the familiar surrounding world. This does not mean that the future and the present would have to be completely absent from the pathological temporality; the case with them is rather that they undergo a change in which the understanding being-ahead-of-itself turns into an escape from an indistinct catastrophe and being-together-with beings into concealing this or that area of beings, in which individual existence finds its possibilities. The pathological temporality, understood in the unity of three temporal ecstasies, could thus be characterized as *escape*, *repeated exposure*, and *concealing*. Insofar as the future temporally establishes the existential projecting, the having-been enables the existential thrownness and the present discloses concerned being-together-with beings, the pathologically disturbed existence escapes the threat of its death indicated in the uncanniness of anxiety, to which it is repeatedly exposed, which it tries to prevent by concealing from itself all

---

[46] Binswanger. *Schizophrenie*, 424–34 (the case of Suzanne Urban).

aspects of being-together-with innerworldy beings, and the consequential possibilities of existence that could induce a new onslaught of anxiety.

Nevertheless, even if we do regard psychopathological phenomena in the light of the third mode of temporality which, unlike authentic and inauthentic temporality, temporalizes itself from the dimension of the having-been, it still remains unclear whether the essence of psychopathological disorders shall reveal itself in its abysmal fearfulness. For the abyss of madness to appear in all its bottomless depth, we need to comprehend not only the temporal structure of existence that conceals its actual situation from itself in order to escape at any cost the threat of death uncovered in the repeated onslaughts of anxiety, but also that from which the pathologically disturbed existence seeks to save itself, which is nothing else but utter disintegration of its individual being. The real nature of a pathologically disturbed existence cannot appear until we take into account the disintegration of the individual being this existence must face.

This applies especially to cases of severe psychotic disorders, where the disintegration of individual existence not only looms, but actually takes place. How are we then to address the disintegration of individual being occurring in schizophrenia together with the breakdown of the significative structure of the surrounding world? Can we expound it otherwise than as a privation, i.e. as a relative weakening of the self-consistent and self-subsistent individual being tied by Heidegger to the authentic temporalizing of temporality? Insofar as the authentic mode of existence is regarded as the most primordial ontological form of sojourning in disclosedness, the pathologically conditioned disintegration of individual being needs to be addressed in a similar way as the inauthentic inconsistency and dependence of individual being, that is to say, as a privative modification of authentic temporalizing. A really radical disintegration of individual existence cannot actually take place within the framework of the ontological project of being-there, because as long as being-there exists, the existential integrity of its individual being sustains itself on the basis of the ecstatic unity of temporality that always temporalizes itself as a whole.

This impression, however, can easily vanish if we look more closely at the temporal analysis of anxiety as provided in *Sein und Zeit*. Although no temporal ecstasy can *de iure* fall out of the integral unity of temporality, what is *de facto* missing here is the dimension of the present that establishes concerned being-together-with beings. What shows itself in anxiety is the connection between thrownness and the existential project that is ontologically grounded in the bond between the having-been and the future. The disintegration of the referential and significative structure of the surrounding world occurring in anxiety, precludes, in Heidegger's opinion, the inauthentic being-together-with innerworldly beings that is grounded upon making present without automatically leading to a resolute takeover of the transitory being in disclosedness and the correspondent modification of concern with beings. Anxiety merely makes us ready for a possible resolution, to whose temporal constitution belongs the moment as the authentic modus of the present. However, anxiety alone "does not as yet have the character of the Moment."[47]

---

[47] Heidegger. *Sein und* Zeit, 344. English edition: Heidegger. *Being and Time*, 316.

In the uncanniness of anxiety, being-there is exposed to nothingness and void into which beings present-at-hand and ready-to-hand fall. Of course, this does not mean that beings themselves should simply disappear in anxiety; what happens is rather a lapse of concerned being-together-with beings that is not to be mistaken for a mere occurrence in the presence of beings present-at-hand. Anxiety exempts us from our concern with beings, since beings themselves cease to address us in uncanniness. In anxiety, beings fall into total insignificance that reveals to being-there the empty openness of its being-in-the-world. The uncanniness brings being-there back to its very own thrownness, giving it to understand the utter unanchoredness of its being in disclosedness. The only thing being-there understands in uncanniness is the sheer "that" of its thrown being in disclosedness.

Thus, in anxiety, being-there gains the terrible experience of the loss of the firm ground in which the having-been of thrownness joins the future of projecting. The foundation of being-in-the-world heralded in anxiety is given not in the dimension of the present, but only in the dimensions of the having-been and the future. Even though the disposition of anxiety presents a unique mode of "finding one's self" (*die Befindlichkeit*), being-there here is not simply present to itself. The existential phenomenon of anxiety proves that one cannot meet one's own being in disclosedness in the mode of pure self-presence; the encounter with disclosedness exposes one to the bottomless abyss in which the having-been of thrownness sinks deeper and deeper as existential projecting follows it. This temporal vertigo makes one feel the abysmal character of one's own being in disclosedness. However, what becomes primarily manifest in the vertigo of anxiety is the disjointedness and disconnection of the ecstatic unity of temporality that carries the ontological whole of thrownness, projecting and being-together-with beings. It is as if here, in the very center of the romantic arrangement that marks the character of the ontological project of being-there, we confront the bottomless abyss which opens the pathway toward modern thought addressed by Deleuze and Guattari.

In any case, the temporal disjointedness revealed in the phenomenon of anxiety defies the premise that temporality temporalizes itself always as a whole. And it is not only a question of psychopathological disorders. Had Heidegger taken the phenomenon of anxiety with all the implications that spring from the factual lapse of concerned being-together-with beings, he would have had to abandon the idea of the inseparable temporal unity, upon which the individual character of being-there is founded. He would have had to admit that not only is the awareness of a possible disintegration of the ecstatic unity of temporality rooted in anxiety, but that this disintegration virtually occurs therein.

Since anxiety is not a marginal state, but a fundamental disposition in which the true nature of being in disclosedness is revealed, what could follow from a consistent exposition of anxiety would be a new view of the ontological structure of being-there as such. In *Sein und Zeit*, the phenomenon of anxiety serves as a ground upon which our relation to being is addressed. To concede the fact that anxiety is accompanied by vertigo in which the whole ecstatic unity of temporality falls apart would therefore entail a change of the whole conception of one's own relation to the disclosedness of being. Advancing from discoveredness of beings to disclosedness of being could then occur only at the cost of a disintegration of the individual structure of existence. Disclosedness of being could reveal itself only to the disintegrated individual being. Going beyond the familiar surrounding world would imply not a simple return back to one's own being but rather the rupture of the unified structure of the individual being. The indivisible unity of individual existence would have to be sacrificed to the bottomless abyss of uncanniness, and it would be substituted by an uncertain process of the consolidation of the shattered individual being.

Thus, Heidegger would get substantially closer to the vision of bottomlessness (*sans-fond*) and of loss of ground (*effondement*), related, in *Différence et répétition*, to the revelation of the finitude of thought. His conception of a transitory existence would include in its scope not only the idea of death as one's very own, ultimate and non-relational possibility of individual being, but also that aspect of death that shows it as an impersonal process of dying to which the existing individual can assume no attitude, as it is no longer involved.[48]

Death, notes Deleuze with reference to Blanchot, can be conceived of either as a possibility of a definitive end that the existing individual foreknows in one way or another or as a process of dying in which the existing individual is not involved, since dying remains in itself as an abyss without the present, as "time without a present." Whereas in the first case, death is still regarded from the viewpoint of unity and constancy of the individual existence, in the other case it appears as "the state of free differences when they are no longer subject to the form imposed upon them by an I or an ego, when they assume a shape which excludes *my* own coherence no less than that of any identity whatsoever."[49]

On the basis of death thus conceived, it is thus possible to address the finitude of thought that manifests itself in the pathological disintegration of individual being without the necessity to degrade it to a deficient form of a self-subsistent and self-consistent individual existence. In the light of dying that is not governed by the logic of unity, but rather opens space for multiplicity, even the most extreme, delusion- and hallucination-ridden forms of madness can appear in their own positiveness and fullness. An indispensable condition for elucidating the pathological states as original, non-derived phenomena is to see that multiplicity is not only a medium that determines the nature of the schizophrenic break, but constitutes the process of thought in its essential finitude.

However, all these possibilities are laid aside in *Sein und Zeit* where the focus is rather the idea of the temporal unity of individual existence that corresponds to the spirit of the romantic arrangement as depicted in *Mille plateaux*. The apriori conviction concerning the indivisible unity of the future, the having-been and the present that must be preserved in each of the existential moments of being-there, including the disposition of anxiety thus leads to a schematic and purposive exposition of the present, by means of which the anxious individual is brought "back to one's

---

[48] Deleuze. *Différence et répétition*, 148–51. English edition: Deleuze, Gilles. 1995. *Difference and Repetition* (trans: Patton, Paul). New York: Columbia University Press, 113.

[49] Deleuze. *Différence et répétition*, 149.

ownmost thrownness."[50] The modus of the present peculiar to anxiety has allegedly nothing to do with concerned being-together-with beings. Insofar as the individual is still concerned with beings, it is for Heidegger troubled not by anxiety, but by a mere fear.

However, does not that "held" (*gehaltene*) present of anxiety fall rather into the dimension of the having-been? Is not bringing back to the facticity of one's own being in disclosedness grounded upon the dimension of the having-been? Heidegger himself admits only that anxiety is primordially anchored in the having-been, out of which the future and the present temporalize themselves, which corresponds to the premise that "temporality temporalizes itself completely in every ecstasy."[51] Since anxiety brings one back to thrownness as to that which can be repeatedly retrieved (*wiederholen*), having-been is attributed to the character of the retrievability (*die Wiederholbarkeit*). "*Bringing before the [retrievability] is the specific ecstatic mode [of the having-been that constitutes the disposition of anxiety].*"[52] Anxiety thus regarded entails the possibility of restorative takeover of one's own existence that characterizes the authentic being in disclosedness.

Thus, anxiety becomes the vanishing point of the authentic existence, from whose perspective anxiety seems the condition enabling the self-consistent, self-subsistent and constant individual being. With regard to the authentic existence, through which the true nature of individual being manifests itself, Heidegger accordingly neglects not only the possibility of an irreversible fall into the bottomless abyss of anxiety, but also, and more importantly, the factual disintegration of the temporal unity of existence that takes place in the uncanniness. It is this concealment of the ever-imminent disintegration of the ecstatic unity of temporality that allows him to regard the possibility of leaving anxiety as something granted. All this is an expression of the fact that disclosedness of being that is most primordially manifested in anxiety is thought of throughout *Sein und Zeit* from the viewpoint of the temporal unity of individual existence.

References

1. Binswanger, Ludwig. 1957. *Schizophrenie*. Pfullingen: Neske.
2. Deleuze, Gilles. 1963. *La Philosophie critique de Kant*. Paris: PUF.
3. Deleuze, Gilles. 1968. *Différence et répétition*. Paris: PUF. English edition: Deleuze, Gilles. 1995. *Difference and Repetition*. Trans. Paul Patton. New York: Columbia University Press.
4. Deleuze, Gilles, and Félix Guattari. 1980. *Mille plateaux: Capitalisme et schizophrénie*. Paris: Minuit. English edition: Deleuze, Gilles, and Félix Guattari. 1987. *Thousand Plateaus*. Trans. Brian Massumi. Minneapolis: Minnesota University Press.

---

[50] Heidegger *Sein und Zeit*, 344. English edition: Heidegger. *Being and Time*, 316.

[51] Heidegger *Sein und Zeit*, 350. English edition: Heidegger. *Being and Time*, 321.

[52] Heidegger *Sein und Zeit*, 343. English edition: Heidegger. *Being and Time*, 316.

5. Deleuze, Gilles, and Félix Guattari. 1991. *Qu'est- ce que la philosophie?*. Paris: Minuit. English edition: Deleuze, Gilles, and Félix Guattari. 1994. *What is Philosophy?* Trans. Hugh Tomlison and Graham Burchill. New York: Columbia University Press.
6. Heidegger, Martin. 1983. *Die Grundbegriffe der Metaphysik: Welt, Endlichkeit, Einsamkeit.* Frankfurt am Main: Vittorio Klostermann. English edition: Heidegger, Martin. 1995. *The Fundamental Concepts of Metaphysics. World, Finitude, Solitude.* Trans. William McNeill and Nicholas Walker. Bloomington: Indiana University Press.
7. Heidegger, Martin. 1987. *Zollikoner Seminare. Protokolle, Gespräche, Briefe,* ed. Medard Boss. Frankfurt am Main: Vittorio Klostermann. English edition: Heidegger, Martin. 2001. *Zollikon Seminars.* Trans. Franz Mayr and Richard Askay. Evanston: Northwestern University Press.
8. Heidegger, Martin. 1993. *Sein und Zeit*, 17th ed. Tübingen: Niemeyer. English edition: Heidegger, Martin. 1996. *Being and Time.* Trans. Joan Stambaugh. Albany: SUNY Press.
9. von Herrmann, Friedrich-Wilhelm. 1985. *Subjekt und Dasein.* Frankfurt am Main: Vittorio Klostermann.

Chapter 4
The Problem of Mental Disorder

4.1 The Concept of Illness in *Zollikoner Seminare*

This chapter returns to *Zollikoner Seminare* and to its sketch of the notion of illness. Considering the fact that every illness deprives us of certain existential possibilities, Heidegger explains every pathological state as a phenomenon of privation. This applies not only to mental disorders, but also to somatic disorders. As to the notion of privation, Heidegger explains it with a reference to Plato's concept of relative non-being (τὸ μὴ 'ὸν), which appears in the dialogue *Sophist*, but it seems that his usage of the term "privation" owes much more to Aristotle's notion of στέρησις. It is perhaps no accident that in his *Metaphysics* Aristotle explains the meaning of στέρησις by means of the example of illness (blindness). In any case, Heidegger concretizes his view of psychopathological phenomena suggesting that they bear all signs of the entanglement in the world, and thus of the inauthentic existence. Saying this, he actually makes an analogy between mental illness and the inauthentic existence on the one side, and mental health and the authentic existence on the other. The authentic existence is thus placed in the position of the normative ideal of health, while the inauthentic existence serves as a model explaining all psychopathological phenomena. Nevertheless, it is questionable whether the same applies to the somatic sphere of existence, as well.

Since *Zollikoner Seminare* and *Sein und Zeit* are divided by more then 30 years during which Heidegger's thought went through a substantial change, it is logical that the ontological structure of being-there is viewed in a different light and with different accents. Above all, *Zollikoner Seminare* reconsiders the phenomenon of disclosedness in which being-there dwells. In contrast with *Sein und Zeit*, where disclosedness of being is thought from the viewpoint of the temporal unity of individual existence, disclosedness is no longer understood in the later work from the viewpoint of being-there. On the contrary, being-there is perceived from the perspective of disclosedness, called the clearing of being in *Zollikoner Seminare*. Thus, the statement that the disclosedness of being is not a quality or a component of

© Springer International Publishing Switzerland 2015
P. Kouba, *The Phenomenon of Mental Disorder*, Contributions to Phenomenology 75, DOI 10.1007/978-3-319-10323-5_4

individual existence gains its full force. "Clearing is not an *existentiale*," claims Heidegger; rather, the open being-there "stands out into the clearing."[1] Being-there "is not the clearing itself ... nor is it identical with the whole of the clearing as such."[2] At the same time, being-there is incessantly determined and focused, as it is always open for the concrete surrounding world.[3] Being-there is thus to be conceived of as "standing-within the clearing, as sojourn with what it encounters, that is, as disclosure for what concerns it and what is encountered."[4]

In its relatedness to encountered beings, being-there always maintains the structure of *Jemeinigkeit*, and therefore the question of its individuality can be answered only by demonstrating certain modes of its behavior.[5] But even though the turn in the understanding of the openness of being involves revisions in the view of being-there, the ontological project of individual existence does not change in every respect. Heidegger does not feel any need to challenge the ontological unity and constancy of individual existence. On the contrary, *Zollikoner Seminare* again emphasizes that the "self (*das Selbst*) is what constantly endures as the same in the whole, historical course of [being-there], [it is] what exists precisely in the manner of being-in-the-world."[6] Naturally, the existential constancy of the self is not to be confused with the identity of a substantial self. "The constancy of the self is proper to itself in the sense that the self is always able to come back to itself and always finds itself still the same in its [existence]."[7] However total the alienation from itself and however deep the falling prey to what is available may be, individual existence cannot be kept from being itself.

In Heidegger's opinion, a classic example demonstrating the constancy of individual existence is the experience of awakening in which an individual returns to itself and its everyday world.[8] Individual existence could not awaken into the state in which the world maintains its referential structure along with the innerworldly beings retaining their persistent identity and the discernability of others, unless it were still the same even in sleep. In dreaming one can turn to something else, but this dream world does not change the fact that every dream is "always someone's". It follows that even the dream world forms an integral component of historicity in which the permanence and constancy of individual existence is maintained. Despite their structural difference, the waking and dream modes of being-in-the-world are significantly related, both belonging to one single whole of the existential historicity. On no account can one surmise that apart from the waking mode of existence, there

---

[1] Heidegger. *Zollikoner Seminare*, 258. English edition: Heidegger. *Zollikon Seminars*, 206.

[2] Heidegger. *Zollikoner Seminare*, 223. English edition: Heidegger. *Zollikon Seminars*, 178.

[3] Heidegger. *Zollikoner Seminare*, 258. English edition: Heidegger. *Zollikon Seminars*, 206.

[4] Heidegger. *Zollikoner Seminare*, 204. English edition: Heidegger. *Zollikon Seminars*, 159.

[5] Heidegger. *Zollikoner Seminare*, 204–205. English edition: Heidegger. *Zollikon Seminars*, 159–60.

[6] Heidegger. *Zollikoner Seminare*, 220. English edition: Heidegger. *Zollikon Seminars*, 174–5.

[7] Heidegger. *Zollikoner Seminare*, 220. English edition: Heidegger. *Zollikon Seminars*, 175.

[8] Heidegger. *Zollikoner Seminare*, 288–91. English edition: Heidegger. *Zollikon Seminars*, 228–31.

is also one more historicity of the dream existence.[9] In that case it would be utterly incomprehensible how someone in a waking state could speak of one's dreams and try to understand their meaning.

The very historicity of the individual existence, however, is ontologically grounded in the ecstatic unity of temporality. Being-there can exist historically only because it is always expecting, making present and retaining (*gewärtigend, gegenwärtigend, behaltend*).[10] What manifests itself in the unity of this expecting, making present and retaining is the original interrelatedness of the future, the present and the having-been. As long as being-there exists, it temporalizes itself in the integral unity of three temporal ecstasies, from which none can be missing. Heidegger puts it in the following way:

> All three dimensions of time are equiprimordial, for one never occurs without the other. All three are open to us equiprimordially [*gleichursprünglich*], but they are never open uniformally [*gleich-förmig*]. First, one dimension is predominant, then the other in which we are engaged, or in which, perhaps, we are even imprisoned. In this way, each of the other two dimensions have not just disappeared at any given time but have merely been modified.[11]

Thus, whether we aim to address the waking or the dream state of being-in-the-world, we must depart from the temporal unity of individual existence, observing how the specific temporal ecstasies are modified in each given case. The same applies also to the pathologically altered modes of being-in-the-world. "In all pathological phenomena too, the three temporal ecstasies and their particular modifications must be taken into consideration," stresses Heidegger.[12] The worst mistake one can commit here is to expound the disturbed relation to time, characteristic of some psychopathological states, from the viewpoint of the conventional concept of time founded upon the idea of time as an infinite uninterrupted sequence of single "nows." It follows from the temporal analysis undertaken in *Sein und Zeit* that this traditional view of time, in which time figures as a calculable quantity, is a mere leveling out of the primordial, ecstatic temporality of being-there, which is in itself utterly unquantifiable.

How misleading the interpretation relying on time understood as a measurable sequence of consecutive "nows" can be Heidegger demonstrates by the case of a young schizophrenic treated in the subacute stage of his illness.[13] According to the clinical record, one patient watching a clock on the wall feels a strong urge incessantly to follow the movement of the clock-hand. For him, the moving clock-hand presents an enigma as unsolvable as Zeno's paradox of the flying arrow. The patient becomes so absorbed in this enigma as to "lose the thread to himself." The difference between him and the clock disappears, which brings him under the impression that he himself is the clock. What he experiences is a "running away

---

[9] Heidegger. *Zollikoner Seminare*, 290. English edition: Heidegger. *Zollikon Seminars*, 230.

[10] Heidegger. *Zollikoner Seminare*, 84. English edition: Heidegger. *Zollikon Seminars*, 78–9.

[11] Heidegger. *Zollikoner Seminare*, 61. English edition: Heidegger. *Zollikon Seminars*, 48.

[12] Heidegger. *Zollikoner Seminare*, 229. English edition: Heidegger. *Zollikon Seminars*, 183.

[13] Heidegger. *Zollikoner Seminare*, 66–70. English edition: Heidegger. *Zollikon Seminars*, 51–5.

from himself," while his being is so volatile as to cease totally to be here and now. What occurs in addition to this is the disintegration of the overall structure of his surrounding world that once clearly articulated the referential relations and differences among various beings ready-to-hand. Therefore, the disoriented patient falls into sheer confusion, out of which he returns to the clock.

If we want to understand this state properly, claims Heidegger, we must not let ourselves be misled by the fact that the ill man's eyes are fixed on the clock hand. His attention is directed not to the measured time or time data, but rather to the clock that is, at first, located on the wall, but immediately goes adrift from its place and from the connected referential context. What is especially peculiar here is the compulsiveness of the patient's relation to the clock which goes so far as to cancel any possibility of a practical detachment. The schizophrenic is absorbed in the clock to the extent that he literally loses himself therein. Together with losing the contact with himself, the schizophrenic is torn out of the familiar surrounding world, in which things have their sense, shape and place. Only when he manages to keep his distance from the wall clock again, can he acquire some certainty that enables him, at least for a brief moment, to rest in the familiar world of practical matters. Therefore, what is crucial for the understanding of the given case is neither the question of the measured time, nor a meditation on time passing, but the difference between the relation to the clock that remains part of the referential context of the surrounding world, and the relation to the clock torn out of the surrounding context. Instead of examining the patient's cognitive relation to time, it is necessary to scrutinize his relation to innerworldly beings that address him and to their referential interconnectedness.

Nevertheless, how are we to interpret this pathological mode of being-in-the-world if we have to expound it on the basis of the inseparable unity of three temporal ecstasies? How are we to understand the disintegration of the schizophrenic personality that loses "the thread to itself", if it is necessary to depart from the integral unity of ecstatic temporality? Since the schizophrenic loss of one's own self cannot lead to a total disintegration of the ontological structure of being-there, it must be, in Heidegger's opinion, understood as a certain mode of individual existence.

With regard to the fact that the fragile and insecure individual being characteristic of schizophrenics is often accompanied by signs of compulsive behavior and of desperate clinging to things that can endow the ill with at least an elementary feeling of security and stability, it is not difficult to conclude that schizophrenia condemns the patient to a considerable loss of freedom. The schizophrenic is substantially restricted in his/her relation to possibilities offered by the world, which applies, albeit to a much smaller extent, to other types of psychopathological disorders as well. The agoraphobic is incapable of entering an open space, whereas a closed room is unbearable for the claustrophobic. Other neurotics are largely limited in their relations to possibilities offered by their being-with others. Accordingly, every mental illness means a restriction of a free and full realization of certain possibilities.

However, the same can be said of pathological disorders of a primarily somatic character. "Each illness," claims Heidegger, "is a loss of freedom."[14] Moreover, the

---

[14] Heidegger. *Zollikoner Seminare*, 202. English edition: Heidegger. *Zollikon Seminars*, 157.

division between psychic and somatic disorders is as such unacceptable from the phenomenological viewpoint, since it is grounded upon the Cartesian dualism of *res extensa* and *res cogitans*. Refusing to divide human existence into the corporeal and the spiritual part, Heidegger perceives every illness on the basis of the psychosomatic whole given by being-in-the-world. His notion of the lived body (*der Leib*) makes it possible to understand that illness does not afflict only the corporeal or the spiritual sphere, but the whole being-in-the-world, which is prevented by illness from implementing this or that possibility. The sense of the doctor's question: "*Was fehlt Ihnen?*" lies in the ascertainment of which possibility of the individual being-in-the-world is precluded and what impact this has on one's own relation to the open realm of the world.

The restriction of freedom which characterizes all pathological states brings Heidegger to the view that both somatic and psychic disorders can be subsumed under one common denominator, the phenomenon of *privation*.[15] Every pathological disorder is viewed in *Zollikoner Seminare* as a specific lack, as a specific privation of health. To be ill basically means not to be healthy. Insofar as health is understood as the ability to freely avail oneself of all possibilities shown in the open realm of world, illness represents a certain negation of this ability. The phenomenological interpretation of illness is thus grounded upon the definition of health which is, in one way or another, negated by a specific illness.

This negation, however, is no utter denial and exclusion of the healthy state, but rather a privative form of health which is, in this view, attributed to an entirely positive sense. Since every privation encompasses the essential relatedness to the positive that is lacking, Heidegger claims that everyone dealing with an illness is „actually dealing with health in the sense that health is lacking and has to be restored."[16]

When elucidating the peculiar character of the phenomenon of privation, Heidegger refers to Plato's dialogue *Sophist*, where this phenomenon is revealed in the connection with the question of the relative non-being (τὸ μὴ 'ὸν). Apart from the absolute non-being that simply does not exist, this Platonic dialogue addresses, for the first time in the history of Western philosophy, the possibility of the relative non-being that still in some sense *is*. In other words, the non-being is grasped here not only as the mere opposite to the existent, but also as that which has its own reality. The essence of the relative non-being is found in difference, that is to say, in that by means of which specific beings differ from each other. Every existent manifests itself as the non-being once viewed in relation to other beings, that is, to that which it is not.

Yet, in comparison with Plato's concept of the relative non-being, Heidegger's exposition of the privative negation is much narrower, as it emphasizes lack and shortage instead of difference. At least, that is what all the examples adduced in connection with privation attest to: rest is the privation of motion, shade is the lack of light, shard is the privation of tumbler. The same supposition is also corroborated by the following statement: "If we negate something in the sense that we don't simply deny it, but rather affirm it in the sense that something is lacking, such negation

---

[15] Heidegger. *Zollikoner Seminare*, 58. English edition: Heidegger. *Zollikon Seminars*, 45–6.

[16] Heidegger. *Zollikoner Seminare*, 58–9. English edition: Heidegger. *Zollikon Seminars*, 46.

is called a *privation*."[17] This clearly posits that privation means not just a difference
but above all a deprivation.

Using the notion of privation thus determined, Heidegger's exposition evinces its
debt not so much to Plato's concept of the relative non-being, but rather to Aristotle's
notion of privation (στέρησις), placed in *Metaphysics* into the focal point of the hyle-
morfic doctrine.[18] In the frame of this conception, privation is expounded as lack in
which the specific being is short of what it could or should have. For example,

> blindness is a privation, but one is not blind at any and every age, but only if one has not
> sight at the age at which one would naturally have it. Similarly, a thing suffers privation
> when it has not an attribute in those circumstances, or in that respect and in that relation and
> in that sense, in which it would naturally have it.[19]

Although illness is not the only case of privation, one cannot fail to notice the
fact that in *Metaphysics* it receives mention as a typical example thereof: "The substance of a privation is the opposite substance, e.g. health is the substance of disease; for it is by its absence that disease exists."[20]

This is precisely how the essential character of illness is interpreted in *Zollikoner
Seminare*: illness is explicated as privation that immediately refers to the healthy mode
of existence. That this reference is not fully reciprocal is confirmed by the fact that what
Heidegger says of illness he does not admit in the case of health; in other words, whereas
illness, according to him, is the privation of health, health can hardly be the privation of
illness. Even though it might be said that healthy is he/she who is not ill, this changes
nothing about the fact that in comparison with health, illness is a deficient mode of being.

The privative conception of illness does not, however, relate only to ontic
symptoms of pathological disorders, but defines the ontological status of illness as
such. Illness conceived of as a privative mode of existence is understood as an
"ontological phenomenon" of being in disclosedness. As a lack of health, illness
presents a certain possibility of being-there, i.e. a certain modus of its being.[21]

In this manner, Heidegger demarcates the ontological status of illness without having to produce a taxonomical table of all pathological disorders and their symptoms.
Since every pathological disorder has, in addition, got an individual character that
reflects the factual mode of being-in-the-world, *Zollikoner Seminare* mentions,
instead of a summarizing enumeration of specific illnesses, only a couple of roughly
sketched illustrative examples. It would certainly be a mistake to assume that a specific illness is the same in all individuals; an illness is always different in that it is
determined by means of possibilities whose realization is limited in an ill individual.

The view that illness is a "privative mode of existence," which renders its essence
ungraspable without a preliminary definition of what it means to be healthy, is

[17] Heidegger. *Zollikoner Seminare*, 58. English edition: Heidegger. *Zollikon Seminars*, 46.

[18] See Vetter, Helmuth. 1993. Es gibt keine unmittelbare Gesundheit des Geistes. *Daseinsanalyse* 10/ 65–79.

[19] Aristotle. 1984. *Metaphysics*, ed. Jonathan Barnes, revised Oxford Translation, Oxford: Princeton University Press, book 5, chapter 22, 1615.

[20] Aristotle. *Metaphysics*, book 7, chapter 7, 1630.

[21] Heidegger. *Zollikoner Seminare*, 59. English edition: Heidegger. *Zollikon Seminars*, 46–7.

nevertheless not as self-evident as it might seem at first sight. By taking this view, Heidegger stands in opposition to those who understand illness as a point of departure for comprehending health. Not the least of them is Freud who derives methodical impetuses for normal psychology from psychopathology. The concept of illness adumbrated in *Zollikoner Seminare* is by contrast grounded in the phenomenon of health, against which illness stands as a certain deficiency. This deficiency does not in the least mean only the objectively ascertainable failure of this or that vital function; rather, it is a deficient mode of existence, in which individual existence is deprived of one of the essential possibilities of its being-in-the-world.

Be that as it may, one still cannot resist the impression that such an approach to illness is possible only at the cost of a certain simplification. Is it really certain that illness always brings only a decrease of possibilities that are otherwise normally accessible to us? Could not illness also open up certain possibilities that would remain forever inaccessible without it? To take the example of a blind man Aristotle speaks of: it is obvious that a blind man loses the possibilities opened by means of sight, but he adapts to this disorder by compensating in his capacity for hearing or a tactile orientation that is much more acute and differentiated than in those who see. As far as the possibilities connected with the senses of hearing and touch are concerned, a blind man is much better off than a person with good eyesight, in whom these possibilities are dimmed and pushed into the background. In the case of a blind man, one can thus say that just as illness is deficient as compared to health, health is also deficient in relation to illness.

Heidegger, however, is by no means willing to concede this. For him, illness is nothing but a deficient mode of being and, as such, cannot bring any new possibilities. How a deficient mode of being-in-the-world is to be understood Heidegger demonstrates by the example of the phenomenon of the immaterial and insubstantial openness constitutive of being-there. Unlike things present-at-hand, being-there exists in that it always stands open in the relation to present beings. This standing-open (*die Offenständigkeit*), thanks to which all beings can become evident and understandable, is the basic ontological peculiarity of its existence. As long as being-there stands amidst the clearing of being so that it is open for the encounter with beings, it can nevertheless close itself off from the impulses and claims of the present, which is particularly evident in the case of psychopathological disorders, where certain possibilities of being-in-the-world are factually blurred. In this respect, perhaps the severest disorder of being-open to present beings is represented by schizophrenic unapproachability. But even though the schizophrenic may close himself/herself off from the impulses and claims of the surrounding things so much as to cease to be affected by anything, one still cannot conclude that his/her existence has no longer the character of being-open. "In schizophrenia the loss of [this] contact is a privation of being-open, which was just mentioned. Yet this privation does not mean that being-open disappears, but only that it is modified to a 'lack of contact,'" observes Heidegger.[22] Even when he/she entirely loses contact with his/her surrounding, the schizophrenic does not cease to exist openly, but rather fulfils this openness in a deficient way.

---

[22] Heidegger. *Zollikoner Seminare*, 95. English edition: Heidegger. *Zollikon Seminars*, 73.

As long as being-there is characterized by its being-open to beings encountered in the frame of the significative context of the surrounding world, the schizophrenic is capable thereof only to a very restricted extent. Unlike the healthy individual who is so intimately bound with surrounding things and his/her loved ones that they immediately address him/her and motivate his/her behavior, the schizophrenic is not able to come to terms with his surrounding and adequately respond to it in his/her behavior. The deficient mode of schizophrenic existence is marked by the impossibility to relate to the beings one encounters without helplessly falling prey to them. The schizophrenic in the acute stage of his disease is at the mercy of all he/she encounters to the extent of being totally absorbed and overwhelmed by it. Thus, every contact with the surrounding things or others presents for him/her a direct jeopardy of his/her own being. In order to save himself/herself, to preserve integrity of his/her individual being, the schizophrenic closes himself/herself off from everything that could subjugate him/her by its requirements. This explains the "autistic" traits shown by the schizophrenic being-in-the-world. Yet, since individual being cannot be realized unless one relates to others as well as to surrounding things, the schizophrenic closing-off offers no real recourse from the illness, but merely deepens the ongoing self-alienation and depersonalization.

Despite the far-reaching depersonalization occurring in schizophrenic individuals, however, the radical loss of one's own self is barely thinkable within the framework of the phenomenological project of being-there. Therefore, Heidegger insists that some rudimental individuality is still preserved even in the severest cases of schizophrenia. Just as the schizophrenic unapproachability is a privative mode of openness to present beings, the schizophrenic disintegration of personality is a privation of the original individual being. In the case of schizophrenics, one can thus speak only of their incapacity for integrating their being-in-the-world to a self-collected and self-subsistent existing, but not of the end of their individual existence.

When the schizophrenic whom Heidegger refers to, "loses the thread to himself," he does not cease to be himself, but rather experiences his individual being in a way so alienated that he can mistake himself for the clock he watches. Even this deficient mode of individual existence is a certain modification of being-there that temporalizes itself in the inseparable unity of the three temporal ecstasies. It is precisely the ecstatic unity of the future, the having-been and the present that ultimately forestalls the total disintegration of individual existence. As long as sojourning in disclosedness is carried by the ecstatic temporal unity, the absolute disintegration of its individual being is utterly impossible. Once, however, the ecstatic unity of temporality has fallen apart, being-there draws to its definitive end. Once being-there has turned into no-longer-being-there, the openness of being turns into impenetrable closedness whose ungraspable otherness stands in contrast to all that is familiar and commonly accessible. Since schizophrenia itself must necessarily perish together with being-there, Heidegger cannot comprehend it against the background of the absolute closedness brought forth by death. Therefore, schizophrenia can be nothing but a deficient mode of open standing in the clearing of being.

If schizophrenia is viewed in *Zollikoner Seminare* as a deficient mode of open being-in-the-world, there also must be a correspondent explanation of such phenomena as hallucination and delusion. Many schizophrenic patients in the acute phase of their illness are exposed to uncontrollable hallucinations whose intensity surpasses the impressions and perceptions of everyday being-in-the-world. This does not mean, however, that hallucination couldn't be interpreted as a certain mode of being-in-the-world. Heidegger demonstrates how hallucinatory experiences are to be expounded by the example of a schizophrenic whose illness reached its acute phase when he woke up in the middle of the night to find the rising Sun with a man lying underneath it on the opposite wall.[23] In order to understand such a hallucination, it is necessary to be aware that even a schizophrenic exists in a certain significative and referential context, albeit a highly insecure and unstable one. Therefore, Heidegger claims that "in understanding hallucinations, one must not start with the distinction between 'real' and 'unreal,' but rather with an inquiry into the character of the relationship to the world in which the patient is involved at any given time."[24]

The way the above mentioned schizophrenic relates to his world is marked primarily by extreme un-freedom. What the hallucinating encounters in his world, subjugates him and deprives him of his freedom.[25] But even this utter un-freedom resulting from the inability to move within the polarity between the presence and the absence of something must still be understood as reflection of primordial openness. Only in the light of the original openness and freedom characteristic of being-there is it possible to explicate the deep deficiency of free will to which the schizophrenic is doomed by his illness.

If what Heidegger says about pathological states of the schizophrenic type is valid, it is only logical that the same should also be applied to those mental disorders that pose a far less serious threat to a free and independent existence. As long as the open being-in-the-world and integral individual being don't perish even in the uttermost form of mental disorder, it is clear that other psychopathological states can be explicated only on the basis of a primary openness and individual constancy of existence, either. Whether they be disorders of the psychotic or the neurotic character, it is necessary to view them as privative forms of integral individual being and as deficient modes of open being-in-the-world.

The defining difference among various pathological disorders thus lies in the extent to which the patient lacks the independence of individual being and in the degree of deficiency displayed by the essentially open and free being-in-the-world. From an ontic viewpoint, compulsive behavior could seem to have nothing to do with openness or freedom; on the ontological plane, however, we can see that even this unmanageable compulsiveness does express the fundamental openness and freedom that open the very possibility of the lacking free will. All compulsive action, obsessive rituals, and actually every inability to behave differently in a given situation must therefore be approached as deficient forms of the essentially open and free being-in-the-world.[26]

---

[23] Heidegger. *Zollikoner Seminare*, 195–6. English edition: Heidegger. *Zollikon Seminars*, 151–2.

[24] Heidegger. *Zollikoner Seminare*, 196. English edition: Heidegger. *Zollikon Seminars*, 152.

[25] Heidegger. *Zollikoner Seminare*, 195. English edition: Heidegger. *Zollikon Seminars*, 151.

[26] Heidegger. *Zollikoner Seminare*, 210. English edition: Heidegger. *Zollikon Seminars*, 164–5.

Unless someone "mentally ill" preserves, at least to a rudimentary degree, his/her individual being, unless this human being has the ontological character of open standing in the cleared area of the world, the therapeutic help will stand no chance of opening a way out of his deficient mode of being. Both the pharmaco-therapeutic and the psychotherapeutic help can be, according to Heidegger, beneficial only to someone who remains essentially the same and who retains an elementary openness to possible impulses. In order to be cured, the ill individual must always have the ability to return to itself and make use of the possibilities offered by the world. Only thus can the individual existence in the course of its treatment obtain a freer relation to what it encounters, learn how to accept this relation and bear responsibility for it.[27] As all psychopathological disorders are "disturbances in adjustment and freedom," the aim of the therapeutic intervention is to help the patient to overcome the deficit of adjustment and freedom and to bring him/her to free existence within the requirements given by his/her factual situation.[28] Thus, in *Zollikoner Seminare* the phenomenologically understood treatment proves to be both adaptation and liberation.

In *Zollikoner Seminare*, however, pathological un-freedom and dependence gain their distinct contours only when brought into connection with the inauthentic existence which flees its very own possibilities, alienating itself from its original individual being. What can serve as an illustrative example thereof is Heidegger's exposition of compulsive behavior occurring in patients with bipolar affective disorder.[29] Manic states in which the patient is compelled to incessant euphoric activity, in which he wants to throw himself in ten directions at once, are understood as expressions of the inauthentic existence. The ceaseless fluttering about and headlong seizing of whatever is available at the moment tends to be accompanied in these cases by the feeling of absolute happiness and fullness of life, but that is possible only because "the inauthentic always has the appearance of the authentic. Therefore, the manic human being believes that he is authentically himself or that he is [really] himself."[30]

Inauthenticity escalated into the utmost extreme, in which individual existence deprives itself of a free and independent realization of its possibilities, is an importunate guide of other mental disorders as well. This is best corroborated by the unusually high degree to which the phenomenon described in the context of fundamental ontology as falling prey (*das Verfallen*) asserts itself in these. Both neurotically and psychotically burdened people are affected, to a larger or lesser extent, by falling prey that encloses individual existence into the subjugation to inherited prejudices, ready-made opinions and family schemata governed by nobody and everybody. The oblivion of the original and unique individual being that occurs

---

[27] Heidegger. *Zollikoner Seminare*, 199, 212. English edition: Heidegger. *Zollikon Seminars*, 154–5, 167.

[28] Heidegger. *Zollikoner Seminare*, 199. English edition: Heidegger. *Zollikon Seminars*, 154.

[29] Heidegger. *Zollikoner Seminare*, 219. English edition: Heidegger. *Zollikon Seminars*, 173–4.

[30] Heidegger. *Zollikoner Seminare*, 219. English edition: Heidegger. *Zollikon Seminars*, 174.

amidst public anonymity is also accompanied by the tendency to fall prey to the surrounding world and its parts.

Heidegger documents the way falling prey to the innerworldy beings impacts the concrete character of pathological behavior in the case of a girl suffering from a phobia of the possible breaking of her shoe heel.[31] The panic that renders the girl dependent on something as banal as her high heels is to be understood in the light of entanglement in beings ready-to-hand that are disclosed within the referential structure of the surrounding world. The existence of this girl "is absorbed in a particular, everyday world," but this does not mean that her individual being should disintegrate. "It is a question of [being] an uninterrupted self" whose entanglement in things sentences it to the inauthentic existence.[32]

Under the given circumstances, therapeutic treatment must be directed toward enabling the patient to overcome the inauthentic mode of existence and obtain an open relation to beings that address her in the significative context of the surrounding world without falling prey to them. However, does not the freedom and independence of a healthy existence acquire the status that is reserved in *Sein und Zeit* for the authentic mode of being? Is not health put on a par with the authentic existence? If mental illness represents a privative phenomenon, it is viewed as an inauthentic mode of existence that is, as follows from the existential analytic of being-there, also a privative form of being-in-the-world. Against the inauthentic existence stands the authentic mode of existence in which the primordial form of being in disclosedness manifests itself. In relation to the inauthentic mode of being, the authentic existence plays the same role that health plays in relation to illness.

In this context, one must not forget that the phenomenon of privation, according to Heidegger's conception, is connected not with a value-based devalorization but rather with ontological derivation that manifests itself against the backdrop of the primordial unity and integrity of individual existence. The incoherence and inconsistency of individual being that mark the inauthentic existence is a mere modification of the unity and integrity achieved by the authentic individual being. The same applies to the dependence and lack of freedom of pathological modes of individual existence, whose deficiency is reflected against the background of a free, open relatedness to beings that marks the healthy existence.

If, however, health is put on a par with the authentic way of being in *Zollikoner Seminare*, this cannot occur without a change in the understanding of some constituent moments connected with the free, self-subsistent and self-consistent existence. Unlike the authentic mode of existence as described in *Sein und Zeit*, health is not grasped as heroic readiness for anxiety or as obedience to the voice of one's own conscience. Health as such is entirely extricated from the relation to the uncanniness and existential guiltiness heralded in the voice of conscience. The point is that the relation to the world stripped of all pathological constraints and blocks must be primarily joyful and relaxed. "The being-free for something is a serene and joyful

---

[31] Heidegger. *Zollikoner Seminare*, 256. English edition: Heidegger. *Zollikon Seminars*, 205–6.

[32] Heidegger. *Zollikoner Seminare*, 256. English edition: Heidegger. *Zollikon Seminars*, 206.

mood in itself," claims Heidegger.[33] Insofar as anxiety does appear in *Zollikoner Seminare*, it is only in the forms of sheepishness and imbalance that mark the pathologically narrowed relation to the world. Anxiety is no longer the key to the free and independent existence, but, rather on the contrary, a proof of un-free and dependent existence. The anxiety a young woman suffers is perceived as an expression of hysterical un-freedom, but once the patient has supplanted the anxiety by a joyful mood it is regarded as the proof of her having been cured, i.e. of her having managed to overcome pathological inhibitions and attain a truly free relation to the world.[34] Hence, anxiety is no longer to be regarded as the ontological foundation of individual existence, but rather to be done away with by therapeutic means.

Nevertheless, the fact that anxiety is understood as a pathological phenomenon does not mean that Heidegger explicates psychopathological phenomena in the light of temporality whose defining dimension is the having-been. This possibility remains beyond the horizon of his meditations which imply nothing more than the link between psychopathological disorders and the unauthentic existence whose temporality temporalizes itself primarily out of the dimension of the present. More than to anything else, the shift in the understanding of anxiety attests to the change Heidegger's thought underwent between *Sein und Zeit* and *Zollikoner Seminare*. Even though a more or less identical terminology is used in both texts, the ontological project of being-there undergoes a certain change, which is revealed also by the fact that the phenomenon of anxiety loses the preeminent position it used to have within the existential analysis of being-there and becomes utterly marginal. The only ideas that remain unaltered within the ontological project of being-there are the concept of the existential constancy of individual being, maintained on the ground of the ecstatic unity of temporality, and the phenomenon of privation that is connected with illness and inauthentic existence.

4.2   Boss's Daseinsanalytic Concept and Its Critique

With respect to Boss's therapeutic Daseinsanalysis which is to be discussed in this Chap. 1 can say that it is nothing but a reflection and specification of the notion of mental disorder that is outlined in *Zollikoner Seminare*. Boss fully adopts Heidegger's view of mental disorder and further elaborates on it in detailed clinical studies. He also accepts the idea of the elementary unity of human existence that cannot be disrupted by any psychopathological disorder. All disruptions of individual existence including the schizophrenic dissociation of the self are then viewed as mere privations of the fundamental integrity of the self. Yet, even though Heidegger himself affirmed Boss's psychiatric conception, this conception has met with a considerable critique. Recently, it has been especially Alice Holzhey-Kunz who criticized Boss's therapeutic Daseinsanalysis because of its normative character.

---

[33] Heidegger. *Zollikoner Seminare*, 212. English edition: Heidegger. *Zollikon Seminars*, 167.

[34] Heidegger. *Zollikoner Seminare*, 211–2. English edition: Heidegger. *Zollikon Seminars*, 165–7.

In opposition to Boss, Holzhey-Kunz has created her own hermeneutic concept of psychopathology, in which she stresses the finitude of human existence as the basic ontological character that makes possible a non-normative approach to psycho-pathological phenomena. Since the finitude of human existence has – in Heidegger's eyes – no positive counterpart, it can be seen as the ontological foundation explaining all sorts of psychopathological phenomena. However, even Holzhey-Kunz is not able to put a question mark over the individual integrity of human existence, as she sticks to the common understanding of *Sein und Zeit*. This is why she can explain merely the psychopathological disorders of neurotic character leaving the psychotic disorders aside.

If we are to grasp the viewpoint professed by *Zollikoner Seminare* in its entirety, we must not neglect Heidegger's friend, organizer of the Zollikon seminars and subsequent editor of the seminar proceedings – Medard Boss. Although Boss met such personages as Freud, Goldstein or Jung during his studies and his ensuing professional career, the direction of his scientific development was particularly influenced by Binswanger's psychiatric *Daseinsanalysis*. Later, he abandoned this theory as well, when he created his own psychotherapeutic conception of "therapeutic *Daseinsanalysis*," which consisted in the rigorous effort to understand the ontic phenomena manifested in the realms of psychopathology and psychotherapy on the basis of Heidegger's philosophical views.

Just as psychiatric *Daseinsanalysis*, therapeutic *Daseinsanalysis* relies on the ontological project of being-there, but unlike Binswanger's concept, it is firmly grounded upon the foundations established during the Zollikon lectures and seminars. It is especially by virtue of these that Boss managed to evade the anthropological schemata by which psychiatric *Daseinsanalysis* obfuscated the original sense of the ontological analysis of being-there. Conversations with Heidegger and attendance at his lectures enabled Boss not only to grasp the significance of the fundamental notion of disclosedness, but also to comprehend the change in the concept of the ecstatic being in disclosedness that occurred once this disclosedness had been understood out of itself as the clearing of being. This is corroborated already by the fact that Boss's view on the ontological constitution of being in disclosedness derives much more from *Zollikoner Seminare* than from *Sein und Zeit*.

Correspondingly, in therapeutic *Daseinsanalysis* the disposition of anxiety plays almost no role at all. Instead, what becomes the primordial disposition that reveals the true character of sojourning in disclosedness is cheerful calmness (*die heitere Gelassenheit*) or calm cheerfulness (*die gelassene Heiterkeit*) in which the individual experiences the original openness and freedom of its being. Unlike all other moods by which being-in-the-world is both opened and closed, the disposition of cheerful calmness brings the openness and freedom of sojourning in the clearing of being to their full revelation. Being-there is always already somehow situated within the frame of significative and referential relations between beings, but only the disposition of cheerful calmness enables it to face all uncovered beings without closing itself off from them or wanting to subjugate them to its power. Individual existence attuned to calm cheerfulness lets everything be what it is and thus is addressed by it. By enabling it to remain in the broadest responsiveness, calm cheerfulness brings to individual existence consummate happiness. Boss understands this happiness as a feeling that appears when the realization of all essential possibilities of behavior has been opened for individual existence.

Although such a disposition opens individual existence for grasping the immediately revealed givens, the majority of moods also closes it off in a certain manner. In extreme cases this is conspicuous in affects such as anger and wrath, in which human existence becomes blinded to certain aspects of its present situation. As disposition offers us specific possibilities of behavior, being-in-the-world is always more or less open in a given disposition. Insofar as being-in-the-world is understood as an open comprehension of the significative richness of the world, the individual differences in the maintenance of the open and cleared area of the world can be detected and described. The ideal is thus seen in the maximum openness by virtue of which being-there can encounter the significative richness of beings, and thus completely fulfill its "standing-open." A specific individual can exist in a way adequate to being-there (*daseinsgemäß*) only when it stands open to the challenges and claims of what is announced in the significative and referential context of its world.

Specific individuals differ from each other especially in the degree and extent of reduction in their open relation to the significative richness of the world. This extent highlights the individual norm, marked by both natural constitution and the personal history. The specific individual exists normally as long as it realizes possibilities available to it in an adequate way. The differentiation of the individual extent of openness to the possibilities of perception and action, however, is sensible only provided that, on the ontological plane, being-there still maintains its individual being. Should it not exist as individual being, it couldn't avail itself of the possibilities of maturing and growing, and thus of broadening the field of its own possibilities. The psychotherapeutic help whose sense is seen by Boss in removing restraints created by pathogenic upbringing in the childhood, as well as in giving access to the possibilities hitherto excluded, would thus also become impossible.

Since an instrumental part of the therapeutic *Daseinsanalysis* is played by the interpretation of dreams, it must, understandably, also reflect the structure of individual being. In "*Es träumte mir vergangene Nacht...*," Boss departs from the presupposition that being-there preserves its individuality both in waking and dreaming. Even the dreams of schizophrenics, who experience in them the world's doom and disintegration of their existence, present no exception. Even though they indicate the dreadful loss of one's self, these dreams cannot, in Boss's opinion, cast doubt on the fact that even schizophrenics, who witness their own psychophysical undoing, still preserve their individual being. For, "even waking schizophrenics retain some rudimentary sense of self, and of their dwelling in the world, for otherwise they could never experience a loss of those things, waking or dreaming. And if the loss of those essential human traits were in fact total, such persons would no longer be human beings."[35] Thus, the fact that both dreaming and waking belong to one whole

---

[35] Boss, Medard. 1970. "*Es träumte mir vergangene Nacht*". Bern: Verlag Hans Huber, 146. English edition: Boss, Medard. 1977. "*I Dreamt Last Night...*", (trans: Conway, Stephen). New York: Gardner Press, 191.

of individual existence is not refuted, but rather corroborated by the extreme experience of these patients.

By making this claim, Boss utterly identifies himself with the exposition of the dreaming being-in-the-world as propounded in *Zollikoner Seminare*. Like Heidegger, he also supposes that the discontinuity between the dream and the waking must be understood on the ground of the constantly maintained individual existence and its historicity.

However, *"Es träumte mir vergangene Nacht…"* is not the only work marked by the influence of Zollikon seminars. Their inspiring effect is observable also in Boss's chef-d'oeuvre entitled *Grundriss der Medizin und der Psychologie*. What is attempted here is the ambitious project consisting in a general revision of the ontological foundations of Western medicine and psychology – what is confronted with Descartes's and Galilei's conceptions of science upon which both the theory and practice of the classical medicine are grounded is a phenomenological method which shall enable a much more adequate view of human health and illness. Boss tries to adumbrate the basic phenomenological plan of the medical science by using Heidegger's ontological project of being-there, thanks to which it becomes possible to thematize all phenomena revealed to the medical gaze as aspects of our standing open in the clearing of being. What is merely sketched and illustrated by a few examples in *Zollikoner Seminare* is thus given its systematic form in *Grundriss der Medizin und der Psychologie*.

In order to show the limits of the Cartesian mode of thought and display the phenomenological view on human health and disease, Boss offers a detailed casuistry, which features the case of his patient Regula Zürcher. This casuistry reflects a whole scale of health problems including, apart from psychic disorders, also those of a somatic and psychosomatic nature.

Since early childhood, Regula Zürcher had suffered from severe eczemas, joined in her pubescence by chronic constipation and unbearable pain in her bosom. In the process of psychotherapy, all of these primarily somatic symptoms gradually subsided, until they completely disappeared. However, the interdependence of psychic and somatic symptoms cannot be adequately explained by medicine of the Cartesian orientation, since it remains imprisoned in the dualism of *res extensa* and *res cogitans*; although it can allow for a certain connectedness between the body and the soul, the essence of the psychosomatic phenomena necessarily eludes its grasp. On the contrary, Boss reveals the psychic and somatic phenomena as principally indivisible. Once it has been comprehended not as *Körper*, but as *Leib*, the human body becomes integral part of being-in-the-world. As such, the lived body plays a crucial role in the human sensuality. Each of the five senses that belong to the lived body covers a certain sphere of our openness. This openness, however, does not arise from piecing together the specific sensual spheres. On the contrary, the openness of being-there is what constitutes the unity of all senses. Since the fundamental feature of sojourning in disclosedness, that is, its standing-open, is realized in the dynamic unity of sight, hearing, touch, smell and taste, it is also possible to substitute one sense by another (e.g. sight by touch).[36]

---

[36] Boss, Medard. 1975. *Grundriss der Medizin und der Psychologie*. Bern, Stuttgart, Wien: Verlag Hans Huber, 282.

The extent of the sensual openness can, however, substantially vary in different situations, which can be documented by the example of the pain phenomenon. When Regula Zürcher broke her leg in a car accident, her sensual openness was reduced to one single point, out of which an excruciating pain radiated.[37] Not even after the acute pain had subsided and Regula Zürcher was hospitalized was the openness of her existence the same, as it had been before she was hit by a car. During the time she had been confined to bed, Regula's open sphere of possibilities had been substantially narrowed down. Since the broken leg considerably disrupted the performance of the patient's possibilities, her injury not only pertained to the somatic sphere of her existence, but also limited the overall performance of her open being-in-the-world.

According to Boss, the same applies to other types of injury and illness. Every illness restricts in a certain way the openness of being-in-the-world, thus forming the character of overall being-ill (*das Krank-sein*). Once the pathological disturbance has affected one of the essential moments of being-in-the-world, be it the lived body, disposition or being-with others, all other moments are necessarily impacted as well. It therefore comes as no surprise that the eczemas and constipations Boss's patient had suffered were connected with the restriction of her openness and freedom, and disappeared once she managed, with the help of psychotherapy, to broaden the sphere of her possibilities.

There are also other respects in which Boss clings to the instructions for medical thought indicated in *Zollikoner Seminare*. His *Grundriss der Medizin und der Psychologie* is based upon the conviction that illness is nothing but a specific privation of health. And since health is grasped as the maximal openness to the appearing givens of the world, illness must be articulated as a privation of this very openness. Nevertheless, as a privation, illness is characterized not by complete cancellation of the primordial openness of being-there but merely by the lack thereof. „If all illness," claims Boss, "is in fact the lack of the condition of health, then illness is necessarily always related to, and understandable only in terms of, the state of health. The reverse is never true, for health cannot be constructed from what is its own deficient state."[38] In other words, all pathological phenomena encountered by both organic and psychiatric medicine must be understood, with regard to health, as signs of a deficient sojourning in disclosedness.

Health, understood as uttermost openness to the possibilities of being-in-the-world, thus gets to play the role of the norm, in comparison to which pathological disorders are judged. All manifestations of health are perceived as complying with the norm (*normgemäßene*), whereas pathological symptoms as opposed to the norm (*normwidrige*). This normativity follows not from the findings of comparative anatomy or culturally conditioned rules of social life, but only from the ontological project of the sojourning in the clearing of being.

---

[37] Boss. *Grundriss der Medizin und der Psychologie*, 427–9.

[38] Boss. *Grundriss der Medizin und der Psychologie*, 441. English edition: Boss, Medard. 1994. *Existential Foundations of Medicine and Psychology* (trans: Conway, Stephen, and Cleaves, Anne). New Jersey: Jason Aronson Inc., 198.

On the basis of health, which is the synonym for the maximal openness toward appearing givens, it is then possible to distinguish among various types of pathological disorders depending on which essential feature of human existence is disturbed in its realization. Although it is always more than only one of the existential traits of being-there that is affected by an illness, what comes to the fore is the impact on those that are the most obstructive of the development of an open and free relation to the world. Therefore, Boss can elaborate on his system of general pathology that corresponds to the essential constitution of sojourning in disclosedness. This system differs from the classical nosological table in that it divides illnesses not as entities belonging to this or that category, but as the various forms of being-ill, in which occurs the disturbance of some of the fundamental moments of being-there. Thus, illnesses with the primary disorder of the lived body stand next to illnesses affecting disposition, e.g. depression and bipolar affective disorder, or disorders disturbing spatio-temporal self-positioning of human existence.

The last category comprises, apart from other disorders, also senile dementia, in which the sphere of temporal and spatial relations that the patients are capable of maintaining is severely limited.[39] In these cases, the restriction of the spatial context is marked by gradual disorientation, which is accompanied by obfuscation of the temporal extension of existence. The temporal being of patients suffering from senile dementia is reduced to existence in the present, onto which memories of the past are freely projected. This does not, however, mean that the ecstatic unity of their temporality would disintegrate. According to Boss, one cannot speak of anything but uttermost deficiency that marks one's own embedding in the having-been, the present and the future. The ecstatic unity of the future, the having-been and the present cannot disappear as long as we speak of human existence.

Not only senile dementia, but in effect every form of being-ill is conceived of in *Grundriss der Medizin und der Psychologie* as a privation of health, i.e. as a lack of openness in the relation to the world and its givens. Whichever of the essential traits of human existence, it is always also the overall openness of being-in-the-world that becomes affected.

The fulfillment of openness is nevertheless most clearly disturbed in patients suffering from schizophrenia. Since, particularly severe disorders of the fundamental feature of human existence (i.e. its standing-open) take place in schizophrenia, Boss terms it "the most human and inhuman of all illnesses."[40] Human existence shows itself from the phenomenological perspective as openly standing being-in-the-world which can, by virtue of its responsiveness, immediately comprehend that which reveals itself in the world. The schizophrenic disorder undermines the capability of maintaining open responsiveness to what one encounters within the frame of referential and significative relations of the world. In contrast to healthy individuals, schizophrenics are much less able to adequately respond to the challenges and requirements of their surrounding. Schizophrenic patients cannot relate to the surrounding beings or to others without becoming absorbed or overcome by them; they

---

[39] Boss. *Grundriss der Medizin und der Psychologie*, 467–8.

[40] Boss. *Grundriss der Medizin und der Psychologie*, 483 (translator's translation).

are exposed to the world to the extent that in relation to it they lose their independent and self-subsistent individual being. In order to preserve at least some remnant of their individual existence, they must keep obstinate distance from everything that somehow concerns them. This distancing from things and others brings about total obfuscation and narrowing of the open existence. The schizophrenic who closes himself/herself off in isolation thus pays an exorbitant price for preserving at least a faint shadow of his/her individual being.

All ontic symptoms of schizophrenic disorders, featuring especially the incoherence of thought processes, hallucinations, disorders of affectivity and advancing depersonalization, have to do with the fact that the patient loses his/her independence in relation to the world and has to exert enormous effort to maintain at least remnants of his/her individual being. The schizophrenic is incapable of asserting himself/herself as an independent individual being that keeps up in open responsiveness to what it encounters and responds accordingly. The freedom and independence of his/her individual being disintegrates whenever the sphere of significative and referential relations, within which he/she finds his/her possibilities, broadens to the extent that he/she is no longer able to respond to them adequately.

What occurs together with that is, according to Boss, the psychotic loosening (*die Entschränkung*) of the being-in-the-world, in which the significative and referential structure of the world becomes freely permeable for delusions and hallucinations. The pathological loosening, harbingering the outbreak of schizophrenia, occurs most often in pubescence, post-pubescence and, with women, after childbirth, when one's own openness for the possibilities and claims of being-in-the-world becomes markedly expanded. This psychotic loosening can totally disappear, however, once the patient retreats into the significative and referential context in which he/she is capable of adequately facing the claims and challenges of surrounding.

Thus, for instance, one of Boss's female patients, who demonstrated more and more schizophrenic symptoms when having to exist as a wife and mother of three children, rid herself of all troubles once she stopped being exposed to excessive requirements and began to lead the life of a lone laboratory assistant.[41] Analogically, some chronic schizophrenics can divest themselves of their delusions and hallucinations if the psychotherapist manages to bring them to entrust themselves to his/her hands as a helpless, dependent children, who they in fact still are, and to immerse themselves in the possibilities of an infant to which they can adequately respond without losing their individual being. On the basis of these findings, Boss draws the conclusion that the schizophrenic existence is to be understood as "a radically incomplete manifestation of the free and [authentic] selfhood that normally characterizes human being."[42]

Thus, we get to another level of the phenomenological interpretation of being-ill, departing from the ontological project of sojourning in the clearing of being. As

---

[41] Boss. *Grundriss der Medizin und der Psychologie*, 506. English edition: Boss. *Existential Foundations of Medicine and Psychology*, 236.
[42] Boss. *Grundriss der Medizin und der Psychologie*, 507. English edition: Boss. *Existential Foundations of Medicine and Psychology*, 236.

long as schizophrenics lack the capacity for an independent and free individual being, their existence is to be comprehended as a *privation* of authentic existence. The independence and self-subsistence of the authentic existence then becomes the norm of health. Conversely, the dependence and lack of freedom that mark the inauthentic mode of existence assert themselves wherever the patient pathologically succumbs to the claims of surrounding and to the behavioral models of others.

That does not, however, mean that all forms of inauthentic existence are necessarily pathological. As a privative mode of sojourning in the clearing of being, inauthenticity has both pathological and non-pathological forms. It is beyond all doubt that pathological self-alienation and self-oblivion are much deeper than those of non-pathological states. Arguably, the most extreme form of inauthentic existence is schizophrenia, in which the privation of the authentic individual being goes so far as to render the patients incapable of integrating their existence into an independent, coherent performance. Therefore the schizophrenic mode of being-ill is thematized in *Grundriss der Medizin und der Psychologie* purely *negatively*. "The pathology in such patients is their *lack* of the possibility available to the healthy person to assemble his responses and behavior to be self-reliant, free, open and enduring in the face of whatever may be encountered."[43] Instead, schizophrenics fall prey to possibilities offered in the social relations or in the form of beings-ready-to-hand and present-at-hand.

For instance, Boss mentions a young schizophrenic who could not bear the sight of a chair without feeling the compulsion to sit on it.[44] By the same token, he felt compelled to imitate a gardener at work. The patient fell prey especially to the claims of being-with-others imposed on him by the opinions and intentions of his parents. Owing to their dictatorial oppression, he never learned to exist in his own time. The patient had always lived the "time of the other," i.e. time not of his own. His existence reached such an extreme degree of depersonalization that his limbs seemed to him inanimate appendages belonging to someone else. This depersonalization, according to Boss, related to nothing but "extraordinarily high degree of inauthenticity of his whole being-in-the-world."[45]

Albeit to a much lesser extent than in the case of schizophrenia, inauthenticity appears also in the behavior of patients suffering from bipolar affective disorder. Even though they irresistibly fall prey to everything they encounter in their manic phases, they are not depersonalized and their individual being turns out undisturbed. On the contrary, a manically excited individuals gets the feeling of being themselves more than ever in their omnipotence. Their falling prey to the offered possibilities, each of which diverts them from what they have just uncovered and rivets them to itself, also does not lead to the loosening of the structure of the world, observable in schizophrenics. All the world's givens rather stay in their place without disruption

---

[43] Boss. *Grundriss der Medizin und der Psychologie*, 507. English edition: Boss. *Existential Foundations of Medicine and Psychology*, 236.

[44] Boss. *Grundriss der Medizin und der Psychologie*, 489. English edition: Boss. *Existential Foundations of Medicine and Psychology*, 226.

[45] Boss. *Grundriss der Medizin und der Psychologie*, 492 (translator's translation).

in their significative and referential bonds. The hegemony of the surrounding beings over the manic individual being is reflected "merely" in the unfree succumbing to all possible excitements and stimuli. This unfree succumbing is understood in *Grundriss der Medizin und der Psychologie* as an expression of falling prey (*das Verfallen*), in which the individual existence robs itself of its freedom and independence. From the perspective of the intact existence that independently displays its openness, falling prey seems a "deficient mode of fundamental being-in-the-world."[46]

Yet, falling prey is harbingered not only in bipolar disorders, but also in other disorders of the psychotic or the neurotic character. Both psychotic and neurotic patients are marked by the phenomenon of falling prey that prevents them from fully developing their independent, free and totally open existence. Therefore, Boss brings this phenomenon into the focus of his exposition of psychopathological disorders, grasping it as a privative mode of a primarily independent, free and open existence. Measured by the norm of authentic existence, falling prey appears as lagging behind the ideal of an independent, free and open sojourning in disclosedness. Thus, authenticity becomes the synonym for an intact, mature and healthy existence, whereas falling prey and inauthenticity are found wherever the psychiatric gaze reveals a pathologically disturbed and immature performance of being-in-the-world.

As long as authenticity prescribes the norm of health and maturity, whereas inauthenticity serves the understanding of the various forms of pathological dependence, lack of freedom and closure, all this has impact on the direction of the *daseinsanalytically* oriented therapy. The objective of therapeutic treatment is to help the patient to attain a fully authentic existence. *Daseinsanalytically* oriented therapy is to be understood as a path from the privative mode of being-in-the-world toward the primordial, intact form of sojourning in disclosedness. To achieve full recovery, it is not enough to merely remove the pathological symptoms that plague the individual at the given moment, but it is necessary to bring the individual back to himself/herself in the sense of an independent, free and open existence. This requires that individual existence overcomes both the pathological blocks and hindrances that prevent it from developing its very own possibilities, as well as the unfree falling prey to the possibilities that are not its own. Patients can accept their individual existence only by gradually getting rid of their dependence on adopted opinions and attitudes foisted upon them by their pathogenic upbringing and embracing instead those modes of behavior that always already belong to them, and yet still remain concealed in their illness.

For this reason, Boss adjusts the fundamental question of "big psychotherapy" to the need for liberating patients from the pathological narrowing of their relations to the world and bringing them to such individual being that is utterly free and of their own. Instead of the classical question of "why?" by which the psychoanalyst seeks to unveil the hidden sense of psychopathological symptoms, what is preferred in the *daseinsanalytical* therapy is the formulation "actually, why not?" ("*Warum denn eigentlich nicht?*"). This question aims to cast doubt on the pathological restraints

---

[46] Boss. *Grundriss der Medizin und der Psychologie*, 475 (translator's translation).

and adopted models of behavior that hold sway over the patient's existence. At the same time, the patient is given to understand that there are ways of behavior much more open and independent than what his/her relation to the world has been so far. Naturally, a prerequisite indispensable for the patient's ability to attain a truly independent and open relation to the world is the free and safe area provided by his/her relationship with the therapist. Without an open, balanced affability with which the therapist accepts all the meaningful givens unveiled by his patient, the patient would hardly pluck up the courage to enter into an independent and free relation to possibilities he/she has thus far evaded for various reasons.

As long as he qualifies recovery by the norm of authentic existence and perceives illness in the light of falling prey, it is clear that Boss does not understand authenticity and inauthenticity in the spirit of *Sein und Zeit*. In *Grundriss der Medizin und der Psychologie*, authenticity denotes maximal openness, freedom and independence of individual existence, whereas pathological closure and dependence are regarded as proofs of inauthentic existence. Thus, authenticity is devoid of its heroic pathos connected with the anticipation of death, with the resoluteness to hearken to the voice of conscience or with the readiness to face the uncanniness of anxiety, becoming rather the ideal of autonomous existence that is able, by virtue of its openness and independence, fully to meet the claims imposed by the surrounding world.

This corresponds to the way the phenomenon of anxiety is interpreted in *Grundriss der Medizin und der Psychologie*, as well. In contrast to the phenomenological description of being-there undertaken within the framework of fundamental ontology, anxiety belongs not to the free and independent performance of individual being, but to the privative mode of being in which both the independence and the openness of sojourning in disclosedness are restricted. Hence, in the process of therapy, the proneness to anxiety is to be removed and replaced by the feeling of cheerful calmness that attests to the maximal openness and freedom of being-in-the-world.

Although he must have been more aware than anyone else that this picture of authentic and inauthentic existence is not in accord with the project of fundamental ontology, Heidegger had no reservations about Boss's exposition of health and illness. On the contrary, therapeutic *Daseinsanalysis* met with his unconditional support, of which the preface to *Grundriss der Medizin und der Psychologie*, where the author thanks Heidegger for not only inspiration, but also active cooperation in the creation of the work, bears the clearest proof. This help consisted in outlining the overall structure of the whole work, as well as in a critical revision of the written text, whereby Heidegger did not deny his attention to "one section of 'philosophical' import."[47] This, after all, is further confirmed by the later publication of *Zollikoner Seminare*, where several passages can be found containing specific pieces of advice and recommendation concerning Boss's oeuvre.[48] With regard to the fact that *Grundriss der Medizin und der Psychologie* adopts the privative conception of illness and the ensuing strategy of the exposition of pathological phenomena, it can be conceived of as a work of two authors, albeit signed by one. But

---

[47] Boss. *Grundriss der Medizin und der Psychologie*, 9.
[48] Boss. *Grundriss der Medizin und der Psychologie*, 273–5, 279–80.

even if Heidegger's co-authorship were to be restricted to a mere friendly help, this still suffices for therapeutic *Daseinsanalysis* to pass for the only "officially acknowledged" doctrine of a *daseinsanalytically* oriented investigation in the realm of medicine and psychology.

Even the supreme philosophical sanctification couldn't ensure, however, that *Daseinsanalysis* be generally and unreservedly accepted. Despite the weight of authority Heidegger naturally assumes in the realm of phenomenological investigation, there are some doubts concerning the correctness of the way the phenomenological method asserts itself in the fields of medicine and psychology. In this connection, we must mention especially the name Alice Holzhey-Kunz, who emphasizes the difficulties posed by some aspects of Boss's concept. The medical project adumbrated in *Grundriss der Medizin und der Psychologie* is, in her opinion, one-sidedly focused on the notion of health which is attributed the role of a preliminary guideline in determining all the various types of pathological disorders.[49] As long as health is understood as utmost openness and freedom, as supreme ability to realize the various modes of behavior, illness cannot present anything but a lack of such openness and freedom. Thus, illness seen as a mere privation of health is denied any positive meaning it could have for human existence.

Daseinsanalytical pathology consequently becomes a purely descriptive examination of deficient modes of being-in-the-world. What is at stake therein is nothing but a description of how the individual existence is restricted in its relations to the world. A pathological deficiency of being-in-the-world can then be judged on the basis of a certain scale, since it expresses the degree of lagging behind the maximal possible openness. With regard to the fact that all disorders are measured against healthy and intact existence, *daseinsanalytical* investigation acquires an outspokenly normative character.

Hence, despite coming up with an ambitious project of a new foundation of medicine and psychology, Boss never leaves the ground of modern medicine which, as Foucault claims in *Naissance de la clinique*, is marked not only by the emphasis on the individual dimension of illness, but also by a certain tendency toward normativity. Modern medicine that supplants classificatory medicine of natural species brings about a certain shift in the understanding of health and illness: illness is no longer the mere opposite to health, but is understood as a pathological disturbance of the normal state. Health is not a mere contrary to illness, as it becomes the norm against whose backdrop the nature of pathological processes is determined. Medical knowledge must therefore in the first place encompass the knowledge of healthy human being who states the norm from which the ill person more or less diverges.[50]

Even though it differs from the rest of modern medicine in that it relies neither on biological knowledge concerning the functioning of the human organism, nor on social norms of the healthy life, *daseinsanalytical* pathology still avails itself of a

---

[49] Holzhey-Kunz, Alice. 1988. Die Zweideutigkeit seelischen Leidens. *Daseinsanalyse* 5: 81–3.

[50] Foucault, Michel. *Naissance de la clinique*. English edition: Foucault, Michel. 1973. *The Birth of the Clinic* (transl. Sheridan. A.M.). London: Tavistock Publications Limited., 34.

normative approach. The phenomenological criterion for distinguishing between the normal and the pathological consists in the integrity of open existence, which is seen by Boss in the most open and independent performance of all possibilities of being-in-the-world.

In reply to this, one could with a certain mischievousness raise the objection: as long as it is the degree of openness to appearing givens that really determines whether one exists in a healthy way, i.e. the way adequate to the nature of being-there, it means that the bisexual is healthier and more adequate to being-there than the heterosexual, simply because he/she opens himself/herself to meanings and possibilities of love life that are inaccessible to the heterosexual. In order to avoid this absurd conclusion, Boss can only complement the "ontological" criterion of health with that of normality, oriented toward social adaptability.

Together with Holzhey-Kunz, one can also ask whether the ideal of an independent, self-subsistent and maximally open existence, with which the therapeutic *Daseinsanalysis* stands or falls, does not correspond to the modern ideal of an autonomous, balanced and flexible individual that is fully *"fit for life."*[51] Should that really be the case, it merely corroborates that *Grundriss der Medizin und der Psychologie* does not transcend the frame of modern medical thought, but only elaborates on its epistemological possibilities.

What is more, the phenomenological description of being-ill does not even take full advantage of the possibilities offered by the modern episteme, which becomes especially conspicuous in its comparison with Freudian psychoanalysis. Whereas Boss contends himself with creating "psychiatry and psychotherapy adequate to being-there," and thus adopts the normative attitude of modern medicine, Freud turns the normative view inside out by regarding pathological phenomena as a springboard for understanding normal life. Instead of the normative distinction between health and illness, it is the other side of modern medicine, i.e. the problem of the finitude of human existence, which gets into the forefront here. As long as human being is understood on the basis of its finitude, illness ceases to be a mere faint shadow of health, and appears in its positive fullness. Once brought into the relation with death, which is the limit as well as the fundamental principle of human existence, illness manifests itself as an original phenomenon, and not as a negative state of a pathologically disturbed nature.

Nevertheless, Boss does not pay any special regard to the finitude of human existence vis-à-vis pathological phenomena. Even though his conception of pathology departs from the ontological project of the temporary being-there, his reflection on mental disorders never gets beyond the general assertion of the "fragility" of human existence. Consequently, the question of why the human individual can go insane, i.e. the question of the conditions enabling its overall breakdown, remains utterly unclear in the framework of *daseinsanalytical* concept. The aim of the therapeutic *Daseinsanalysis* is not to uncover the conditions of psychopathological phenomena; its only goal is the description of disturbed and non-disturbed modes of being-in-the-world.

---

[51] Holzhey-Kunz, Alice. 1992. Psychoterapie und Philosophie. *Daseinsanalyse* 9, 161.

The finitude of being-there asserts itself within the framework of this description only in the sense that death remains the extreme possibility of a *bodily* being-in-the-world.[52] As the extreme possibility of sojourning in disclosedness, death is the ultimate limit of that mode of being to which belongs the existing body. It is, however, not to be taken for granted that death should be the end of everything. "[Death] could also mean having one's previous existential manner of bodily existence transformed into an utterly different sort of being, one that is inaccessible to a mortal's perception while he is still alive. It is even possible that in death existence enters into something that is *prior* to all being; the dead may attain a relationship to Being-ness as such that is hidden from the living."[53] Boss infers from this that the possibility of death needs not be unveiled only in the disposition of anxiety, as is the case of *Sein und Zeit*, but can also be accepted with cheerful calmness (*die heitere Gelassenheit*). Those who relate to the possibility of their death with cheerful calmness allegedly prove the essential openness of their existence under such circumstances which make others drown in the empty nothingness of anxiety or seek an escape in their concern with beings and their socialized coexistence with others. Both anxious contraction and evasive escapism from the possibility of death attest to insufficient bearing of openness, in which human existence dwells. Even deep sorrow, in which some, usually exceptionally gifted, individuals are provided with a fundamental "insight into the finite limits of existence and its essential separation from the absolute and unconditional," is a mere corroboration of the fact that what they lack is a different, "more primordial recognition" of the finitude of human existence; that is to say, knowledge permeated by cheerful calmness.[54]

Insufficient openness in the relation to the possibility of death appears in states of "melancholic" sorrow, in which the irrecoverable breach of the finitude of individual existence is experienced to an insufferable degree.[55] "Melancholic" persons are exposed to the excruciating realization of the finitude of their existence, and yet their feelings of inferiority, nothingness and guiltiness spring only from the fact that they "weren't able to gather their existence into a reliable, genuine self and carry it to fulfillment."[56] Instead of giving way to their unique individual being, they have always denied and violated themselves for fear of losing the love and favor of their close ones. It is thus not the finitude of human existence that is the true reason for "melancholic" sorrow, but rather the extremely high degree of dependence that marks those affected by this feeling. Once, however, the "melancholic" has been given the courage to change his/her existential view, to stop defying himself/herself

---

[52] Boss. *Grundriss der Medizin und der Psychologie*, 309.

[53] Boss. *Grundriss der Medizin und der Psychologie*, 310–1. English edition: Boss. *Existential Foundations of Medicine and Psychology*, 120.

[54] Boss. *Grundriss der Medizin und der Psychologie*, 298–9. English edition: Boss. *Existential Foundations of Medicine and Psychology*, 114.

[55] Boss. *Grundriss der Medizin und der Psychologie*, 480. English edition: Boss. *Existential Foundations of Medicine and Psychology*, 221.

[56] Boss. *Grundriss der Medizin und der Psychologie*, 478. English edition: Boss. *Existential Foundations of Medicine and Psychology*, 220.

for fear of losing love, and to accept his/her very own nature that he/she can bring to realization in his/her relations with others, both the sorrow and the feelings of nothingness and guiltiness vanish into thin air.[57]

What is characteristic of Boss's explication of "melancholic" sorrow is the fact that the key to its understanding is the phenomenon of falling prey in which individual existence turns away from its very own individuality. The lack of independence, of constancy and of integrity that marks the "melancholic" existence is the privation of the original, integrated and independent individual being, which also encompasses the disposition of cheerful calmness that enables being-there to take a balanced and open attitude to all its possibilities, including the possibility of its own death.

However, such open and balanced relation to the extreme possibility of being-there is possible only under the condition that death is perceived as a transition to some other mode of being inaccessible to mortals, as an "introduction into the womb of all beings." It is thus possible to grasp anxiety or deep sorrow as deficient modes of the relation to death, which are opposed by the disposition of cheerful calmness. In such an interpretation, however, death becomes completely devoid of its urgency. The fact that in *Grundriss der Medizin und der Psychologie* death loses the meaning that the existential analysis in *Sein und Zeit* ascribes to it is conspicuous especially in instances where the question of its relation to individual being is raised. First of all, Boss notes that in face of death everyone remains absolutely alone, since dying rids individual existence of the support provided by others and things of concern. Therefore, being-toward-death enables individual existence to break out from its lostness and entanglement in the surrounding world. Yet, the existing individual is enabled to come to terms with loneliness brought by dying by virtue of the awareness that death pertains to merely the bodily being-in-the-world. What is certain for Boss is only that "existence after death is no longer in the world in the same [bodily] way as before."[58] In other words, death is no absolute end, but rather a change in the existing being-in-the-world. What is tacitly assumed is that one who has ceased to be-there still in some sense remains himself/herself, because otherwise there would be no sense talking of his/her transition to other mode of being.

This assumption, however, is in stark contrast to the analysis of being-toward-death as put forward in *Sein und Zeit*, where the relation to death is linked with the awareness of a possible end of individual being. Death as conceived of in the context of the existential analysis offers no possibility of a further continuation of individual being. As Heidegger claims, death "offers no support for becoming intent on something, for 'spelling out' the real thing that is possible."[59] Strictly speaking, death means the end of being in disclosedness, and as such it brings utter closedness. Death itself is something ungraspable and impenetrable; it is inaccessibility

---

[57] Boss. *Grundriss der Medizin und der Psychologie*, 481. English edition: Boss. *Existential Foundations of Medicine and Psychology*, 221.

[58] Boss. *Grundriss der Medizin und der Psychologie*, 310. English edition: Boss. *Existential Foundations of Medicine and Psychology*, 120.

[59] Heidegger. *Sein und Zeit*, 262. English edition: Heidegger. *Being and Time*, 242.

and closedness *par excellence*. As absolute closedness, death is what individual existence, grasped as being-toward-death, always somehow relates to.

It is on the basis of this understanding of being-toward-death that the difference between the authentic and the inauthentic existence is thematized in *Sein und Zeit*. Whereas the authentic existence advances toward the possibility of its non-being that is heralded in the uncanniness of anxiety, the inauthentic existence evades not-being-at-home and strangeness, into which anxiety casts it, preferring the familiar, inhabited world, in which things of concern and those who deal with them enable it to forget about the essential jeopardy of its being. The authentic existence that anticipates its extreme and unparalleled possibility thus fulfills the transitory character of being in disclosedness, whereas the inauthentic existence lags behind it.

Such lagging behind, however, connotes not the pathologically deficient mode of being-in-the-world, but merely the mediocre, tranquil existence that fulfills with ease the various tasks and duties of its everydayness. Insofar as there is something characteristic of our falling prey, it is especially the feeling of relief that is nowhere similar to the fatigue and burden that we suffer in every ill. Also, authenticity can hardly serve as a paradigm for the undisturbed, balanced existence if the authentic existence opens itself to the weight of its lot and of its essential jeopardy that springs from its own being in disclosedness.

As long as Boss uses openness and independence as the norms of health against which illness shows itself as a privative mode of being, one can further ask whether that pertains not only to psychic, but also to somatic disorders. If so, a broken leg or pneumonia would then necessarily condemn the ill to inauthentic existence, rendering him/her dependent on his/her surrounding and restricting his/her sphere of possibilities. If not, doubts arise concerning the psychosomatic view of health and illness that was supposed to be the main asset of therapeutic *Daseinsanalysis*.

Since neither of these possibilities offers a satisfactory solution, it becomes increasingly conspicuous that the conceptual differentiation between authenticity and inauthenticity cannot imply any norm for distinguishing health from illness. The exposition of the two fundamental modes of existence as given within the context of fundamental ontology provides no normative guideline that could be utilized within the field of medical and psychological examination.[60] As long as he does so and perceives all pathological phenomena in the light of the self-alienation/self-appropriation polarity, Boss willy-nilly draws the conclusion that falling prey, which forms an indispensable part of the overall ontological constitution of being-there in the context of fundamental ontology, can be, with the help of effective therapy, overcome and replaced once and for all by the coveted authenticity. This, however, clearly contradicts Heidegger's statement that "[t]he ontological-existential structure of falling prey would also be misunderstood if we wanted to attribute to it the meaning of a bad and deplorable ontic quality which could perhaps be removed in the advanced stages of human culture."[61]

---

[60] Holzhey-Kunz, Alice. 1992. Psychotherapie und Philosophie. *Daseinsanalyse* 9, 159.
[61] Heidegger. *Sein und Zeit*, 176. English edition: Heidegger. *Being and Time*, 165.

The question remains, however, how Heidegger could have possibly tolerated such a misleading interpretation of his ontological views, let alone actively promoted it. He himself must have seen most clearly that to tie authenticity and inauthenticity with the normative distinction between sanity and insanity means to extricate both fundamental modes of being in disclosedness from the dramatic context of *Sein und Zeit*. In the context of fundamental ontology, the search for one's integrity is bound with the decision to move beyond the mediocrity of everydayness, with the resolution not to cover up the not-being-at-home and uncanniness that form the foundations of being-in-the-world, and not with the ability to respond adequately and independently to the demands of the surrounding world. The point is the courage to accept the transitory character of individual existence, the heroism of the advance toward one's own ultimate, irredeemable possibility, and not the search for the strength to lead a normal, adapted life. Why, then, use the moments of authenticity and inauthenticity in order to describe normal and pathological phenomena?

One of the reasons for the decision to utilize authenticity and inauthenticity in the framework of medical and psychological discourse may be the mutual relation of both fundamental modes of being in disclosedness that are adumbrated in *Sein und Zeit*. As long as inauthenticity is understood as a privation of the ontologically more primordial mode of being that is the authentic existence, it is in the same position as illness in the relation to health. Both inauthenticity and illness are privative modes of being that can be thematized only in the light of the more primordial mode of being. Authenticity, on the other hand, cannot be ontologically grasped from out of inauthenticity, just as health cannot be derived from illness. If inauthenticity is a mere privative mode of the authentic existence, it is only one step away from being identified with the deficiency of openness, freedom and independence that mark being-ill. The problem with the idea of privation, however, is that it does not permit illness to be thematized in any way other than as a negative mode of being in openness. All the special modes of behavior and feeling encompassed in being-ill must be interpreted as a lack of openness, integrity and independence that mark the healthy existence. The concept of illness, based on the Platonic notion of the relative non-being, or rather on the Aristotelian notion of privation, thus adopts the traditional metaphysical method, in which negation appears as a lack or absence of something positive.

However, does not the above-mentioned mode of thematization contradict the fundamental rule of phenomenological examination, according to which phenomena are to be expounded out of themselves? "This rule," reads *Zollikoner Seminare*, "requires us to let each phenomenon show itself explicitly in its unique features."[62] Is it not necessary in that case to thematize pathological phenomena as they manifest themselves, instead of interpreting them on the basis of something they lack, namely being-healthy?

After all, being-ill does not necessarily mean only the loss of certain possibilities, but also the discovery of new ones that enable the ill to come to terms with his/her illness. Having learned to spatial orientation through touch and hearing, the

---

[62] Heidegger. *Zollikoner Seminare*, 82. English edition: Heidegger. *Zollikon Seminars*, 64.

blind man gains possibilities that the healthy individual enjoys only to a very limited degree. Nor are mental disorders to be regarded purely negatively. A mental disorder can also coerce human existence to search for new possibilities; it can enrich it and render it more open to what otherwise remains beyond its horizons. From this viewpoint all modes of behavior by which neurotic or psychotic patients react to incessantly imminent onslaughts of anxiety are to be perceived. The behavior of the "mentally ill" is not only a sign of insufficient openness, dependence and of falling prey to the surrounding world; it is rather a herald of the essential finitude of sojourning in disclosedness that does not mean a denial or lack of something originally positive. With regard to the fact that the uncanniness of anxiety is the basic expression of the finitude of being-there, it is possible to thematize all psychopathological phenomena on its basis without necessarily reducing them to privative forms of being-healthy.

As long as the psychopathological states are to appear as original phenomena, we must realize that death does not have to mean only the possibility of physical death, but that it can also take the shape of psychic destruction of being-there. Being in disclosedness can come to an end not only in physical, but also in psychic death. The possible end of being-there is reflected in e.g. extreme forms of schizophrenia, which leave not a vestige of the existential openness and individual being. Although the states in which being in disclosedness slips into utter closedness present the limit of being-there that is not attained in other types of mental disorders, they are not to be treated lightly. In relation to other psychopathological phenomena, they have the same position as death has in relation to primarily somatic illnesses. Extreme states of schizophrenia present the fulfilment of the ultimate possibility of being-there: the possibility of no-longer-being-there. Insofar as they should be thematized out of themselves, and not out of lacking health, psychopathological disorders are to be perceived against the backdrop of the overall disintegration of the open and self-subsistent sojourning in the clearing of being, against which the "mentally ill" defend themselves in all possible ways.

The fact that Heidegger did not see the possibility of explicating psychopathological phenomena out of themselves, that he did not manage to perceive them as immediate expressions of the existential finitude, probably has to do with the fact that he had no objections against the passage in *Grundriss der Medizin und der Psychologie*, where death is reduced to the physical being-in-the-world. Boss's normative hierarchization of the ways in which one can relate to the possibility of physical death is however only a rough reflection of a much more subtle problem.

Insofar as death is the departure [*Abschied*] from beings," as *Zollikoner Seminare* posits, what is inscribed in the relation to death is also the relation to being that itself is no-thing.[63] The finitude of being-there lies in the fact that in our relation to death we are exposed to what is different from all beings, that is, being.[64] Nevertheless, the relation to being, as we know already, defies the reach of the lived body. *Zollikoner Seminare* explicitly states that the lived body as such plays no role in the explicit

---

[63] Heidegger. *Zollikoner Seminare*, 230. English edition: Heidegger. *Zollikon Seminars*, 184.
[64] Heidegger. *Zollikoner Seminare*, 230. English edition: Heidegger. *Zollikon Seminars*, 184.

relation to being. As for the clearing of being, to which we relate with understanding, "we see it only in [reflective] thinking," not by means of sensuality that belongs to the lived body.[65] But does not the thought of being thereby turn back to the difference between the body and the soul? Is not the contrast between sensual perception and pure contemplation merely transposed onto the level of standing amidst the clearing of being? It really remains questionable how far Heidegger surpasses the Cartesian dualism when he claims that the understanding of being is not a matter of the lived body, but only of pure thought. Under these circumstances, a passion for the wisdom of Eastern religions is enough to make an orthodox Heideggerian entertain the notion an after-death transition to pure being, as indeed Boss did.

It must be noted that the contradiction between pure thought and sensuality marks not only the approach to the finitude of being-there, but also the way Heidegger understands the difference between human existence and the animal mode of being. This difference is elaborated especially in his *Die Grundbegriffe der Metaphysik*, which features, besides the ontology of being-there, also the ontology of living nature. In comparison with human existence the animal appears as unfree since it is instinctively bound to what concerns it, whereas human existence always surpasses all that immediately surrounds it, relating to the openness of the world as such. The animal might be open to its environment, but is never freely related to the world as such; its relatedness to the surrounding beings has merely got the character of disinhibition (*die Enthemmung*) that allows it to react to certain stimuli. Conversely, human existence uncovers beings *as beings*, i.e. dwells in the discoveredness of beings, for it relates to the very being of beings. It is therefore impossible to comprehend human existence from the animal mode of being, but only from itself. Human being must not be understood as *animal rationale*, i.e. as an animal that is, unlike others, endowed with reason, because all its phenomenal structures are to be explicated from its own mode of being. Nevertheless, a thematic consideration of animality from the standpoint of being-there is admissible for Heidegger. The ontology of life can be gained from the ontology of being-there under the condition that one embarks on the method of the *privative* interpretation. Here, once again, the Aristotelian idea of privation emerges in that the animal mode of being is ontologically determined as the privation of being-there. Being-there is in its essence world-forming (*weltbildend*) because it is related to being of beings, whereas the animal is poor in the world (*weltarm*), since it has an access to beings only in the frame of its instinctive predetermination.[66]

The idea of privation also suggests that the phenomenological thematization of the difference between human being and animal can be of relevance in the realm of pathological disorders, too. On the basis of the privative logic, one can say that the ill approximate, in some respect, the animal state, since illness restricts the freedom and independence of his/her existence. Illness reduces one's own freedom by tying

---

[65] Heidegger. *Zollikoner Seminare*, 244–5, 254. English edition: Heidegger. *Zollikon Seminars*, 196–7, 204.

[66] Heidegger, Die Grundbegriffe der Metaphysik, 263, 284. English edition: Heidegger. *Fundamental Concepts of Metaphysics. World, Finitude, Solitude*, 176–8, 192–3.

individual existence to the present situation. In extreme cases, the dependence on the surrounding and falling prey to givens that show themselves to the senses can reach such a degree as to render the ill capable of merely some animal vegetation. Even though one cannot fully sink to animality, the ill can display the openness of his being-in-the-world in such a deficient way as to become similar to the animal. The actual privation of the open being-in-the-world means not that the openness of being-there has completely perished, but only that it is not fulfilled in an adequate way. It follows from Boss's medical conception that only those who display to the maximum degree their being-free and openness to appearing beings exist in a way adequate to being-there; conversely, every lagging behind the essential freedom and openness of being-there is to be regarded as a privation. However, neither pathological phenomena nor animal confinement to the surrounding beings can be fully elucidated in a merely privative way, which was already demonstrated by Jiří Němec and Petr Rezek, who stated that this mode of thematization did not make possible the phenomenologically strict view of illness and animality.[67]

A similar objection against the idea of privation is raised also by Holzhey-Kunz. According to her, the privation-based distinctions between an adequate and an inadequate, an undisturbed and a disturbed mode of existence preclude the question whether illness may be something more than a merely deficient mode of independent and self-subsistent being-in-the-world.

In the realm of psychopathological phenomena, the approach that seeks in a mental disorder nothing more than a lack of the presupposed health is all the more doubtful in that it applies a normative standpoint that is typical of modern psychiatry. Despite strictly opposing the natural scientific orientation of modern medicine, Heidegger and Boss never demur at the normative discourse of psychiatry in which all behavior is divided into ill and healthy, disturbed and undisturbed, immature and mature, and accept it without any second thought.

However, Holzhey-Kunz raises the objection against such an approach to human behavior, claiming that behavior which is usually regarded as deranged is not ill in itself. It can be regarded as such only when perceived in the light of health; only when the presupposed and required health is brought into play can illness enter the stage, where it represents the privation of health. Yet, taken as it immediately manifests itself to us, deranged behavior can only be said to be unreasonable and nonsensical. Behavior that appears as deranged does not correspond to the given circumstances, does not fit in the significative context of a given situation, and thus remains primarily incomprehensible for us. Unlike behavior adapted to circumstances, deranged behavior is perceived as disturbing, since it doubts the significative and motivational context of the world we share with others. Once someone reacts to a given situation in a non-adequate way without doing so out of his/her own volition, i.e. once someone regards one's own deranged behavior as adequate or is unmanageably compelled to it, a pathological disorder is said to have broken out.

---

[67] Němec, Jan, Rezek, Petr. Fenomenologický přístup k lidské animalitě. In Němec, Jan, Patočka, Jan, and, Rezek, Petr. 1976. *Vybrané filosofické problémy psychopatologie a normality*. Prague: Archiv Jana Patočky.

The psychiatric view of the pathological disorder lies in the primary nonsensicality of a deranged behavior being regarded as an inability to act in an adequate and free way, which turns it into an expression of a deficient performance of human existence. Un-reason and non-sense are thus interpreted as privations of the balanced and adapted mode of existence. If that is the case, the disquieting otherness of deranged behavior is not regarded out of itself, but adjudicated on the basis of health, which makes it possible to state the seriousness and scope of any given pathological disorder. As long as they approach neurotic and psychotic disorders in the same way as modern psychiatry, Heidegger and Boss can thematize them merely as more or less serious privations of health, but never understand what appears as un-reason and non-sense out of itself. Instead of searching for the sense hidden in what appears at first sight as nonsensical behavior, they can merely describe how far a specific individual lags behind the possibilities offered by the whole, independent and free performance of human existence.

On the contrary, Holzhey-Kunz distances herself from the normative discourse of modern psychiatry, replacing it with the effort to unveil the original sense of pathological behavior. She does not content herself with the primary unreasonableness of deranged behavior, from which she would conclude that the patient's existence is of a deficient character. According to her, the goal of psychopathological examination is to unveil the hidden significative relations, out of which the pathological experience itself is comprehensible. To make psychopathological phenomena graspable in their original fullness, it is necessary to penetrate to the significative context that endows the initially incomprehensible and nonsensical expressions with their meaning.

Rather than a privative mode of being-healthy, the pathological experience is one of suffering (*das Leiden*) whose positive significative content can be deciphered by means of a suitable interpretation. By stating this, Holzhey-Kunz avows her indebtedness to Freud's legacy, even though she otherwise prefers phenomenological method to psychoanalytical jargon, burdened with natural scientific notions and constructs. For her, the revelation of the hidden meaning of pathological symptoms is not the cognizance of metapsychological structures, but rather a hermeneutic performance led by the ontological structure of being-there. Hermeneutic psychopathology as conceived by Holzhey-Kunz in her *Leiden am Dasein* relies primarily on the fact that being-there is a being that cares about its own being. Since everyone of us relates with understanding to his/her own being, every psychopathological disorder basically consists in suffering from one's own being.[68] Unless being-there cares about its own being, it could never be exposed to mental suffering. The realization that the existential openness to one's own being enables and conditions mental suffering thus opens the path to a non-normative view of the psychopathological phenomena, reduced in Heidegger and Boss to privative modes of being-healthy.[69]

---

[68] Holzhey-Kunz, Alice. 1994. *Leiden am Dasein: die Daseinsanalyse und die Aufgabe einer Hermeneutik psychopathologischer Phänomene*. Wien: Passagen-Verlag, 15.

[69] Holzhey-Kunz. *Leiden am Dasein*, 149–50.

With regard to the fact that the understanding relation to one's own being is thematized especially in *Sein und Zeit*, Holzhey-Kunz reverts to fundamental ontology in order to cleanse it from the normative exposition of the phenomena of authenticity and inauthenticity, and to develop her own hermeneutics of psychopathological disorders on its basis. Hermeneutic psychopathology that is to rely on fundamental ontology must, in the first place, take into account the fundamental disposition of anxiety, in which individual existence is brought back to itself in its original not-being-at-home and insecurity. In anxiety, individual existence understands the uncanniness and loneliness of its being-in-the-world. As long as it evades anxiety in its everydayness, it is because individual existence has always got some inkling about uncanniness that is the fundamental condition of its being. Mental suffering that is immediately manifested in the form of nonsensical behavior also presents a certain mode of coming to terms with existential insecurity that appears in the uncanniness of anxiety.

A primarily nonsensical mode of behavior, claims Holzhey-Kunz, receives a certain sense once we realize that mental suffering is marked by sensitivity to what anxiety gives one to understand. Those who suffer from a certain mental disorder are open to their anxiety-ridden being, evincing it with words and gestures that don't correspond with the generally shared significative context, but rather reply to the urging of uncanniness. Thus, mental disorder is no expression of the inauthentic mode of being in which we remain within the frame of the familiar surrounding world; its essence consists rather in the extraordinary, albeit non-thematic, sensitivity for the not-being-at-home and unanchoredness of sojourning in disclosedness. Mental suffering cannot be understood from the tranquilized, superficial being-together-with beings, since it is accompanied by perceptivity (*die Hellhörigkeit*) for the fundamental truth of being in openness which usually remains concealed in the course of normal everyday existence.[70] The concealment of empty openness into which the existing individual is thrown ensures the smooth course of everyday existence, as well as easy interaction with others within the frame of what is called "common sense." If there is, however, someone who loses this common sense, who moves away from the others, taken away by the ontological experience of the sheer "that" of his/her being in disclosedness, it cannot be simply concluded that his/her existence is deficient. Thanks to their heightened susceptibility to the openness of being, individuals suffering from mental disorders touch the very experience that becomes explicitly thematized in philosophy, poetry and art in general.

Even Boss does admit that his schizophrenic patients display an outstanding openness to what is otherwise accessible only to poets and philosophers, but he adds in one breath that this heightened impressionability primarily attests to the deficient character of their existence that has not grown up to its own openness.[71] Schizophrenics don't owe their heightened impressionability to gradual maturing and opening to what is different from all beings and what shines through them; their openness to what lies hidden behind the stable and narrowly determined world of

---

[70] Holzhey-Kunz. *Leiden am Dasein*, 159–60, 186.
[71] Boss. *Grundriss der Medizin und der Psychologie*, 503.

everydayness is a consequence of psychotic loosening (*die Entschränkung*) that rids them not only of their firm ground, but also of all their self-subsistence and independence. As they are incapable of coming to terms with the boundless responsiveness to what lies beyond the sphere of everydayness, their broadened openness to being is accompanied by a severe disturbance of the performance of individual being.

Therefore, Boss claims that schizophrenics are unable to stay in the cleared dimension of being adequately to the nature of being-there. The fact that the psychotic loosening brings not a higher, but a lower degree of freedom and openness of the existence is, in his opinion, corroborated by both the helpless exposure to hallucinations the schizophrenic falls prey to, and the desperate clinging to those ontic givens that promise at least provisionary refuge from the dreadful revelation of the hidden side of everyday being-in-the-world. The loosening of the existential openness is thus nothing but a privative mode of an independent, free and balanced staying in openness. In *Grundriss der Medizin und der Psychologie*, even perceptivity for the fundamental truth of being is thus taken as a ground for a normative differentiation of a self-subsistent, open mode of existence and its privative forms.

Although she never in the least doubts the Sisyphean effort psychotic or neurotic patients must exert in order to obscure the unbearable ontological experience of being by the use of ontic means, Holzhey-Kunz still refuses to see in their heightened impressionability a mere proof of a privative mode of existence. Since perceptivity for what is not commonly evident and still lies at the bottom of all everydayness reveals to the mentally ill something that healthy individuals generally ignore, mental suffering, in *Leiden am Dasein*, is not understood from being-healthy, but out of itself. The reason that leads to the realization of the necessity to thematize every psychopathological disorder from what becomes manifest therein lies in the fact that heightened impressionability renders one more perceptive to not only the open dimension of being, but also one's own nothingness consisting in thrownness into the openness of being. As long as it is to be understood in the spirit of *Sein und Zeit*, this nothingness cannot mean any sort of deficiency or privation of something positive. The existential nothingness has no conceptual counterpart. Sojourning in disclosedness is fundamentally imbued with nothingness and negativeness one encounters in such phenomena as guilt and conscience. Existential negativeness and nothingness can therefore never be therapeutically done away with. The irremediable insubstantiality of one's own existence cannot be measured by any criterion of some fuller and more successful existence, which is why it can be used as a point of departure of a non-normative approach to psychopathological phenomena. It is this irremediable insubstantiality that is the source of all mental suffering the psychotic and neurotic individuals try to cope with by means of various cover-ups.

The primary presupposition of the non-normative view of mental suffering is the realization that existential nothingness has to do with the finitude of individual existence. Being-there is final not only because "one day it shall die and then be no more", but also because it is thrown being in disclosedness. That is to say, it can never revert to the state preceding the facticity of its existence, it cannot but accept and bear it. Hence, the finitude of being-there as explicated in *Leiden am Dasein* not only encompasses the possibility of physical death, but rather imbues the whole existence that can be disrupted at any time from the familiar world and brought to face the sheer "fact" of being in disclosedness.

This happens especially in anxiety, where one falls from the being-at-home into the not-being-at-home and the uncanniness of being-in-the-world. Since being in disclosedness is finite, is individual existence is incessantly jeopardized by anxiety that can without any clear stimulus shatter its familiarity with the world and socialized coexistence with others. In this sense, being-there is exposed to jeopardy that comes not from somewhere outside, but from within its very own disclosedness. It is imbued down to its very bottom with anxiety that can surface at any moment.

The vague and yet harrowing apprehension of this danger can then explain a host of pathological phenomena, including, for instance, sadism and masochism.[72] Whereas the sadists, claims Holzhey-Kunz, seek to cover up their nothingness and limitedness by subjugating the other and rendering him/her a helpless tool of their own will, the masochists want to rid themselves of their guilt and loneliness by surrendering their own will and becoming a mere objects for the other. Nevertheless, neither of these ontic ways of tackling the ontological finitude can lead to a complete fulfillment of its goal, since neither can get individual existence rid of the painful comprehension of the fact "that it is and has to be" a lonely sojourning in disclosedness. Therein lies the basic tragedy of all pathological attempts at coming to terms with the ontological experience of one's own finitude.

In any case, the realization that the finitude of human existence is connected with its thrownness into empty disclosedness opens the theoretical possibility of thematizing mental suffering not on the basis of inauthentic or authentic temporality, but on the ground of that third mode of temporality that temporalizes itself from the dimension of the having-been. Even though Holzhey-Kunz does not explicitly elaborate on this possibility, one can assume that the temporal sense of mental suffering lies not in the temporality whose determining dimension is the present or in one whose determining dimension is the future, but in that mode of temporalization oriented primarily to the having-been.

As a temporal dimension that ontologically conditions the thrownness into disclosedness, the having-been is the dimension out of which anxiety comes. By means of anxiety, individual existence is thrown into uncanniness that reveals to it the most original character of disclosedness, in which it already dwells in one way or other. This dwelling has, initially and for the most part, the character of familiarity with the surrounding world, but its most original character appears in the uncanniness of anxiety. And in this uncanniness lies the root of the suffering to which the mentally ill individual is exposed. The suffering from one's own being is given by the heightened impressionability for the urge of the uncanniness of anxiety and by the perceptivity to what this uncanniness, despite all the familiarity with the world and innerworldly beings, gives one to understand.

However much the suffering from one's own being issues from existential thrownness into empty disclosedness, it wouldn't be possible without the understanding of one's own being and without the relation to things of concern in which

---

[72] Holzhey-Kunz. *Leiden am Dasein*, 104–5.

it becomes incarnated and concretized. It is thus clear that suffering can sever the temporal dimension of having-been that ontologically determines the existential thrownness from neither the temporal dimension of the future that ontologically carries and establishes the understanding nor the temporal dimension of the present in which the concern with beings is ontologically constituted. Even in the suffering from one's own being, temporality temporalizes itself as a whole in that having-been determines the sense of the other two temporal ecstasies. Even in the most excruciating suffering from one's own being, the subsistence of individual being is thus preserved, since the ecstatic unity of temporality essentially guarantees the integral unity of individual being.

From here, however, follows the fundamental doubt about the solidity of the conception put forward in *Leiden am Dasein*. As long as she intends to make mental suffering accessible on the basis of the temporal unity of individual existence, it remains a mystery how Holzhey-Kunz wants to thematize not only neuroses, but also the severe personality disorders and psychotic states in which individual being disintegrates. Insofar as schizophrenic depersonalization, for instance, is to be explicated on the basis of the ontological structure of *Jemeinigkeit* that characterizes being-there, can it be shown in any other way than as a privative mode of individual being whose ground is the ecstatic unity of temporality? Although this view of the schizophrenic break-down of the personality contradicts the fundamental requirement according to which every psychopathological phenomenon must be explicated out of itself, *Leiden am Dasein* never takes into consideration the possibility of a radical disintegration of individual being, since that would demand taking into account the possibility of the temporal disintegration of being-there. On the contrary, the individual structure of being-there is considered utterly unchallengeable, since the very concept of mental suffering stands or falls with the ontological statement that being-there is *in each case mine*.

Under these circumstances, one cannot but accept the fact that the psychotic depersonalization can appear only as a privation of the primordial individual being, and not as an original, non-derived phenomenon in which the disintegration of the individual being combines with the effort to reintegrate it. Once we take into account that in *Sein und Zeit* the original constancy of individual being is characterized by means of the self-subsistence of authentic existence and the correspondent future-oriented temporality, we must draw the necessary conclusion that although mental suffering is indeed different from the inauthentic existence in that it is carried not by present-oriented temporality but by a temporality oriented toward having-been, in its extreme forms it nevertheless presents an even higher degree of privation of the autonomous and integrated individual being that marks authentic existence than is the case with the non-autonomous self-oblivious individual being, typical of inauthentic existence. Therefore, the privative conception of the phenomenon of mental disorder appears an unavoidable fate of a conception in which the existential finitude is comprehended with no regard to the eventuality of the temporal and personal disintegration of being-there.

Since in her approach to mental suffering Holzhey-Kunz departs not from the temporally conditioned disintegration of individual being, but from the basic structure of *Jemeinigkeit* that implies the understanding of one's own being, the question arises whether the concept of finitude employed by hermeneutic psychopathology is sufficient for yielding an adequate perspective on un-reason and non-sense as such. As long as behavior that immediately appears unreasonable and nonsensical gains its meaning on the basis of the understanding of one's own being, does not this mean that un-reason is thematized on the basis of primary understanding?

It seems that hermeneutic psychopathology which finds the meaning of mental suffering in the fact that individual existence suffers from its own being is unsatisfactory as compared with Foucault's concept of non-sense that offers no final reconciliation of reason and un-reason. In *Maladie mentale et psychologie* or *L'Histoire de la folie*, un-reason appears as a sign of the finitude of our reason, and not as its derivate. Non-sense stands there outside reason as that which is other and strange. Un-reason that forms the very own dimension and ultimate truth of mental disorders can be grasped by means of medical and psychological notions, but only at the cost of becoming alienated from itself and discretely silenced. Therefore, Foucault understands psychiatric discourse as reason's monologue about un-reason. Even though reason may try to enter into a dialogue with un-reason, this still does not mean that it recognizes therein its own denial and terminus. However, such is the precondition for un-reason to appear in its empty fullness and barren positivity.

Nevertheless, it is not only the case that the disputability of the attempt to explicate un-reason on the basis of the understanding of being disqualifies Holzhey-Kunz's concept, but also a critical approach to the hermeneutic psychopathology sheds light on the whole range of possibilities of utilizing the ontological project of being-there in the realm of psychopathological examination. Since the hermeneutic approach to psychopathological experience draws its understanding of mental suffering from fundamental ontology, we have all reasons to assume that neither *Sein und Zeit* nor *Zollikoner Seminare* can offer an ontological basis on which un-reason and non-sense could appear as original phenomena.

References

1. Aristotle. 1984. *Metaphysics*, ed. Jonathan Barnes. Oxford: Princeton University Press.
2. Boss, Medard. 1975. *Grundriss der Medizin und der Psychologie*. Bern/Stuttgart/Wien: Verlag Hans Huber.
3. Foucault, Michel. 1963. *Naissance de la Clinique*. Paris: PUF. English edition: Foucault, Michel. 1973. *The Birth of the Clinic*. Trans. A.M. Sheridan. London: Tavistock Publications Limited.
4. Foucault, Michel. 1966. *Maladie mentale et psychologie*. Paris: PUF.
5. Heidegger, Martin. 1983. *Die Grundbegriffe der Metaphysik: Welt, Endlichkeit, Einsamkeit*. Frankfurt am Main: Vittorio Klostermann. English edition: Heidegger, Martin. 1995. *The Fundamental Concepts of Metaphysics. World, Finitude, Solitude*. Trans. William McNeill and Nicholas Walker). Bloomington: Indiana University Press.
6. Heidegger, Martin. 1987. *Zollikoner Seminare. Protokolle, Gespräche, Briefe*. ed. Medard Boss. Frankfurt am Main: Vittorio Klostermann. English edition: Heidegger, Martin. 2001.

Zollikon Seminars. Trans. Franz Mayr and Richard Askay. Evanston: Northwestern University Press.

7. Heidegger, Martin. 1993. *Sein und Zeit*, 17th ed. Tübingen: Niemeyer. English edition: Heidegger, Martin. 1996. *Being and Time*. Trans. Joan Stambaugh. Albany: SUNY Press.
8. Holzhey-Kunz, Alice. 1988. Die zweideutigkeit seelischen Leidens. *Daseinsanalyse* 5: 81–95.
9. Holzhey-Kunz, Alice. 1992. Psychotherapie und Philosophie. *Daseinsanalyse* 9: 153–162.
10. Holzhey-Kunz, Alice. 1994. *Leiden am Dasein: die Daseinsanalyse und die Aufgabe einer Hermeneutik psychopathologischer Phänomene*. Wien: Passagen-Verlag.
11. Němec, Jan, Jan Patočka, and Petr Rezek. 1976. *Vybrané filosofické problémy psychopatologie a normality*. Prague: Archiv Jana Patočky.
12. Vetter, Helmuth. 1993. Es gibt keine unmittelbare Gesundheit des Geistes. *Daseinsanalyse* 10: 65–79.

Chapter 5
Mental Disorder and the Finitude of Being-There

In order to overcome the limits given by the understanding of the finitude, which determines the ontological structure of the individual existence presented in *Sein und Zeit* or *Zollikoner Seminare*, without leaving the context of Heidegger's thought, it is possible to turn to his *Die Grundbegriffe der Metaphysik* and above all *Beiträge zur Philosophie*, where we can find a radicalized exposition of existential finitude. In this respect, Heidegger introduces the concept of being-away (*Weg-sein*) that functions as an internal opposite to being-there (*Da-sein*). Being-away which is closely related to the finitude of being-there includes not only the possibility of physical death, but also the possibility of mental burn-out. Being-away that is accompanied by a complete destruction of the self can thus shed some light on extreme states which mentally ill people try to evade at all costs. From the perspective of being-away, we can understand not only the dark regions of psychoses, but all the lifesaving maneuvers with the help of which the mentally ill react to the fundamental peril of the total self-disintegration.

However, is it at all possible to perceive mental disorders as non-privative phenomena? Is not what first appears as un-reason and non-sense essentially always a certain privation of the understanding which characterizes being in disclosedness? If un-reason is to be seen as an expression of the finitude of being in disclosedness, and not as its privative modus, it is first of all necessary to understand that the destructive invasion of non-sense can bring being-there to its end just as its physical death, with which all sense and openness are brought to their end. This invasion must be grasped as the ultimate possibility of sojourning in disclosedness whose fulfillment means that being-there has turned into no-longer-being-there. Only thus can we see the finitude of being-there as a condition that enables mental disorders, in which modern psychiatry sees a privation of sane reason instead of encountering, in it and through it, the abysmal dimension of non-sense and un-reason.

As long as *Zollikoner Seminare* considers merely the privative approach to psychopathological phenomena, whereby un-reason is prevented from appearing out of itself, and if even *Sein und Zeit* offers no possibility to encounter non-sense

P. Kouba, *The Phenomenon of Mental Disorder*, Contributions to Phenomenology 75, DOI 10.1007/978-3-319-10323-5_5

as such, all we can do is to seek support elsewhere. In order to prove that the non-privative view of un-reason is not just a pious wish, we do not have to refer to only Foucault or Deleuze, but we can also focus on other Heidegger's texts, beginning with *Die Grundbegriffe der Metaphysik*. These lectures, which were given at the University of Marburg less than 3 years after the first publication of *Sein und Zeit*, deserve our attention especially because here the notion of being-away (*das Weg-sein*) appears for the first time, functioning as a conceptual complement and counterpart of being-there (*das Da-sein*).[1] The ontological project of being-there adumbrated here is not only restricted to the phenomenon of being-there, but also allows for the possibility of being-away. The very difference between being-there and being-away, claims Heidegger, has nothing in common with the presence or absence of some thing. Being-away does not mean that some being present-at-hand has been removed, since what is at stake here is an essential possibility of the human existence. Being-away is thus to be strictly distinguished from being-not-at-hand, just as being-there is not to be confused with the determination of a place in which some thing occurs.

Nor does the difference between being-there and being-away correspond to the opposition between consciousness and unconsciousness. The reason for this is that being-away is not necessarily connected with unconsciousness; in many instances, it can be brimming with clear consciousness. For example, in a situation where we do not pay attention to what is going on, lost in thought instead, we are "away," and yet still not totally unconscious. Even though we find ourselves outside of the context that springs from the immediately given circumstances, we can occupy ourselves with something much more important, which keeps us in full consciousness.

Even the extreme form of being-away, presented, according to Heidegger, by insanity, does not rule out consciousness. "Think of the extreme case of madness, where the highest degree of consciousness can prevail and yet we say: The person is de-ranged, displaced, away, and yet there."[2] The madman appears de-ranged, since he is displaced from the significative connections that are obvious to everyone else. A being present-at-hand, such as the stone, cannot be "absent" in the same way a de-ranged individual can be, because it is either at-hand, or not-at-hand. Not even the animal, despite perceptively relating to its environment, can truly be "away." The reason is that the animal is instinctively bound to the givens of its momentary situation. Conversely, human being, who exists as being-there, almost incessantly advances ahead of the context of the given situation, and therefore is always "away" in a certain sense. Being-away is no random occurrence that sometimes happens to anyone; it is rather an essential characteristic of the human existence. Thus, only human being can go insane. The possibility of going insane – such is the rueful privilege of human existence.

---

[1] Heidegger. *Die Grundbegriffe der Metaphysik*, 94–9.

[2] Heidegger. *Die Grundbegriffe der Metaphysik*, 95. English edition: Heidegger. *The Foundational Concepts of Metaphysics*, 63.

Since the madman is displaced from the context which determines the meaning of a given situation, his behavior seems unfathomable and nonsensical. This displacement, which heralds the immediate coming of un-reason and non-sense, is no mere privation of an open being-there, but an extreme mode of being-away that essentially belongs to the human existence. Whereas the privative concept of mental disorder shows total disregard for the question of why human being can actually go insane, the ontological project of being-there undertaken in *Die Grundbegriffe der Metaphysik* gives the impression that the enabling condition of insanity is the potentiality-of-being-away (*das Wegseinkönnen*) bound with being-there. The possibility of being-away is what enables the peculiar detachment that occurs non-sense and un-reason.

However, even the specific not-being-there that is being-away cannot be regarded as a privative form of being-there. Human being can be away only on condition that its existential character is that of being-there, but this does not mean that being-away is a privative mode of being-there. Being-away is something more than a merely deficient form of being-there. The peculiar absence that lies in being-away is an original phenomenon, since the fact that we have to be-there in order to be-away is valid also the other way round.[3] Being-away cannot be judged by means of a normative criterion of being-there mainly because the one cannot be separated from the other: "In the end, this being-away pertains to the essence of [being-there]," claims Heidegger.[4] Being-away is no accidental quality, but a feature constitutive of being-there. As being-there, human being is at the same time also not-being-there, since it always already advances beyond the context of the situation in which it is immediately located. Never fully bound in its being-there to the immediately given situation, human being is also constantly exposed to the danger of displacement and de-rangement concealed inside its being-away. This view is important, not only for the understanding of the essence of insanity, but also for the right determination of the transitory character of being-there. For the possibility of de-rangement and displacement is essentially connected with transitoriness, i.e. with the transitivity and finitude of being-there.

Some of the possible consequences of the phenomenon of being-away have already been pointed out by Helmut Vetter in his article, "Es gibt keine unmittelbare Gesundheit des Geistes."[5] However, his analysis of being-away is by far not exhaustive. Leaving aside the problem of the existential finitude, Vetter's consideration of the phenomenon of insanity cannot provide us with an answer to the question of how being-away relates to the transitoriness of being in disclosedness.

---

[3] Heidegger. *Die Grundbegriffe der Metaphysik*, 98. English edition: Heidegger. *The Foundational Concepts of Metaphysics*, 65.

[4] Heidegger. *Die Grundbegriffe der Metaphysik*, 95. English edition: Heidegger. *The Foundational Concepts of Metaphysics*, 63.

[5] Vetter, Helmuth. 1993. Es gibt keine unmittelbare Gesundheit des Geistes. *Daseinsanalyse* 10: 65–79.

In *Die Grundbegriffe der Metaphysik* the transitoriness of being-there is seen in its ex-sistence, i.e. in that it goes beyond itself without ever leaving itself.[6] It is not from some interior that being-there advances, but from its own possibilities offered by the uncovered beings, toward the being of beings to which it always stands open. More precisely, being-there is in transit from the specific and limited sphere of beings to its own ontological openness for being as such. Since being-there dwells on the border between beings and being, its existence has the character of transition. As existing, being-there "is *enraptured* in this transition and therefore essentially 'absent.'"[7] This absence, however, must not be understood as mere not-being-at-hand of things present-at-hand. Being-there is absent in the sense that it lies not only in the present, but is also enraptured (*entrückt*) into the having-been and the future. Being-there can be-away because it is ecstatically enraptured into its present, into its having-been and into its future.

In this ecstatic rapture (*die Entrückung*) there always lies concealed the possibility of pathological de-rangement that is the extreme form of being-away. Pathological de-rangement is the basic possibility of the transitory existence and as such attests to the abysmal dimension of its finitude. Yet, as follows from the comparison between human being and the animal or the being present-at-hand, the finitude of being-there, and thus also the possibility of being-away, is not an expression of its imperfection, but, conversely, an inner corroboration of its very own ontological quality.

However, this view of the existential finitude is not in itself satisfactory either. To perceive the relation between being-there and being-away in the full light, it is necessary to abandon *Die Grundbegriffe der Metaphysik* and to turn to *Beiträge zur Philosophie*, where Heidegger substantially deepens his exposition of the phenomenon of being-away. Here the peculiar not-being-there tied with being-there is no longer examined against the backdrop of a certain specific situation we can either participate in or disregard. The difference between being-there and being-away is seen from the perspective of the appropriating event, the so called "enowning" (*das Er-eignis*) of being as such, to which and into which our ex-sistence belongs. Since in *Beiträge zur Philosophie* the openness of being is no longer thought from the structure of the human existence, as is still the case in *Die Grundbegriffe der Metaphysik*, but from itself, i.e. from how it gives itself to us and simultaneously holds itself back, it becomes possible to understand being-there as open involvement in the clearing of being. Being-there thus conceived must be distinguished from deliberate attention to what goes on around, since this "there" corresponds, not to some specific situation in which we find ourselves, but to the openness of being as such.

Being-away is thus no inattention of someone absent-minded at the moment, but non-involvement in the self-giving and self-withholding openness of being.

---

[6] Heidegger. *Die Grundbegriffe der Metaphysik*, 531. English edition: Heidegger. *The Foundational Concepts of Metaphysics*, 365–6.

[7] Heidegger. *Die Grundbegriffe der Metaphysik*, 531. English edition: Heidegger. *The Foundational Concepts of Metaphysics*, 365–6.

Being-away defines a certain mode of relating to the openness of being, that is, ignorant non-involvement in it. Human being is given the possibility to either perceptively sustain the openness of being, or turn away from and forget about it. These two possibilities maintain, albeit on another level, the parallel with deliberate involvement and ignorant non-involvement in a certain specific situation. Viewed from the perspective of the clearing of being, the difference between being-there and being-away appears as a difference between involved openness to the secret of being and non-involved closedness in which we, absorbed in beings, forget about being.

The fact that we are, initially and for the most part, absorbed by beings we deal with leads Heidegger to call being-away "the *more originary* title for [being-there's] *disownedness* [*Uneigentlichkeit*]," which is in *Sein und Zeit* taken as a counterpart of the authentic mode of existence.[8] Due to its clinging to things of concern and forgetting of the openness of being, the ordinary everyday existence is not being-there, but being-away without necessarily ceasing to belong to the clearing of being.

Being-away, however, is not exhausted only in the inauthentic entanglement in beings and matters we initially and for the most part deal with, but is also heralded wherever human being radically veers away from its everyday cares and other people, since what occurs is its displacement (*die Verrückung*) from the openness of being. Displacement, in which human being not only swerves from the context of the immediately given situation, but also moves away from its being-there, can be detected in the form of madness. Being-away, manifested in madness, is no doubt much more radical than common entanglement in beings that still preserves its inner relation to the possibility of being-there. This extreme shape of being-away is not-being-there to such an extent that its final stages are closer to death (i.e., no-longer-being-there) than to being-there.

With regard to the fact how deeply the human existence is imbued with the possibility of being-away, it is clear that being-there is no anthropological constant that would characterize man as such.[9] Being-there presents no quality given to the human existence; rather, it is its task and promise. For this reason alone, being-there cannot be something as simple and effortless as sound health. On the contrary, to involve oneself in sustaining the clearing of being is the most difficult role human existence can fulfill. It is because being-there is our most difficult task that it can be missed so easily, in two different ways: either in the common everyday existence in which the openness of being is forgotten the more we cling to beings, or in madness that appears as one of the possible forms of death. Both these possibilities are subsumed by Heidegger's term "being-away."

Although both these modes of being-away present certain distraction and deviation from the openness of being, the one must be distinguished from the other. Not-being-there, manifested in madness and other forms of death, is not to be mistaken for being-away, in which lies the essence of inauthentic existence. Death-ridden

---

[8] Heidegger, Martin. 1989. *Beiträge zur Philosophie (vom Ereignis)*. Frankfurt am Mein: Vittorio Klostermann, 324. English edition: Heidegger, Martin. 1999. *Contributions to Philosophy (From Enowning)* (trans: Emad, Parvis, and Maly, Kenneth). Bloomington: Indiana University Press, 227.
[9] Cf. Ibid, p. 300.

not-being-there is an extreme concealed in the openness of being, i.e. in the "there" in which dwells being-there. In *Beiträge zur Philosophie*, this extreme of openness is sketched as follows:

> What belongs to the t/here as its utmost is that shelteredness-concealedness in the open that is ownmost to the t/here, the *away*, being-*away* as constant *possibility*; man knows being-away in the various shapes of death. But wherever [being-there] is to be grasped primarily, *death* must be determined as the utmost possibility of the t/here. If *here* one speaks of "end" and if before all else and in all keenness [being-there] is differentiated from every manner of being-extant, then "end" here can never mean the mere ceasing and disappearing of an extant. If time *as* temporality is [rapture], then "end" here means a "no" and an "otherwise" of this [rapture], a total [displacement] of the t/here as such, into the "away".[10]

What follows from the passage above is that death is not to be understood in merely the physical sense of the word. As long as it implies utter displacement from the clearing of being, death may also have the form of madness. More accurately, death in its extreme otherness from being-there is what makes madness possible in the first place. It is only because death belongs to the open sphere of being that human existence can become displaced and de-ranged.

In order to understand the possibility of psychopathological disorder, we must therefore expound it from the perspective of absolute concealment, which is our very own extreme of the openness of being. This concealment, in which lies the constant possibility of no-longer-being-there, is no privation, no shadow of the clearing of being, but its radical otherness that belongs to it. Since *Beiträge zur Philosophie* approaches madness on the basis of concealment and closedness that are inherently bound with the openness of being, madness is not a mere privation of sane reason, but something much more ominous. Madness is what rises out of the abysmal openness of being as "something" that belongs to it, and yet is totally different.

Despite never specifying various forms of madness in the extreme possibility of displacement and understanding them only from the appropriating event of being that leaves in the openness of being space for radical concealment, Heidegger might be said to come much closer to the phenomenon of insanity than he had managed to in *Zollikoner Seminare* and in his cooperation with Boss. In this respect, it is doubtlessly significant that instead of normative psychopathology, *Beiträge zur Philosophie* considers the special role that Hölderlin, Kierkegaard and Nietzsche play in modern thought. It is probably no coincidence that all these thinker-poets, whose experience of the fate of modern thought was the deepest and most agonizing, "had to depart from the brightness of their days prematurely."[11] Out of the three it is especially Hölderlin who determines the direction of Heidegger's own meditations. Although he predated both Kierkegaard and Nietzsche, he remains for Heidegger the one who went furthest in his poetry. It is for this alone that one cannot

---

[10] Heidegger. *Beiträge zur Philosophie*, 324 (meditation 202). English edition: Heidegger. *Contributions to Philosophy*, 227–8.

[11] Heidegger. *Beiträge zur Philosophie*, 204. English edition: Heidegger. *Contributions to Philosophy*, 143.

overlook that Hölderlin's ruminating poetry is connected with the madness in whose darkness this poetic work perished.

Madness is not only an imminent possibility accompanying the act of poetic creation, but also a region governed by the all-pervading death. As long as human existence is finite, the madman's speech displays death in its nakedness. When human speech becomes the expression of death, when not-being-there that withholds all sense speaks through it, what comes into play is un-reason. The voice of un-reason thus unveils the essential bond between death and sense-less speech. This sense-less speech is not privation of a sensible utterance, as modern psychiatry would have us believe, but an immediate expression of concealment and closedness tied with the openness of being. The relation of reason and un-reason, into which we are situated by means of the confrontation with madness, is thus a relation between the openness of being and ultimate closedness. It is this relation that Hölderlin rendered conspicuous to a much higher degree than modern psychology or psychiatry has ever managed to.

What is also clear from Hölderlin's tragic end is that the danger of madness has nothing to do with inauthentic entanglement in beings and the corresponding being-away, but that it springs from the ecstatic rapture (*die Entrückung*) into openness as such. Insofar as temporality is the ecstatic rapture into "there," that is, into the openness of being, it must be incessantly jeopardized by the possibility of a radical displacement (*die Verrückung*) into "away." Such displacement and the ensuing being-away is the innermost possibility of the rapture into the openness of being.

In other words, the ex-sisting being-there, through its relation to the clearing of being, is exposed also to the impenetrable concealment that belongs to it. As long as human being is to be really being-there, it must accept and sustain also the all-withholding concealment as something that has always already appropriated it. Only the one who breaks free from common ideas about death and accepts the ultimate, final withholding of all sense that issues from concealment as such can fulfill his/her being-toward-death in a way that is adequate to the character of being-there. This *running ahead into death*, claims Heidegger, does not mean nihilism or resignation from the search for some sense, but coincides with the involved sustaining of the sense-giving openness of being.[12] Running ahead into death that characterizes being-there means entering into the changeable, essentially uncertain relation between the openness and impenetrable closedness.

What is necessary for the understanding of the shaky relation between the clearing of being and its inseparable absolute otherness is the realization that this relation is beyond the power of being-there, and that it happens by the grace of the appropriating event that leaves closedness to persist as both the extremity and the innermost possibility of the open realm of being. Thus, death is no longer merely our ultimate and very own possibility of individual existence, as is the case in *Sein und Zeit*, but presents the most extreme limit of openness as such.[13] In *Beiträge zur Philosophie* death is thought from the perspective of closedness itself, and not from out of

---

[12] Heidegger. *Beiträge zur Philosophie*, 285, 324–5.

[13] Heidegger. *Beiträge zur Philosophie*, 324.

individual existence that relates to it as to its ultimate possibility. Being-there is not what enables its relation to death, but, on the contrary, death is what appropriates being-there, and thus makes it into being-toward-death. Being-there, as Heidegger understands it now, is being-toward-death not because it relates with understanding to death as its possibility, but because it is already in advance released into absolute concealment. Only out of this concealment is it possible to see the deepest essence of nothingness to which being-there, as being-toward-death, is exposed.[14] This nothingness is connected, not only with ontological difference, i.e. with the difference between the discoveredness of beings and the empty disclosedness of being, but more importantly with the difference between the openness of being and closedness, which opposes it as concealment does unconcealment.

How crucial ramifications for the thematic grasp of the possibility of un-reason and non-sense issue from the misunderstanding of the abysmal nothingness into which being-there stands out can be best illustrated by Boss's case. Even though *Grundriss der Medizin und der Psychologie* does briefly mention concealment that yields to unconcealment, the "pre-temporal, pre-spatial and pre-human" concealment is never in the least related to psychopathological phenomena.[15] These are expounded merely against the background of the open clearing of being one sustains in a more or less deficient way. However, unless psychopathological phenomena have been related to concealment that belongs to the unconcealment of being without any sort of dependence, justice cannot be done to their phenomenal fullness. Nothing but this concealment makes it possible to grasp that which stands at the root of pathological displacement and what the "normal," everyday mode of being-away avoids as much as possible when sinking into things of concern.

If madness is to be seen in its unreduced fullness, displacement into concealment as such must be comprehended as a radical breach in the ecstatic rapture into the openness of being. This ecstatic rapture, Heidegger adds, is where individual being, which marks being-there, is established.[16] Individual being is not given as a particular "I" that is defined against some "you" or "us." Every division into "I," "you" and "us" is secondary in relation to individual being, which happens as ecstatic rapture into the clearing of being.[17] The blurring and crumbling of the boundaries among "I," "you" and "us," which happens as part of the mass, anonymous mode of existence can then be understood as an expression of the inauthentic being-away that is oblivious to the clearing of being. Once, however, the ecstatic rapture into the openness of being has turned into displacement, a deep disruption and disintegration of individual being must follow. Utter displacement from openness into closedness must therefore be accompanied by a total demise of individual being.

Insofar as the disintegration of individual being should not only be philosophically postulated, but also documented on specific clinical cases, we can point to casuistries that are presented in Binswanger's treatise on schizophrenia. Unlike

---

[14] Heidegger. *Beiträge zur Philosophie*, 325.

[15] Boss. *Grundriss der Medizin und der Psychologie*, 353 (translator's translation).

[16] Heidegger, *Beiträge zur Philosophie*, 303.

[17] Heidegger. *Beiträge zur Philosophie*, 320–1.

Boss's *Grundriss der Medizin und der Psychologie*, it is to a much lesser degree subjugated to a preordained philosophical platform and leaves much more room for detailed clinical observation which has some value in itself. When describing the final stages of schizophrenia, Binswanger talks of a total disintegration of individual being that springs from the overall renunciation of being-there. According to him, in the case of total schizophrenic "detachment", one cannot discern any "self" that would close itself off from the world, since here no individual being remains. The schizophrenic is uprooted from himself/herself and his/her being-there. "Where [being-there] no longer temporalizes and spatializes, where it has ceased to be a self and to communicate with others, it no longer has a [there] (*da*). For it has its [there] only … in [disclosedness] (*Erschlossenheit*), which is only a comprehensive term for temporalization, spatialization, being a self, etc."[18] Since in such a case no rapture into openness takes place, what occurs is not being-there, but no-longer-being-there.

Although Binswanger himself never uses the term being-away, it is possible to interpret his clinical observation of schizophrenic "detachment" as a total displacement from the openness of being, and thus endow it with a completely new philosophical grounding. Also the lighter forms of psychopathological disorders can be understood from concealment as such, despite the fact that being-there does not completely perish in them. The displacement into concealment and closedness of all sense is especially conspicuous in the case of depression, but its traces are to be found wherever this displacement is faced with a defense against the eminent danger of total loss of individual being. Unmistakable traces of self-defense that concerns not only the relation between "I" and "you," but individual being as such, can be found in Binswanger's description of neurotic and pre-psychotic states, whose structures and mechanisms cannot be fully explicated, as long as they are derived from the normal, balanced mode of behavior. In order for them not to be trivialized as privative modes of being-healthy, these defensive mechanisms must be regarded in the light of the deadly danger to which the mentally ill is exposed. To understand the un-reasonable and meaningless behavior as the expression of the deficit of sane reason would be mistaken especially because this behavior refers to concealment and closedness that the "normal" everyday existence does not want to take into account, which, on the other hand, ensures for it the feeling of safety, balance and security.

Only when we discard the self-assured haughtiness and understand the disintegration of individual being as our very own possibility that arises from our exposure and inclination to concealment can we approach those whose fate has become un-reason. That does not mean to surrender our own reason, but rather to open ourselves to the truth about ourselves that madness tells us. What is at stake is to understand that the exposure to concealment is our shared lot that puts us in the

---

[18] Binswanger, *Schizophrenie*, 311. English edition: Binswanger, Ludwig. 1958, The Case of Ellen West: An Anthropological-Clinical Study. In Mendel, Werner M. (trans), Lyons, Joseph (trans) May, Rollo (ed), Angel, Ernest (ed), Ellenberger, Henri F. (ed). *Existence: A new dimension in psychiatry and psychology*. New York, NY, US: Basic Books, 288.

precarious position between reason and un-reason, sense and non-sense. Since we are enraptured into openness to which belongs all sense-withholding concealment, we must never give in to the feeling that madness and un-reason apply only to the other. As long as this happens, as long as "scientific" distance from madness is kept, we prevent the encounter with un-reason which Foucault calls for in his early works. This encounter does not mean standing in resigned awe of the fact of un-reason; the essence of a true confrontation with un-reason is rather the ability to advance into the dimension that opens to us through the primary experience of non-sense. The reason's confrontation with un-reason does not thus deprive us of the duty to try to understand and help the other, but on the contrary brings us to the start of an endless journey. Since they keep incessantly undermining and doubting each other, it would be definitely naïve to think that reason and un-reason can ever be definitively reconciled. If we may believe what *Beiträge zur Philosophie* implies, then the contention between sense and non-sense must last for at least as long as the tension between the openness of being and closedness that is its extreme as well as its denial.

References

1. Binswanger, Ludwig. 1957. *Schizophrenie*. Pfullingen: Neske.
2. Binswanger, Ludwig. 1958. The case of Ellen West: An anthropological-clinical study. In *Existence: A New Dimension in Psychiatry and Psychology*. Werner M. Mendel (Trans.), Joseph Lyons (Trans.), Rollo May (ed.), Ernest Angel (ed.), Henri F. Ellenberger (ed.). New York: Basic Books.
3. Boss, Medard. 1975. *Grundriss der Medizin und der Psychologie*. Bern/Stuttgart/Wien: Verlag Hans Huber.
4. Heidegger, Martin. 1983. *Die Grundbegriffe der Metaphysik: Welt, Endlichkeit, Einsamkeit*. Frankfurt am Main: Vittorio Klostermann. English edition: Heidegger, Martin. 1995. *The Fundamental Concepts of Metaphysics. World, Finitude, Solitude*. Trans. William McNeill and Nicholas Walker. Bloomington: Indiana University Press.
5. Heidegger, Martin. 1987. *Zollikoner Seminare. Protokolle, Gespräche, Briefe*. ed. Medard Boss. Frankfurt am Main: Vittorio Klostermann. English edition: Heidegger, Martin. 2001. *Zollikon Seminars*. Trans. Franz Mayr, and Richard Askay. Evanston: Northwestern University Press.
6. Heidegger, Bartin. 1989. *Beiträge zur Philosophie (vom Ereignis)*. Frankfurt am Mein: Vittorio Klostermann. English edition: Heidegger, Martin. 1999. *Contributions to Philosophy (From Enowning)*. Trans: Parvis Emad, and Kenneth Maly. Bloomington: Indiana University Press.
7. Heidegger, Martin. 1993. *Sein und Zeit*, 17th ed. Tübingen: Niemeyer. English edition: Heidegger, Martin. 1996. *Being and Time*. Trans. Joan Stambaugh. Albany: SUNY Press.
8. Vetter, Helmuth. 1993. Es gibt keine unmittelbare Gesundheit des Geistes. *Daseinsanalyse* 10: 65–79.

Chapter 6
Poetic Experience as a Point of Departure for a New Approach to Insanity

In the preceding chapter, we adumbrated the relation between concealment and unconcealment of being, while the question was left aside as to how the running ahead towards death, in which being-there becomes vulnerable to the strife between unconcealment and concealment, can turn into absolute not-being-there. What way actually leads from being-there, as exposed to both the clearing of being and absolute concealment, to total displacement and de-rangement? The answer to this question could be provided by Heidegger's interpretation of the oeuvre whose author attained in his poetic rapture the self-annihilating de-rangement. This poet is of course none other than Friedrich Hölderlin.

Besides, the phenomenon of being-away points to the region of mental death, but it cannot explain all the suffering of the mentally ill. To come closer to this suffering we need to pay attention to Heidegger's elucidation of Hölderlin's poetry where the phenomenon of suffering plays a decisive role. Contrary to *Sein und Zeit*, in *Erläuterungen zu Hölderlin's Dichtung* suffering is not viewed on the basis of the integral ontological structure of being-there, but marks the point of its disintegration. Suffering is here understood as the suffering from the disintegration of the self. Moreover, the disintegration of the self is not a mere accident, for it corresponds to the temporal split in which and through which the openness of being opens itself to being-there. Suffering thus reflects the radical finitude and contingency of our being in openness.

Besides the temporal disjointedness of the self suffering is also marked by the collapse of the integral order of experience which issues from the fact that the openness of being is in *Erläuterungen zu Hölderlin's Dichtung* understood as the chaotic openness in which all order of experience perishes and reappears. The openness of being is here adumbrated as chaos from which all order arises and in which it perishes. In the light of such chaotic openness, Heidegger uncovers the meaning of suffering that is different both from the conventional clinical concepts and from his own privative notion of illness. But seeing the openness of being as the open abyss of chaos allows not only a new view of illness and health, but also a new view of being-there as such. Since being-there is essentially situated amidst the

© Springer International Publishing Switzerland 2015
P. Kouba, *The Phenomenon of Mental Disorder*, Contributions to Phenomenology 75, DOI 10.1007/978-3-319-10323-5_6

openness of being, its overall ontological structure, as it is depicted in *Erläuterungen zu Hölderlin's Dichtung*, must differ from the ontological structure outlined in *Sein und Zeit*. Considering the radicalization of the finitude of being-there we can presume that Heidegger has made a step from existential analysis to post-existential analysis. By making this step he has exceeded the romantic arrangement of thought and arrived at a position that is much closer to Deleuze and Guattari.

The awareness of this shift in Heidegger's thought explains our approach to his reading of Hölderlin. Contrary to majority of scholars, we are interested neither in the accuracy or inaccuracy of Heidegger's interpretation of Hölderlin, nor in the political issues involved in this interpretation. We are thus leaving aside Paul de Man's polemics with Beda Alleman concerning the question whether there is a homogeneity or rather a heterogeneity between Heidegger's and Hölderlin's thought as well as the criticism of political biases that prevent Heidegger from a proper engagement with Hölderlin's poetry, formulated by Phillipe Lacue-Labarthe or Jennifer Anna Gosetti-Ferencei.[1] What we are interested in are the changes in the understanding of the ontological structure of human existence that appear in Heidegger's confrontation with Hölderlin's poetry. Together with them we must track a new view of the temporality of human existence that is presented in *Erläuterungen zu Hölderlins Dichtung*. The problem of temporality is analyzed, for instance, in Timothy Torno's book *Finding Time. Reading for Temporality in Hölderlin and Heidegger*.[2] But Torno pays attention especially to Hölderlin's understanding of time, while the Heideggerian notion of time remains unthematized. We, on the contrary, intend to focus on the way the ontological structure of being-there and its temporal foundations change in Heidegger's encounter with Hölderlin's poetry.

The importance of Hölderlin's poetic work for the ontological inquiry into the structure of human existence follows from the fact that poetry, in Heidegger's opinion, concerns not only the poet, but all people, for the essence of human existence is characterized by the fact that "poetically man dwells on this earth". The fact that human existence is essentially poetic means that it relates to its own origin, that it, through the medium of language, touches the cleared and clarified area of being. In this respect, the poet is a precursor who shows a poetic way of existence to others. For Heidegger, Hölderlin is thus a poet who thinks the very essence of poetry.

But what exactly is the essence of poetic creation? In one of the letters to his mother, Hölderlin writes that poetry is "the most innocent of all occupations." Poetry appears to be an innocent playing with words. Unlike practical action that

---

[1] See: De Man, Paul. 1983 Heidegger's Exegeses of Hölderlin. In *Blindness and Insight. Essays in the Rhetoric of Contemporary Criticism*, Second Edition, Revised. Minneapolis: University of Minnesota Press. Alleman, Beda. 1954. *Hölderlin und Heidegger*. Zurich: Atlantis Verlag. Lacue-Labarthe, Phillipe. 2007. *Heidegger and the Politics of Poetry* (trans: Fort, Jeff). Urbana and Chicago: University of Illinois Press. Gosetti-Ferencei, Jennifer Anna. 2004. *Heidegger and the Subject of Poetic Language. Toward a New Poetics of Dasein*. New York: Fordham University Press.

[2] Torno, Timothy. 1995. *Finding Time. Reading for temporality in Hölderlin and Heidegger*. New York: Peter Lang.

always has certain consequences and thus also makes us responsible for them, poetry harms no one; on the other hand, it remains without a practical effect. Its only effect is restricted to the fictitious world of pictures arising out of the medium of language.

Nevertheless, according to another Hölderlin's statement, language is "the most dangerous of goods" given to us. Language presents a peril *par excellence* as it establishes the possibility of some danger coming into being as such. Since human being is endowed with language, its existence is open to both the clarity of what manifests itself and the unclarity of what hides itself. By means of language, we are positioned in both unconcealment and concealment whereby beings defy our under-standing by appearing as what they are not. Although language makes possible clarity and obviousness, it also encompasses the possibility of obfuscating all mean-ing – and therein lies its extreme dangerousness. "Language first creates the mani-fest place of this threat to being, and the confusion and thus the possibility even of the loss of being, that is – danger."[3]

The concealment to which language exposes us does not consist only in the pos-sibility of sham or error, but refers to where the utterable falls into the unutterable. How deeply language is imbued with concealment is already implied in *Sein und Zeit*, where Heidegger distinguishes three ways in which a phenomenon can be covered up.[4] In his opinion, this occurs when it has been once discovered, but then covered up again. Distortion occurs when covering up is not total and the phenom-enon is still visible, albeit as a semblance. The third mode of covering up is absolute concealment which one speaks of when the phenomenon has not been discovered at all. Whereas the first two modes of covering up have their place within the inauthen-tic absorption in the public interpretation of the world, the third mode of covering up is much more enigmatic.

Given that phenomenon is what shows itself, can one talk of a phenomenon that has never showed itself? What kind of a phenomenon is it if we have "neither knowledge nor lack of knowledge" about its being? Is there any point in saying that "something" that has never showed itself can arise from concealment to unconceal-ment? If yes, how is one to understand unconcealing of "something" that has never showed itself? If there is any point at all in speaking in this case of unconcealing, it must be understood as creation of something new.

Creation, understood as extracting a phenomenon out of concealment, thus brings us to a more profound level of concealment that essentially surpasses the fogginess that occurs in the frame of falling prey. This concealment is the original concealment inherent to unconcealment understood as the clearing of being. Although absolute concealment reluctantly allows for the creation of what is new, it alone defies the realm of our comprehension, and therefore can never be penetrated or overcome by the light of reason. Creation that is no mere fabrication, but rather

---

[3] Heidegger, Martin. 1951. *Erläuterungen zu Hölderlins Dichtung*. Frankfurt am Main: Vittorio Klostermann, 34. English edition: Heidegger, Martin. 2000. *Elucidations of Hölderlin's Poetry* (trans: Hoeller, Keith). New York: Humanity Books, 55.

[4] Heidegger. *Sein und Zeit*, 36. English edition: Heidegger. *Being and Time*, 32.

an open strife between the utterable and the unutterable, thus has its place in the blurred, indistinct zone between concealment and unconcealment. This zone is nothing else than language, given to us as the "most dangerous of goods."

The strife between concealment and unconcealment makes it possible to see that language is given to us not only as a tool of communication we use in order to tell others our experience, knowledge or decision. Language is no mere means at our disposal, but belongs to us in a much more primordial sense. Insofar as human being, unlike beings whose character is not that of being-there, is endowed with language, it can be in the world as a changeable sphere of possibilities that appear and vanish irretrievably. As it exposes us to both unconcealment and concealment, language must be comprehended as an event that determines the most essential possibilities of our being. Language is a field of strife between the utterable and the unutterable, and as such it establishes the fundamental possibilities of human existence. As being-there, man bears witness to these possibilities, which occurs when he creates and protects or, by contrast, destroys his world.

Nevertheless, the creation and arising of a world, like its destruction and demise, don't primarily happen by means of specific deeds or practical action. These remain on the surface, whereas what is essential is decided in language itself. That is the reason why Hölderlin can claim: "But what remains is founded by the poets." By means of the word, poets found a world in which beings obtain a new shape, measure and relation. In order for beings to show themselves in such a fashion, however, their being must first be taken out of concealment. The task of the poet is to bring being into clearness – there, according to Heidegger, lies the proper character of poetry: "Poetry is a founding: a naming of being and of the essence of all things – not just any saying, but that whereby everything first steps into the open, which we then discuss and talk about in everyday language."[5] Poetry does not name that which is already known, does not rely on what is at hand, but rather sets out on the thin ice of being and non-being on which it establishes the ground for human existence.

Since the founding role of poetry is also accompanied with the possibility of confusion and derangement, poetry in its essence can be both a most dangerous vocation and an "action most innocent." Heidegger does not seek to overcome this paradox but rather intends to maintain its inner tension, since that is the only way the peculiar nature of poetry can be understood. This encompasses both its innocent exterior that distinguishes it from practical action and the highest peril that springs from its peculiar interior.

The greatness of such peril is also attested to by Hölderlin's own fate. Madness, which prematurely and suddenly disrupted his poetic work, belongs to poetry not as a haphazard accident but as that which preserves it from the beginning in an inner tension. Even though he may seem to indulge in a free play with words and ideas, the poet is essentially the one who most primordially testifies to who man is, what the status of his being is; thus, the unutterable excess of what he beholds can easily bring him under the spell of the dark night of madness. The glaring brightness in

[5] Heidegger. *Erläuterungen zu Hölderlins Dichtung*, 40. English edition: Heidegger. *Elucidations of Hölderlin's Poetry*, 60.

which the hidden foundation of human existence is perceived can cast the poet into darkness. The poet, in his concentration on the hidden foundation of human existence, is close to the madman in that he surpasses the horizon of everydayness; like the madman, the poet is "cast out" of the ordinary everydayness in which things have their exactly determined purpose, and placed on the margin of human society.[6] The poet's place is to be found on the very limits of being with others.

The place where the poet finds or loses himself is described in Heidegger's meditation on the elegy entitled "*Heimkunft/ An die Verwandten.*"[7] In this elegy, Hölderlin depicts the lot of a poet who returns home from his stay abroad. The poet's homecoming, however, does not denote an unproblematic return to the close ones and familiar things. Although both people and things give the poet the impression of familiarity, by coming back from abroad he has not reached his home quite yet; he has yet to find his home in the familiar things and people. As the returning poet seeks his home, something tells him: "What you seek, it is near, already comes to meet you." As long as he encounters his home merely through familiar things and faces, the poet remains estranged from it. In order to really return back home, the poet must first recognize that which is the home's peculiar character.

Those who have never left their home cannot profess to really know it. To learn what is peculiar to their home it is not enough to be familiar with the things we use and the people we encounter. In order to experience the home in its unmistakable uniqueness, it is first necessary to go abroad and take on the lot of expatriation; it is necessary to experience the foreignness and exile in what is *unheimish*. It is not until not-being-at-home is experienced that one can understand what makes one's home. That is precisely the sense of the way home for which the poet sets out. The poet's repatriation requires not only a simple return to the familiar environment, but first and foremost the discovery of his own origin (*der Ursprung*). Coming back from abroad, the poet searches for his origin in which the real essence of his home remains. "What is most characteristic of the [home], what is best in it, consists solely in its being this nearness to the origin – and nothing else besides this", claims Heidegger.[8] The origin into whose closeness the poet returns in his homecoming is the clearing of being that clears itself and everything else along with it.

Insofar as the poet's homecoming consists in returning to his origin, it is not to be understood as getting hold and appropriation of the clearing of being. By means of his repatriation, the poet returns merely into the nearness to the origin to which he himself belongs without ever being able to fully attain it. Man cannot penetrate the clearing of being and reveal its secret, since it withholds itself and hides from him. The closer we get, the more the clearing of being recedes from us. Thus, to dwell in the nearness to the origin means to respect its secret and keep it as such. As

---

[6] Heidegger. *Erläuterungen zu Hölderlins Dichtung*, 42. English edition: Heidegger. *Elucidations of Hölderlin's Poetry*, 63–4.

[7] Heidegger. *Erläuterungen zu Hölderlins Dichtung*, 13–30. English edition: Heidegger. *Elucidations of Hölderlin's Poetry*, 23–49.

[8] Heidegger. *Erläuterungen zu Hölderlins Dichtung*, 23. English edition: Heidegger. *Elucidations of Hölderlin's Poetry*, 42.

long as the poet, by means of his word, cherishes the secret of the clearing of being, that is, as long as he accepts it in its self-concealment, his homecoming reaches its goal. This is revealed in the poetic meditation on the movement of repatriation, which is depicted in the elegy *Heimkunft/ An die Verwandten*. Put more precisely: "The elegy 'Homecoming' is not a poem about homecoming; rather, the elegy, the poetic activity which it is, is the homecoming itself....".[9]

Poetry is the homecoming in the profound sense of the word. The essence of poetry, as Heidegger determines it in relation to Hölderlin, consists in returning to the nearness to the origin that gives and withholds itself as the clearing of being.[10] The poet's journey to the origin cannot, however, be taken once and for all, but must be repeated as long as the poet is poet. The poet can dwell in the nearness to the origin only by constantly returning to it. The return to the clearing of being is the poet's unflagging care.

By nurturing the care for dwelling in the nearness of the clearing of being, the poet distinguishes himself from his compatriots who have never left their home. Although they are his compatriots, those who stick only to old habits and everyday matters remain remote from the poet. Since the necessary prerequisite for repatriation is a prior expatriation, those who stay with the familiar beings cannot reach the essence of home that consists in nearness to the origin. The poet's compatriots have yet to learn to listen to his word and muse on the secret of the clearing of being; only thus can they become his true kindred ones. It is only when they learn to heed the nearness to the clearing of being as told by the poet's language that they can become the sort of kindred ones to whom the poem *Heimkunft/ An die Verwandten* is devoted.

The poet addresses others in order to bring them by means of his word to the nearness of their origin and together with them care about the clearing of being. This thoughtful care requires man not to let himself be absorbed by familiar beings, but to remember the clearing of being that lies concealed behind them. Since 'to remember' means to carry remembrance within oneself, Heidegger understands the remembering of the clearing of being as remembrance (*das Andenken*) of the concealed secret of the origin. By preserving this remembrance and remembering the clearing of being, others, like the poet himself, return to the nearness to the origin, albeit in their own way. Even though they are not directly occupied with poetry, by means of remembrance, others become kindred with the poet who returns to the nearness of the origin. "In this remembrance there is a first beginning, which will in time become a far-reaching kinship with the homecoming poet."[11]

As regards the character of the remembrance of the clearing of being as well as the way in which the poet's return to the homeland, to the nearness to the origin, is

---

[9] Heidegger. *Erläuterungen zu Hölderlins Dichtung*, 24. English edition: Heidegger. *Elucidations of Hölderlin's Poetry*, 44.

[10] Heidegger. *Erläuterungen zu Hölderlins Dichtung*, 28. English edition: Heidegger. *Elucidations of Hölderlin's Poetry*, 47.

[11] Heidegger. *Erläuterungen zu Hölderlins Dichtung*, 29. English edition: Heidegger. *Elucidations of Hölderlin's Poetry*, 48.

projected therein, this is further elaborated upon in Heidegger's reflection on another of Hölderlin's poems, which bears the title "*Andenken*." This meditation that dates back to the period of the *Heimkunft/ An die Verwandten* lecture is also included in the *Erläuterungen zu Hölderlins Dichtung* collection, where it presents another, even deeper view on the process of repatriation that belongs to the essence of poetry. The poet is here again understood as the one who experiences expatriation in order to find on his way home the place of the nearness to the origin, but unlike *Heimkunft/ An die Verwandten*, this lecture goes into further detail regarding the necessity of the journey abroad, its significance and the peculiar character of the homecoming.

As long as poetry is understood as repatriation, that is, as settling in the nearness to the origin, it is of primary importance to reflect once again on the secret of this origin. That the clearing of being withholds its secret can be comprehended if we envision the origin as the overflowing source (*die Quelle*).[12] As source, the origin remains concealed because it releases beings that draw all attention to themselves. The origin is a source that conceals itself behind the multitude of beings that it allows to emerge in their presence. It is marked by ceaseless self-withdrawal, as it does not appear as such, but merely through beings that spring from it. This incessant overflowing and self-exceeding of the source makes it impossible for it to appear in its unmediatedness and simplicity. Since the overflowing source ceaselessly recedes into the background of what arises from it, it is insufficient to comprehend it as a well hidden deep down in the ground. Whereas a well can be revealed and ridden of its secret, provided that we penetrate deep enough, the source Heidegger discusses preserves its secret and remains itself in its own self-withholding. Despite giving rise to beings, the source does not disappear or dissolve in them, but rather maintains its difference that guarantees its mysterious permanence.

What is still valid is that home in its very own essence lies not in familiar things or people, but in the nearness to the origin, and thus in the nearness to the source. To remain at home means to dwell in the nearness of the source. Since, however, our sight first addresses beings, and not the clearing of being hidden behind them, the source necessarily remains hidden. Even the poet first focuses on the present beings without clearly realizing the nearness of the source that he merely divines. Even though he senses this concealed source and longs naively to unveil its secret, the poet is incapable of drawing nearer to it; his effort to find the clearing of being vainly drowns in the flood of beings with which he is familiar. No thing can satisfy the indistinct longing after being. Searching for the clearing of being in the richness of impressions and things he knows, the poet is doomed to fail and to despair in vain. Therefore, Heidegger claims that the poet in his unclarified openness to the clearing of being is consumed by the familiarity with what is, initially and for the most part, offered to him from home.[13]

[12] Heidegger. *Erläuterungen zu Hölderlins Dichtung*, 87–8, 138. English edition: Heidegger. *Elucidations of Hölderlin's Poetry*, 116–7, 167–8.

[13] Heidegger. *Erläuterungen zu Hölderlins Dichtung*, 88. English edition: Heidegger. *Elucidations of Hölderlin's Poetry*, 116.

This explains the necessity of going abroad, which opens the possibility of finding home in the nearness to the origin. The poet's not-being-at-home therefore still remains bound to home and to the possibility of settling in the nearness of the clearing of being. This not-being-at-home is not led by a desire for adventure that compels man toward exciting novelties, but rather clings to home as to that which is to be found at the end of the journey.[14] Instead of searching for the exotic, the poet's expatriation and confrontation with a strange environment is a first step toward the realization of the unmistakable uniqueness of home at which he is aiming from the very start. In order to gain a free relation to his origin, to freely dwell in its nearness, the poet must first encounter strangeness and otherness. "This is the law by which the poet, by means of the poetic passage away from home to the poetic land, becomes at home in what is proper to him."[15]

Returning on his way home to the nearness to the clearing of being, the poet cannot impress his will upon it, but must accept it as a source from which his poetry draws its inner veracity and persuasiveness. Despite referring to specific things familiar to everyday existence, what the poem addresses primarily is the clearing of being concealed behind the immediately appearing beings. This concealing, however, results not merely from human carelessness but rather from the character of the clearing itself, which withholds itself from the inquisitive view. That is the reason why the poet must first make his journey abroad and experience the trials and tribulations of exile in order to attain genuine poetic maturity. It is only thanks to his expatriation that the poet can come close to the clearing of being without losing in his relation to it his shyness (*die Scheu*) arising from the recognition of its principal ungraspability. Therefore, shyness is the essential mood of the poetic thought that returns through repatriation to the nearness to its origin. As Heidegger puts it: "This essential shyness is the mood of a homecoming which *commemorates and remembers* the origin. Shyness is the knowledge that the origin cannot be directly experienced."[16]

However, is not what we encounter here an altered form of the fundamental moments of being in disclosedness that we known from *Sein und Zeit*? Are not the poet's original preoccupation with familiar things, his journey to unfamiliar and strange places, as well as the ensuing repatriation, all merely different forms of the authentic existence that exceeds the inauthentic falling prey to the surrounding world even at the cost of having to face the uncanniness of anxiety? As William Richardson observes in his Heideggerian monograph, the poet's naïve openness for the clearing of being that initially falls prey to the sphere of familiar things corresponds to the entangled being-together-with innerwordly beings that marks our

---

[14] Heidegger. *Erläuterungen zu Hölderlins Dichtung*, 129. English edition: Heidegger. *Elucidations of Hölderlin's Poetry*, 158.

[15] Heidegger. *Erläuterungen zu Hölderlins Dichtung*, 83. English edition: Heidegger. *Elucidations of Hölderlin's Poetry*, 112.

[16] Heidegger. *Erläuterungen zu Hölderlins Dichtung*, 124. English edition: Heidegger. *Elucidations of Hölderlin's Poetry*, 153.

existence in its ordinary everydayness.[17] The poet's expatriation and the experience of not-being-at-home as adumbrated in *Erläuterungen zu Hölderlins Dichtung* also corresponds to uncanniness in which individual existence is cast out of the familiar circle of things and its close ones. The poet's repatriation thus has a status similar to the one of the return from uncanniness, which is tacitly presupposed in *Sein und Zeit*, whereas in *Erläuterungen zu Hölderlins Dichtung* it becomes the proper theme of philosophical meditation. All this makes it possible to compare the poetic pilgrimage toward the clearing of being with the phenomenological description of transitory existence in the disclosedness of being.

The mentioned comparison is valid, however, only insofar as we are aware of an important distinction. If individual existence is understood in *Sein und Zeit* on the basis of its transcendence from beings to being, and consequently the disclosedness of being seems as what the transcending existence relates to, the situation in *Erläuterungen zu Hölderlins Dichtung* is quite different: instead of regarding the clearing of being from the perspective of the transcending existence, the poet's pilgrimage is perceived from the viewpoint of the clearing of being. Although the poet's pilgrimage essentially fulfills the transitivity of existence, this transitivity is not a key to the understanding of the clearing of being, but precisely the opposite: the clearing of being determines how the finitude of sojourning in disclosedness is to be grasped. The focus of philosophical inquiry is thus not the transcending existence that relates to the disclosedness of being as to its own ground, but the clearing of being in which human existence is involved: Priority is not given to the individual existence that must advance from entangled being-together-with beings in order to reveal its thrownness into disclosedness, but on the contrary to the clearing of being that withholds itself from us by hiding behind the appearing beings. The poet does have to undergo expatriation in order to overcome the forgottenness of being in which he first dwells, but this forgottenness is a merely different expression of the fact that we are forsaken by being. The clearing of being withholds itself from us, and even if the poet opens himself to it on his journey abroad, this does not mean that he could appropriate it as such. Not even after his homecoming can the poet achieve the clearing of being, but merely attains its nearness; here he allows it to bring him into the essentially poetic disposition in which he understands it by respecting its secret.

All this obtains its full sense in remembrance, through which the poet keeps returning to the clearing of being, for only thus can he really dwell therein. In this remembrance, the poet does not return to the clearing of being as to something past that is to be re-presented in mind.[18] The poet returns to the clearing as to what has already been, and yet this having-been comes to him as something future. It is the strange paradox of remembrance "that it thinks toward what-has-been, in such a way, though, that what-has-been comes back to the one who thinks of it, coming

---

[17] Richardson, William J. 1963. *Heidegger: Through Phenomenology to Thought*. The Hague: Martinus Nijhoff, 450, 468–9.

[18] Heidegger. *Erläuterungen zu Hölderlins Dichtung*, 91.

from the opposite direction."[19] In other words, in remembrance the understanding of the having-been is also the understanding of what is coming. As it clears itself with the advent of the holy, the clearing of being is for the poet not only having-been, but also the future. In his return to the clearing of being, the poet must await the advent of the holy, and so the having-been manifests itself in remembrance as the future. Consequently, remembrance relates not only to the having-been, but also to the future. The present as such, on the contrary, is absent here, since the clearing of being never gives itself in the pure present, but only in its receding and coming.

Thereby, the temporality of remembrance resembles the temporal character of the disclosedness of being that emerges in the uncanniness of anxiety in a way that problematizes the fundamental idea of *Sein und Zeit* – the idea of the ecstatic unity of the having-been, the present and the future. Just as what appears in the uncanniness of anxiety, what appears in remembrance is the temporal unity of the three dimensions in its disjointedness and dis-unity. But whereas in *Sein und Zeit* the factual disintegration of the unity of the three temporal ecstasies that occurs in anxiety is veiled by the emphasis on the inseparable temporal unity of being in disclosedness, this is not the case in *Erläuterungen zu Hölderlins Dichtung*, since the disclosedness of being is here no longer viewed from the perspective of the temporal unity of being-there, but being-there is regarded from the viewpoint of the temporal dis-unity in which the clearing of being gives and withholds itself.

This temporal disunion in being-there can only be overcome if the poet establishes the absent presence by means of his work in which he gives word to the clearing of being. The sense of the poetic work thus lies in the establishment of the present that arises from the having-been and the future of the clearing of being. Since the beings that appear to us in the familiar surrounding of our home are not supposed to serve as the objects of artistic representation in poetry, the poet's present must be preserved especially in his work. It is exactly there that the present lies, the present which together with the having-been and the future of remembrance forms the peculiar temporality of poetry. Only in the unity of such present, having-been and future does the poet thus find his individual being.

In this manner, the remembrance of the clearing of being, out of which arises the present of the poetic work, answers the question of who the poet is as poet. The poet, remembering the clearing of being, must willy-nilly question himself, whereby remembrance itself provides him with an answer. This answer does not lie in a delineation of some isolated "I", or in immediate return to one's self. What is at work here is the understanding of the specifically poetic individual being that sets out on a perilous journey toward the clearing of being; what reveals itself is a peculiar individual being whose precarious and non-self-evident character consists in fulfilling the essence of poetry.

In this context, Heidegger speaks of being-alone (*das Alleinsein*) of the poet who sets about his work by returning to the clearing of being as to what has already been

---

[19] Heidegger. *Erläuterungen zu Hölderlins Dichtung*, 94, 142. English edition: Heidegger. *Elucidations of Hölderlin's Poetry*, 123, 172.

and what simultaneously comes as something future.[20] The poet's work is like an unsteady footbridge that spans across the bottomless abyss of the having-been and the future. What will happen, however, if the poetic work fails and in its non-presence there yawns the bottomless abyss of the having-been and the future that reveals the clearing of being, endlessly receding and withholding all ground? Won't the disintegration of the poetic work also necessitate a breakup of the poet's individual being? Won't the poet's individual being be ruptured between the having-been and the future, no longer connected by any present? Once the poetic work has lost its coherence and disintegrated into poorly chosen words and outcries, the poet is at his end. The immediate doom of the poet's individual being heralded in the unintelligible welter of words and gestures expresses the finitude of human existence, poetic in its essence. This termination is the inner possibility of being-there that becomes truly poetic, when the poet abandons the familiar sphere of things in order to find his home. The breakup of his own individual being is the ultimate peril to which the poet must expose himself as long as he is to be a poet; it is there that the jeopardy of the poetic vocation manifests itself unadorned.

How one should understand the essential jeopardy of poetic existence that springs from its finitude is demonstrated in another of Heidegger's studies contained in *Erläuterungen zu Hölderlins Dichtung*. The study entitled *"Wie Wenn am Feiertage..."* is devoted to the poem that begins with the following words: "As when on a holiday..." The opening words of this poem evoke the festive mood in which everything appears different from what it is like in everyday existence. What is essential for Heidegger is that this diversion from the everyday that belongs to the essence of holiday forms an indispensible aspect of poetry. Poetry as poetry is characteristic by its non-everydayness, i.e. its holiday-ness. Poetry as such is holiday in the deep sense of the word.

For the sense of the word "holiday" to become truly apparent, one must become aware of the fact that holiday does not mean a mere intermission in work.[21] As a diversion from everydayness, holiday is marked by the fact that something uncommon is heralded therein, something that usually cannot be experienced and undergone, since the familiar reality leaves no space for it. Substantially different from all we are familiar with, this extraordinary character can evoke shyness, awe or fear. However, there is nothing marvelous or sensational in the extraordinary which gets revealed during holiday; its uncommonness rather brings man to stop and experience quietude, in which there unfolds a region whose openness determines the essence of his existence. This open realm cannot manifest itself in the familiar beings of everyday life, but only in the uncommonness of holiday. The rapture from ordinary everydayness allows us to witness how the clearing of being, in which we essentially dwell, clears itself through the agency of the holy. Thus, holiday gains its own exceptionality and uncommonness through the holy. The

---

[20] Heidegger. *Erläuterungen zu Hölderlins Dichtung*, 130–1. English edition: Heidegger. *Elucidations of Hölderlin's Poetry*, 160.

[21] Heidegger. *Erläuterungen zu Hölderlins Dichtung*, 97. English edition: Heidegger. *Elucidations of Hölderlin's Poetry*, 125–6.

holiness of holiday has its purpose and origin in the holy by whose advent the clearing of being clears itself.[22]

Understood as holiday, even poetry is thus connected with the advent of the holy by which the openness of being takes place. The poet does not become a poet in the common course of everyday, but in holiday when he lets himself be addressed by the coming of the holy and responds to it in his own word. Holiday is the day of the poet's birth, it is the dawn "in whose light the open clears itself, so that the poet sees the coming of what his verses must say: *the holy.*"[23]

Nevertheless, how are we to understand the holy that becomes the poet's word? An answer to this question is what Heidegger seeks in his interpretation of the poem *"Wie wenn am Feiertage ..."* For us, his meditation on Hölderlin's hymn is especially valid in that it substantially ponders the finitude of human existence that out of itself cannot clear the clearing of being, and thus depends on the advent of the holy, without which the clearing could not open itself at all. To understand the holy in its coming will, then, enable us to comprehend also human existence in its dependence on the opening and concealing of the clearing of being.

In order to accomplish this task, we must depart from that which the holiday disposition brings into a light different from the one of everyday. In Hölderlin's poem, what is heralded in holiday differently from what is known to the practical regard of everyday existence, is "the powerful, divinely beautiful nature." As it appears during holiday, nature is remote from all practical concern, which is why it can show itself in its splendor. On holiday, the poet lets himself be inspired, fascinated and thrilled by the beauty of nature. For him, nature cannot have the character of readiness-to-hand as is the case in *Sein und Zeit*, where the nature of the surrounding world is understood from the viewpoint of what it has to offer to us.[24] In the framework of the surrounding world, natural beings appear not as what they are in themselves, but as what they can serve for: "The forest is a forest of timber, the mountain a quarry of rock, the river is water power, the wind is wind 'in the sails'."[25]

But if we are to adhere to Hölderlin's poetic view, nature cannot fall into the order of beings-present-at-hand either; its beautiful simplicity won't be approached if we understand it as a being-ready-to-hand devoid of its readiness and left in the mode of the simple presence-at-hand. As Heidegger points out, nature is not a whole of beings-present-at-hand, it is not a set of particularities that together form a reality. The whole of reality can never suffice for an understanding of nature, for it is she herself that establishes all reality; it is only through her that beings become reality.[26] Therefore, it can be called not only "divinely beautiful,", but also "powerful." As she

---

[22] Heidegger. *Erläuterungen zu Hölderlins Dichtung*, 99. English edition: Heidegger. *Elucidations of Hölderlin's Poetry*, 127–8.

[23] Heidegger. *Erläuterungen zu Hölderlins Dichtung*, 98. English edition: Heidegger. *Elucidations of Hölderlin's Poetry*, 127.

[24] Heidegger. *Sein und Zeit*, 70–1. English edition: Heidegger. *Being and Time*, 66–7.

[25] I Heidegger. *Sein und Zeit*, 70. English edition: Heidegger. *Being and Time*, 66.

[26] Heidegger. *Erläuterungen zu Hölderlins Dichtung*, 51. English edition: Heidegger. *Elucidations of Hölderlin's Poetry*, 75.

precedes and preconditions all reality, nature is not just an opposite to the creations of man's hand or spirit. Such a delineation would render it a specific sphere of beings, although nature herself is present in all beings, irreducible to any of them: "Nature comes to presence in human work and in the destiny of peoples, in the stars and in the gods, but also in stones, growing things, and animals, as well as in streams and in thunderstorms."[27]

What is clear from this is that Heidegger is not interested in nature in the pastoral sense, whose harmonious beauty would refine the human spirit. *Erläuterungen zu Hölderlins Dichtung* also refuses Schelling's philosophy of identity, in which nature is understood as identical with the spirit.[28] Instead of the conception elaborated by Hölderlin's friend and schoolmate, what is emphasized here is the Greek concept of φύσις, within whose framework nature is demonstrated as a process of arising and growing. The Greek φύσις, φύειν that still resonates in notions such as "physics" or "physiology" does not denote merely increase or accretion, but rather the arising and coming out of concealment. It is a revelation in openness where something at all can appear in its presence. By providing all beings with their presence, the openness itself recedes into background and closes itself off from direct gaze. What is contained in the word φύσις is both the arising of beings into openness and the retreating of this openness into occultation.

It is in the same way that *Erläuterungen zu Hölderlins Dichtung* meditates on the source which releases beings and recedes into their background. However, Heidegger does not only want to revive the pre-Socratic concept of nature. According to him, Hölderlin's word "nature" rather refers to what in the Greek φύσις remains unthought, which is nothing but the clearing of being. It is only by virtue of it that beings can become beings, i.e. to stand in the light as something concrete and nameable. It is only of it that one can meaningfully say that it is previously present in all beings, without being identical with them. The clearing of being in whose light come and go all appearing beings is the nature poeticized by Hölderlin in his depiction of the atmosphere of a holiday. It is this clearing that clears itself in a holiday morning when nature awakens from her sleep.

But even when nature rests peacefully in herself the poet is not absolutely cut off from her. In his divination the poet corroborates his unity with nature that simultaneously gives and withholds herself as the clearing of being. The poet can indeed seem separated from the clearing of being, however, as long as he senses it, he is always a part of it, and thus never absolutely forsaken. By sensing the sleeping nature and awaiting her awakening, the poet relates to her as to what has always already surrounded him and what is still only coming to him. His dwelling in the unity with nature thus places him into a relation to both the having-been and the future. The poetic presentiment of nature is a return to her initial givenness as

---

[27] Heidegger. *Erläuterungen zu Hölderlins Dichtung*, 51. English edition: Heidegger. *Elucidations of Hölderlin's Poetry*, 75.

[28] Heidegger. *Erläuterungen zu Hölderlins Dichtung*, 54. English edition: Heidegger. *Elucidations of Hölderlin's Poetry*, 79.

well as thinking about her coming.[29] Even though "all-present," because providing all beings with the openness in which they can appear as something present, nature manifests itself as remaining in itself and still coming. Nature is never present as something that is present-at-hand, but lets itself be sensed only as having-been and future.

As long as he is to be worthy of his unity with nature, the poet mustn't regard her as something present, graspable and usable for one's own ends; the poet must cease to consider nature as a set of beings ready-to-hand that stand at his disposal, perceiving it instead as a mysterious source that always remains future and having-been. The temporality of nature is the temporality of becoming, which, according to Timothy Torno, is "self-contradictory" and "self-destructive".[30] But only insofar as he maintains an awareness of this becoming, an awareness that in its own temporal character corresponds to how nature comes and at the same time remains in herself can the poet really respond to her. It is the readiness to respond to nature that makes a poet.

Not every poet is a poet in the true sense, however. The capacity for responding to nature and remaining in an inner accord with her is not something the poet is automatically given, but is the fruit of his maturation, during which he learns to hear and heed her. The poet, claims Heidegger, must let himself be "educated" by nature, and yet this education has nothing to do with the search for the concord with beauty and the harmony of nature idyll or with the return to a landscape untouched by civilization.[31] To let oneself be educated by nature means to devote oneself to the clearing of being with the awareness of its inattainability and ungraspability. Since the clearing of being itself never appears in the mode of the present, the poet can respond to it only while returning to its original givenness and anticipating its coming. Only then can the poet witness the awakening of nature that happens on a holiday, when the clearing of being clears itself.

As has been said, holiday has its essence and sense in the advent of the holy, by which the clearing of being clears. This is not to say that on holiday nature only is seen in a light different from the one she is commonly perceived in; rather, as the clearing of being, she opens and clears herself by means of the holy. When on holiday nature awakens from her dream, the clarity and openness of the clearing of being goes out of its occultation and clears again, which happens through the holy that determines it from its very ground. For the holy is nothing extraneous to nature. "The holy," claims Heidegger, "is the essence of nature."[32]

Yet, this is not to say that nature would be some image of divine beauty and wisdom. Nature is not a divine creation, but rather gods themselves are enabled by

---

[29] Heidegger. *Erläuterungen zu Hölderlins Dichtung*, 53–4. English edition: Heidegger. *Elucidations of Hölderlin's Poetry*, 87.

[30] Torno. *Finding Time*, 61.

[31] Heidegger. *Erläuterungen zu Hölderlins Dichtung*, 51–3. English edition: Heidegger. *Elucidations of Hölderlin's Poetry*, 85–7.

[32] Heidegger. *Erläuterungen zu Hölderlins Dichtung*, 58. English edition: Heidegger. *Elucidations of Hölderlin's Poetry*, 82.

nature, for only she endows them with clarified openness, in which they can be what they are. Gods are mere epiphenomena and personifications of the clearing of being that clears itself through the holy. The clearing of being cannot therefore be connected with eternity in the metaphysical sense of the word.[33] The clearing of being has nothing to do with the concept of eternity that defines eternity as *nunc stans* and *totum esse praesens*. What belongs to its essence is rather the peculiar temporality devoid of the present, which temporally stretches further than all temporalities belonging to men and nations. As long as the temporality of nature surpasses all other temporalities, it is because it stretches further than all of them, i.e. because it combines within itself the furthermost having-been with the further-most future. Nature is more having-been than everything that has been and yet more future than everything that is future; she is both the oldest and the youngest, because all that is present arises and perishes in her. Her peculiar temporality enables one to say that she is "*wie einst*," that is to say, she once has been and once will be. All this paradoxical singularity is contained in the way nature awakens. "By awakening, nature's coming, as what is most futural, comes out of the oldest of what has been, which never ages because it is each time the youngest."[34]

However, we still don't know how we are to understand the holy that is the essence of nature. How are we to regard the holy, through which the clearing of being clears and opens itself? Thanks to the clearing of being, all beings can appear in a clear contour and firm shape; all can appear therein as clearly defined and brought into mutual relation. The clearing of being mediates the relations of beings in that they have measure and order. Since it endows beings with their laws, the clearing of being can be said to be law *par excellence*.[35] As this law, the clearing of being is present in all appearing beings, without becoming any one of them. Whereas it mediates for all beings their form and mutual relations, the clearing itself maintains its immediate ungraspability.

However, the νόμος that determines the form of beings as well as their ordered relations would be nothing unless it arose from χάος; what opens its own dimension is – chaos. Insofar as beings revealed in the clearing of being are to have some law, this clearing must consist of chaos. However absurd such a statement might seem, since chaos means nothing but absolute disorder and havoc, Heidegger has a good reason to maintain it. As long as it is thought from the perspective of the clearing of being, and not from the viewpoint of the ordered beings, chaos is not a mere tumultuous mayhem, but "the yawning, gaping chasm, the open that first opens itself, wherein everything is engulfed."[36] This chasm withholds from human thought and

---

[33] Heidegger. *Erläuterungen zu Hölderlins Dichtung*, 57–8. English edition: Heidegger. *Elucidations of Hölderlin's Poetry*, 81–2.

[34] Heidegger. *Erläuterungen zu Hölderlins Dichtung*, 61. English edition: Heidegger. *Elucidations of Hölderlin's Poetry*, 85.

[35] Heidegger. *Erläuterungen zu Hölderlins Dichtung*, 59–60. English edition: Heidegger. *Elucidations of Hölderlin's Poetry*, 83–4.

[36] Heidegger. *Erläuterungen zu Hölderlins Dichtung*, 61. English edition: Heidegger. *Elucidations of Hölderlin's Poetry*, 85.

perception any support for the distinction and recognition of beings, and thus seems a boundless disarrangement. Yet, the chaos addressed in *Erläuterungen zu Hölderlins Dichtung* is no mere privation of law and order, but their essential presupposition. In relation to order in which all ordered relations among beings are anchored, chaos stands not as something deficient, but as a dimension in which all order is born. As long as chaos is conceived of as "gaping out of which the open opens itself," it is evident that it is chaos that eventually enables something discernible, definable, and organizable to appear in the clearing of being.

Thus, chaos and its confused multitude (*die Wirrnis*) must be understood as the genuine essence of the openness of being, which also means that it must be conceived of as the holy that itself clears and opens the clearing of being. "Chaos is the holy itself," claims Heidegger.[37] And, if nature is understood as the arising of order from chaos, the holy is its essence. Nature as the clearing of being is thus no longer a mere static openness, but rather a dynamic process in which order arises from chaos and again collapses into it. Put more precisely, insofar as chaos is unorganized openness, out of which emerges the inexhaustible multitude of possibilities and changeable shapes, order must be a limit of this boundless profuseness. By determining and structuring the unlimited space of the possible, order becomes the concretization of chaos. It is a concretization of endless possibilities that remain ungraspable in the boundless openness of chaos.

Chaos, as gaping opening (*die Aufklaffung*), which opens the endless field of possibilities and transmutations, cannot be preceded by any being, for only in it does all that is real arise and perish, ascend and descend. Since it precedes all appearing beings, chaos is always already older, i.e. more having-been, than all of them; at the same time, however, chaos is also younger, i.e. more future, since it is therein that all reality perishes. In relation to beings, chaos is the first and last; it is what once has been and once will be. Chaos always heralds itself as future and having-been at once; it is the future that comes from the furthermost having-been. By giving itself only as future and having-been, chaos stretches itself as a bottomless abyss, in which there is nothing to hold on to, for the dimension of the present is missing, here. Everything that is present, everything that appears through law and order in clear shapes and organized relations, loses all support in chaos and falls into its bottomlessness.

Despite all differences between *Erläuterungen zu Hölderlins Dichtung* and *Sein und Zeit*, chaos thus plays a role similar to that of disclosedness that shows itself in the uncanniness of anxiety, for chaos, just as uncanniness, deprives the everyday concern with beings of its firm ground. The unproblematic being-together-with beings that occurs in the sphere of familiarity with the surrounding world is shaken and derailed by chaos. Chaos does away with the habitual certainties of thought by ridding it of its familiarity with beings in which it initially and for the most part maintains itself. Since it divests human existence of all its certainties and guarantees, chaos is more awesome than all that is awesome; chaos is "the awesome itself."

---

[37] Heidegger. *Erläuterungen zu Hölderlins Dichtung*, 61. English edition: Heidegger. *Elucidations of Hölderlin's Poetry*, 85.

Yet, chaos does not usually herald itself in its awesomeness, but remains hidden behind beings which the clearing of being endows with constant shape, clear delineation and mutually organized relations.

Everyday experience tells us that the world is a place of order where all has its fixed place and clearly determined sense. However, what proliferates behind or rather in the bottomless ground of this order which we always understand in one way or another, is chaos that defies all understanding. In this gaping chaos, the habitual order of experience can at any moment perish in order to give way to new order. The old order of experience must perish in chaos in order for the new one to appear. Such is the experience veiled by our everyday mode of existence. What eludes us in the world of ordinary everydayness is the fact that all order arises out of chaos and again disintegrates back into it.

Despite this hiddenness that makes possible the uninterrupted course of everyday dealing with beings, human existence always preserves a certain awareness of the gaping openness of chaos. Even the order of everyday world is not immaculate. It always contains a certain ingredient of chaos, albeit suppressed and reduced to the very margin of experience. Although chaos usually does not break out in its annihilating excess, the transition from one order to another is only possible via dis-order. The minimum admixture of chaos is also the prerequisite for any improvisation and random search. The one who must more than anyone else sustain the inkling of chaos, who must not let himself be deluded by the seemingly unshakeable firmness of everyday reality is, according to Heidegger, the poet. It is he who must nurture within himself the presentiment of that to which others turn a blind eye in order to exist "in the normal way." The poet's perception of the awesome character of the gaping openness is reflected in the discovery that chaos does not stand opposite to him as something extraneous, but that it is the abysmal strangeness to which he himself essentially belongs. This presentiment is the expression of the fact that the poet is always already encompassed in chaos. Though the same is valid for his close ones, the poet perceives his inclusion in chaos in an exceptionally intense and direct way, which allows him on the other hand to witness the awakening of nature, in which law and order arise from the bottomless chaos.

As the clearing of being clears itself in that there from out of the gaping chaos arise law and order, the poet is not a distanced observer, but he himself forms part of the process. By essentially belonging to the gaping openness that opens in chaos, the poet is also part of its opening. The poet's own openness happens as a participation in the arising of order out of chaos. It is only thanks to this participation in which the poet's gaze re-opens and clears itself that the poet can abandon the habitual norms and create a truly original work. Without his inclusion in chaos out of which all order arises, the poet could not see anything in a new light and would merely drown in empty mastery instead. Formal education and theoretical knowledge as such are insufficient unless the poet has discovered the true source of his creativity that is the clearing of being which takes place as the arising of order out of chaos. If the poet is to be a true poet, what is needed is more than human knowledge or aptitude; this undeserved surplus is provided by the clearing of being which clears itself and returns to itself with the coming of the holy chaos. As long as he stands within the clearing in that he awaits it as what has always already opened itself, the poet responds to it by his own being.

Even though the poet belongs to the clearing of being that awakens to itself on holiday, he cannot govern or manipulate the arising of order out of chaos; all he can do is to await it patiently. Although the outbreak of chaos can be stimulated by various means, the very arising of order out of chaos is beyond human control. Chaos, out of which a new order arises, defies all manipulation and systematic accessing. "Even a poet is never capable of attaining the holy through his own meditation, or indeed exhausting its essence and forcing it to come to him through his questioning."[38] Chaos remains inaccessible and ungraspable for human existence, as it is always only having-been and future. Thus, the holy chaos in its immediacy can come only as an event, i.e., as what has no present, but only the having-been and the future. It is always too late, or too early. The holy, says Heidegger, gives itself as a unique *event* in which the clearing of being awakens to itself, thus clearing also the poet's gaze that is encompassed within it.[39]

However much the poet's essence belongs to the gaping openness that gives itself as having-been and future, the poet cannot do without a specific relation to the present provided by the appearing beings. Even though poetry itself is initiated by the coming of chaos which has always already opened itself, the poet shouldn't totally abandon the present beings and their reality, since he needs them as a provisional support for his creation. This is not because he would find in them the object of artistic representation, but in order not to lose firm ground underneath his feet. Even though reality as such is not to be represented in poetry, the poet must not lose touch with it unless he wants to follow a path of total self-destruction. As long as the poet's song is not to change into a song of death, the poet must not fully expose himself to the bottomless abyss of chaos, but he must preserve at least a partial sense of reality, albeit in order for it to serve him only as a place in which chaos vicariously heralds itself through beings. Otherwise, he would have to accept "a ton of bricks" that follows from the all-shaking chaos and the excess of sense that arises from it.

In facing the awesomeness of chaos and the "excess of meaning as can scarcely be uttered," the peril of ruination is, however, always relevant. Since the awesomeness of chaos emanates from "the oldest depths" of the clearing of being into which the poet is essentially drawn, it can be finally alleviated not by everyday reality, but only by the poetic work that arises from the cleared openness of being as a new present. The created work mitigates the awesomeness of the gaping openness in that it mediates it without ever possibly grasping it. Despite never being able to subdue the gaping openness as such, the poet finds in his own work rest and peace amid the all-shaking chaos. His work provides him with reassurance and protection from the awesomeness of chaos. Therefore, Heidegger professes: "The shaking of chaos,

---

[38] Heidegger. *Erläuterungen zu Hölderlins Dichtung*, 64. English edition: Heidegger. *Elucidations of Hölderlin's Poetry*, 88.

[39] Heidegger. *Erläuterungen zu Hölderlins Dichtung*, 57, 74. English edition: Heidegger. *Elucidations of Hölderlin's Poetry*, 81, 98.

which offers no support, the terror of the immediate, which frustrates every intrusion, the holy is transformed, through the quietness of the protected poet, into the mildness of the mediated and mediating world."[40] It is in this mediation that the poet's supreme happiness consists, which means not only a successful completion of his work, but also the overcoming of the threat of essential unhappiness. The creation of the work always contains the possibility that the poet shall not be able to bear the excess of that with which he is endowed, and thus it is true that "not always, when a work succeeds, is there good fortune, too."[41]

The possibility of the essential unhappiness clearly points to the fact that the act of poetic creation, despite its focused calmness, does not reduce the threat of ruination, but rather exposes the poet to the ultimate peril. In Heidegger's opinion, all who set out in Hölderlin's footsteps, fulfilling in their work the essence of poetry adumbrated by him, must accept this extreme peril, for "they must stand where the holy opens up more prepared and more primordially."[42] In their confrontation with the bottomless abyss of chaos, these poets must "leave to the immediate its immediacy, and yet also to take upon themselves its mediation as their only task."[43] In other words, it is necessary to let the arising of order out of chaos, in which the poet is involved, flicker in the mediating word without reducing this arising to what it is not. Thus, the immenseness of such a task increases the danger of poetic ruination to such an extent that it becomes "hardly bearable."[44] Once the poetic creation has really turned into a disaster as in Hölderlin's case, all focused calmness disappears into savage muddle of words, gestures and thoughts. Having become thus devoid of the support in the present, the poet also loses his individual being whose temporal unity disintegrates in the yawning abyss of the having-been, and yet always future chaos. Then, not even all support and certainty of everyday are of any help, for their habitual order uncontrollably disintegrates in chaos.

For this reason alone there can be no doubt about the fact that the possibility of unhappiness and ruination is essentially grounded in chaos which is the enabling possibility of the poet's suffering. In *Erläuterungen zu Hölderlins Dichtung*, this suffering (*das Leiden*) is something more than a mere mental illness. The suffering, here, is understood not as a deficiency of good health, but as experiencing the tumultuous forces of chaos that open for human existence its very own dimension. This suffering is no purely pathological phenomenon, but belongs to the very essence of poetry as that which must be experienced by every poet that wants to meet his

---

[40] Heidegger. *Erläuterungen zu Hölderlins Dichtung*, 68–9. English edition: Heidegger. *Elucidations of Hölderlin's Poetry*, 92.

[41] Heidegger. *Erläuterungen zu Hölderlins Dichtung*, 67. English edition: Heidegger. *Elucidations of Hölderlin's Poetry*, 90–1.

[42] Heidegger. *Erläuterungen zu Hölderlins Dichtung*, 69. English edition: Heidegger. *Elucidations of Hölderlin's Poetry*, 93.

[43] Heidegger. *Erläuterungen zu Hölderlins Dichtung*, 69. English edition: Heidegger. *Elucidations of Hölderlin's Poetry*, 93.

[44] Heidegger. *Erläuterungen zu Hölderlins Dichtung*, 69. English edition: Heidegger. *Elucidations of Hölderlin's Poetry*, 93.

belonging to the gaping openness of chaos. The poet must be ready to experience suffering that arises out of his inclusion in chaos without perceiving it merely as an endured harm. Since the belonging to chaos opens the source of poetic creativity, the poet cannot evade it, but rather must be aware of the fact that "this insistent belongingness is suffering, not mere endurance."[45] What is in question is thus not only a resigned bearing with chaos, but the recurrent clinging to the origin of all creation that always comes as future. "Suffering is remaining steadfast in the beginning. For the beginning is an arising, a bestowal, that is never lost or ended, but is always only a more magnificent beginning, a more primordial intimacy."[46] What this means is that chaos as such is marked especially by excess and superabundance, and thus the poet's suffering cannot denote decrease or exhaustion, but rather an insufferable excess; it is the perception of the awesome immenseness of what arises out of the openness of chaos.

It is only suffering thus conceived that enables us to understand the situation of the poet who has gone insane. His suffering is no longer a voluntary affirmation of his own belonging to the gaping abyss of chaos, but rather a helpless falling in which all support and certainty of understanding disappear. Together with the decline of the poetic work and the familiar order of the world, the temporal unity of human existence disintegrates, falling into the having-been and the future of chaos. Insofar as the temporal unity of human existence breaks apart in the bottomless abyss of chaos, what necessarily happens there is also the disintegration of the individual being. Suffering in this case becomes the suffering from the disintegration of one' own individual being. However, once this decomposition has reached the extreme, can one say that it is an individual existence who in its deepest essence experiences suffering? Who is it that actually suffers in chaos where the whole unity of individual being has disintegrated? Strictly speaking, it is no one, or at least no one in the sense of an individual existence. Insofar as it remains in its initial openness, the holy itself is pure suffering. It is the impersonal suffering of the gaping openness, suffering in which nature suffers from itself.

What emerges together with this realization is also the question of whether one can understand suffering as a certain mode of disposition (*die Befindlichkeit*). As long as suffering exposes human existence to the disintegration of its individual being, can one speak of its immediate finding itself? It seems rather that unlike the way *Sein und Zeit* explicates the fundamental disposition of anxiety, that is, as the fundamental moment of individuation in which the lone being-there is brought back to its very own being, suffering must be understood as a peculiar *Un-Befindlichkeit*, i.e., as in-disposition, in which being-there loses rather than finds itself.

The moment that points beyond the individual structure of human existence is also projected onto other states that are thematized in *Erläuterungen zu Hölderlins Dichtung* in connection with the self-giving and self-withholding clearing of being.

---

[45] Heidegger. *Erläuterungen zu Hölderlins Dichtung*, 72. English edition: Heidegger. *Elucidations of Hölderlin's Poetry*, 96.

[46] Heidegger. *Erläuterungen zu Hölderlins Dichtung*, 72. English edition: Heidegger. *Elucidations of Hölderlin's Poetry*, 96.

Whether it is shyness or poetic drunkenness, in each of these states there lurks a reference to the ungraspable character of the clearing of being as well as to the principal jeopardy of the individual existence that follows from the dimension of clearing.[47] However, the most radical expression of the impersonal mode in which the clearing of being gives and at the same time withdraws itself is suffering. Even though the suffering man is confronted with his thrownness into chaotic openness, this thrownness is not a situatedness in which being-there finds itself, but an essential non-situatedness in which the disparity between thrownness and existential project becomes increasingly intensified. It is a strange situation where the bare facticity of impersonal being defies the existentiality of understanding. Therefore being-there thrown into chaos becomes increasingly remote not only from the possibility to understand beings ready-to-hand and others who deal with them, but also from the possibility to understand one's own self.

Though grounded upon the vulnerability to the awesome abyss of chaos that shakes all certainties, suffering does not necessarily have to display chaos as such. Chaos does not, with the possible exception of pathological states that remain practically inaccessible to us, show itself in its immediacy. There are always some beings whose clearly defined shapes and significative relations are being blurred and effaced, whose whole order is dissolving and turning into chaos. Not even when the firm order of the world has lost its contours and begun to be permeated by wild and disordered perceptions do beings as such disappear, but merely cease to provide their support. Despite the incessantly deepening inconsistency of experience, even madness does maintain a certain relation to beings, but these beings appear in confusion and disarray; such beings make suddenly no sense, forcing the madman to desperately seek to find some foothold. Beings themselves cannot, however, offer a secure support any more, since their present is elusive and increasingly recedes into the having-been and the future of chaos. The wider the bottomless abyss of chaos, the more desperately human being strives to hold on to anything that could reintegrate the order of its experience and save its collapsing individual existence. The ultimate limit toward which the whole process of pathological disintegration is directed is impersonal suffering in which the integral individual being is substituted for by random clusters of memories, words and gestures. What remains instead of individual existence is then nothing but a chaotic conglomerate of preindividual singularities. The only possibility of escaping this state lies in emergency measures by which all graspable remnants of sense become consolidated. The critical situation of the madman thus explains for instance the need to create systems of paranoid delusions that are perfectly organized and coherent, yet whose fragility betrays chaos proliferating in their background. The rigidity and fragility of paranoid systems bespeak of chaos that they are to stop and overcome whatever the cost. The same applies also to neurotic defence mechanisms that serve to prevent the annihilating onslaught of chaos upon the integral order of experience.

---

[47] Heidegger. *Erläuterungen zu Hölderlins Dichtung*, 113, 124. English edition: Heidegger. *Elucidations of Hölderlin's Poetry*, 137, 148.

What also becomes clear from this is that health cannot be reduced to a perfectly structured order of experience, but it rather must be attributed also to the ability to open itself to chaos as to that dimension in which all sense and order perish. Health proves itself in the ability to bear chaos and to come to terms with the disintegration of a firmly given order; its essence is the readiness to face situations in which the appearing reality makes no sense. Only in chaos can a new sense and a new order be born. Dwelling in the firmly given frame of a habitual order and certainties demands in some respect less health than exposure to the incertainty of the tumultuous chaos in which a new sense and order can be found.

However, this discovery of new possibilities is still remote from the primordial vigor that is hidden in chaos itself.[48] Chaos, in *Erläuterungen zu Hölderlins Dichtung*, is understood as primordial vigor, in itself pure and intact. As the inexhaustible realm of always new possibilities and transmutation, chaos is absolute vigor out of which all beings draw their own health. At the same time, however, "the primordial [vigor], which thus grants [health], still enshrouds all fulness in itself, as the immediate, and it holds in itself the fabric of the essence of all – thus it is precisely unapproachable by any individual, be that a god or a man."[49]

As far as human existence is concerned, absolute vigor appears not only inaccessible, but outright annihilating for it. Since absolute vigor, that is, the boundless openness to uncalculable possibilities and to their transformations, would be unbearable for human being, we need certain limits and restrictions in order to exist at all. In other words, we need a certain law and order that would enable us to carry only as many possibilities as one can stand. Absolute vigor, insofar as we can speak of it at all, would be actually absolute suffering. As long as there is always for us some admixture of chaos in order, there is no chaos without at least a measure of order either. Order and chaos are not necessarily in a disjunctive relation, since they mutually condition and complement each other. Human health thus can fulfill itself only in the interplay of chaos and order, which also applies to human suffering. Just as human health, human suffering is the question of the relation between chaos and order.

Thus, the way chaos gets thematized in *Erläuterungen zu Hölderlins Dichtung* establishes no normative distinction between health and illness, no measurement of illness through health, but demonstrates that the worst suffering carries within itself a bit of health and the firmest health contains the stinging thorn of suffering. The maximization of health definitely does not entail the minimization of suffering, as Boss thinks. Health can never be quite severed from suffering. Chaos as such, both salubrious and pernicious, is the source of both health and suffering, and thus makes it possible to understand how shaky and changeable is the relation between health and suffering. What now appears to be health supreme can in a moment turn into boundless suffering. This does not have to be just a matter of a progressive

---

[48] Heidegger. *Erläuterungen zu Hölderlins Dichtung*, 61. English edition: Heidegger. *Elucidations of Hölderlin's Poetry*, 85.

[49] Heidegger. *Erläuterungen zu Hölderlins Dichtung*, 61. English edition: Heidegger. *Elucidations of Hölderlin's Poetry*, 85.

pathological evolution in which health inevitably turns into suffering. Examples of such fates as the fate of Hölderlin, Kierkegaard, Nietzsche or Van Gogh clearly prove that the very ability to confront chaos that on the one hand has the affect of supreme health brings boundless suffering on the other. All that matters are minute details and minuscule changes in perspective in which health turns into suffering, happiness into misery, and vice versa.

This uncertainty is all the greater because chaos itself comes as an event that is both having-been and future, but never present. Chaos entirely excludes its being treated and manipulated as something present, and as such assumes a double face for us. Its belonging to chaos provides human existence not only with the possibility of escaping the given significative structures, of getting rid of the habitual modes of action and thought and opening oneself to new significative connections, but also presents an essential jeopardy of its integrity. This is best documented by poetry itself that is exposed to two crucial risks: getting stuck in the poetic description of familiar beings and non-innovative, however formally perfect, repetition of the already established artistic techniques on the one hand, and catastrophic ruination and falling into the bottomless abyss of chaos on the other.

Deleuze and Guattari point to something similar when they warn in their *Qu'est-ce que la philosophie?* against the danger lurking in poetry, or artistic creation as such. Apart from the danger of self-destructive ruination to which the artist is exposed, the other danger lies in the possibility of remaining within the realm of δόξα where the general opinion and cliché assert themselves. The inability to extricate oneself from the subjugation of accepted conventions and clichés is the antipole of the fall into utter incomprehensibility. Both the former and the latter pose a threat faced by every artist. In fact, the escape from the entrapment of conventional ideas and cliché pictures is impossible without the artist taking a risk of being thrown into chaos which human thought fears most of all.

> We require just a little order to protect us from chaos. Nothing is more distressing than a thought that escapes itself, than ideas that fly off, that disappear hardly formed, already eroded by forgetfulness or precipitated into others that we no longer master. These are infinite *variabilities*, the appearing and disappearing of which coincide. They are infinite speeds that blend into the immobility of the colorless and silent nothingness they traverse, without nature or thought. This is the instant of which we don't know whether it is too long or too short for time. We receive sudden jolts that beat like arteries. We constantly lose our ideas. That is why we want to hang on to fixed opinions so much. We ask only that our ideas are linked according to a minimum of constant rules.[50]

However, art must not settle for a preordained opinion and preliminarily fixed patterns. The artist must fight both chaos and opinion, or rather turn the one against the other; his/her task is to find consistency in chaos without falling into conventional opinions and patterns. The task of artist, contend Deleuze and Guattari, is not

---

[50] Deleuze, and Guattari. *Qu'est-ce que la philosophie?*, 175. English edition: Deleuze, and Guattari. 1994. *What is Philosophy?* (trans: Tomlison, Hugh and Burchill, Graham). New York: Columbia University Press, 201.

to represent the seen and heard, but to mediate chaos by rendering it sensible by means of artistic composition.

Nevertheless, the relation to chaos is constitutive not only of art, but also of philosophy. Also philosophy can combat the fixed opinions only by virtue of opening itself to chaos in order to find a certain consistency in it while leaving its immediacy that is given in endless arising and perishing. If philosophy opposes opinion, it does not do so in order to search for some *Urdoxa* common to all opinions, but to provide chaos with consistency that wouldn't be imposed on it from the outside, but would grow out of it. Deleuze and Guattari formulate it so that consistency, created by philosophy, is not to be transcendent in relation to chaos, but rather should permeate it as an immanent plane. Philosophical notions, according to them, serve to create, within chaos that dissolves all cohesion and integrity of thought, an immanent plane of consistency.

> In fact, chaos is characterised less by the absence of determinations than by the infinite speed with which they take shape and vanish. This is not a movement from one determination to the other, but, on the contrary, the impossibility of a connection between them, since one does not appear without the other having already disappeared, and one appears as disappearance when the other disappears as outline. Chaos is not an inert or stationary state, nor is it a chance mixture. Chaos makes chaotic and undoes every consistency in the infinite.[51]

As such, chaos is a virtual realm to which philosophical thought exposes itself and with which it incessantly measures itself. Philosophy, nevertheless, can abandon opinion and settle chaos only by leaving the inhabited territory and setting out for the way of deterritorialization, which also applies, though in a different form, to art. Even though it does not work with concepts, art is a certain mode of thought, and as such connected with the process of deterritorialization and with the complementary process of reterritorialization. Both the thinker and the artist must become exiles who search for their homes and territories.

This is indeed confirmed also by Heidegger who describes the poet's homecoming as repatriation that follows after a previous expatriation. Whereas the poet is he who comes home from abroad to the nearness to his origin, the thinker in *Erläuterungen zu Hölderlins Dichtung* is understood as he who sets out abroad in order to find there that which is worth thinking and to remain with it. "The thinker thinks toward what is un-homelike (*das Unheimische*), what is not like home, and for him this is not a transitional phase; rather, this is his being *at home* (*das Heimische*)."[52] Philosophical thought, unlike the thought of poetry, thus finds its home in the uncanny foreignness. Philosophy settles by means of its concepts that which is alien to it, rendering it its home.

In other words, the difference between philosophy and poetry lies not so much in the act of deterritorialization, which is a prerequisite for thought in both cases, as in

---

[51] Deleuze, and Guattari. *Qu'est-ce que la philosophie?*, 41. English edition: Deleuze, and Guattari. 1994. *What is Philosophy?*, 42.

[52] Heidegger. *Erläuterungen zu Hölderlins Dichtung*, 122. English edition: Heidegger. *Elucidations of Hölderlin's Poetry*, 151.

a different mode of reterritorialization. Thought, however, is always a matter of deterritorialization and reterritorialization. Even if we do take into account science that is thematized in *Qu'est-ce que la philosophie?* as another of the three fundamental forms of thought, thought can be said to be determined by the processes of deterritorialization and reterritorialization that can be either relative, when the constant unity of thought and individual being is maintained in and across them, or absolute, when the unity of thought and individual being is exposed to processes of disintegration and repeated reintegration.

To comprehend under what conditions the absolute deterritorialization and reterritorialization of thought take place presupposes the understanding of the peculiar temporality of the event to whose urgency the artist and the thinker open themselves. Both the artist and the thinker expose themselves to the coming of the event that exceeds its actualization in the states of matters, in bodies and bodily sensations. Despite actualizing itself in the states of things or in sensations, the event is not identical with any state of things. It is immaterial and cannot be experienced as something present. The event, Deleuze and Guattari claim, is different from the state of things in that it is never actual, but always comes without ever having begun or finished.[53] Unlike the state of things, the event has neither beginning, nor end; it is not a duration connecting two moments, but pure becoming that nothing precedes or follows. The event, that is a time without extension and duration.

> It is no longer time that exists between two instants; it is the event that is a meanwhile [*un entre-temps*]: the meanwhile is not part of the eternal, but neither is it part of time – it belongs to becoming. The meanwhile, the event, is always a dead time; it is there where nothing takes place, an infinite awaiting that is already infinitely past, awaiting and reserve.[54]

As a dead time without the present, the event is what is coming, and yet has already happened. It is the meanwhile that is no interval, but an empty time in which nothing happens, and yet everything is shifted into a different light. That is why art and philosophy can understand it better than science that primarily preoccupies itself with the state of things, whereas the event as such escapes it. On the other hand, neither philosophy nor art observe the functions of the state of things; they neither seek the principles of their functioning, nor do they construe systems of their linkage. According to Deleuze and Guattari, their task is simply to capture and seize events that become actualized in the states of matters. Even though never actual as such, the event is not cut off from the states of things, as it could possibly seem at first sight, but rather happens in and through them as pure virtuality. In relation to things, the event is what virtually belongs to their duration, and yet is never identical with it.

The same could be said of the event as conceived of in *Erläuterungen zu Hölderlins Dichtung*. The event in which the clearing of being clears itself comes as what has already happened, as what is both having-been and future. The peculiar temporality of this event does not temporalize itself in the unity of the future, the having-been

---

[53] C Deleuze, and Guattari. *Qu'est-ce que la philosophie?*, 136–9. English edition: Deleuze, and Guattari. 1994. *What is Philosophy?*, 157–60.

[54] Deleuze, and Guattari. *Qu'est-ce que la philosophie?*, 137. English edition: Deleuze, and Guattari. 1994. *What is Philosophy?*, 158.

and the present, but heralds itself as a becoming that lacks the present. The absence of the present, and thus the essential temporal dis-unity of the event, are not privations of some original unity, but rather that which is independent of, or parallel with, every temporal unity. What corresponds to this is the temporal structure of existence that awaits the event as that which has already happened. When awaiting the event that comes as having-been, human existence itself is both having-been and future. If it is stretched also into the ecstasy of the present, this awaiting existence thereby always to some extent betrays the clearing of being that itself is never present, for it can only be mediated by means of beings. But here, the understanding of the temporal character of the event is no longer covered by the emphasis on the inseparable unity of being in disclosedness, as is the case in *Sein und Zeit*. The temporality of human existence is thematized on the basis of the temporal structure of the event, and therefore the ecstatic unity of the having-been, the future and the present can be viewed in its essential non-self-evidence and troublesomeness. The temporal unity of human existence is no longer an *a priori* foundation that in advance guarantees the ontological unity of individual being, but rather something that incessantly disintegrates and what must always be renewed. This unity, and together with it, the structure of individual being, must permanently resist the dis-unity that heralds itself in the having-been and the future of the gaping openness of chaos.

This applies not only to the poet who opens himself to the coming of chaos or to the unfortunate one whose individual being dissolves while confronting the temporal dis-unity proper to this *event*, but to being-there as such. The ontological structure of being-there as laid out in *Erläuterungen zu Hölderlins Dichtung* thus does not allow us to oppose the authentic mode of existence with inauthentic existence that would be a privation of its original unity and integrity; instead, what proves itself as primary is the dis-unity and un-integrity of the event. Unlike the existential analysis elaborated in *Sein und Zeit*, being-there appears here not as basically autonomous, but as essentially heteronomous, which bears in various ways upon the poet's vocation and upon the madman's suffering. Heteronomy is no longer the regrettable quality of the inauthentic existence, but in reverse the fundamental ontological determination of being-there which is marked by it in its own contingency and finitude.

The shift from autonomy to heteronomy eventually follows from the change in the understanding of existential finitude. Whereas existential analysis brings existential finitude into connection with the possibility of death which is the individual's very own, irrevocable and not-to-be-bypassed possibility of existence, our belonging to the gaping openness of chaos makes it possible to understand that death informs our existence in a much more immediate and threatening way. Death thematized on the basis of chaos is no longer only a more or less remote possibility, but something that is always happening, what comes to us as what has long happened and what we are involved in from the very beginning. Dying is thus no longer viewed in the light of an integral ontological constitution of care as is the case in *Sein und Zeit*. The existential analysis of being-there is rather subjugated to the fundamental characteristics of death that is the disintegration of the temporal unity of being-there. Thus we advance from the existential analysis to the post-existential analysis of being-there, within whose framework becoming-dead is understood as temporally conditioned disintegration of the ontological structure of individual existence. Only in this sense is it true that being-there exists as dying. The post-existential conception of dying which reflects the gaping openness of chaos thus completely consummates Hölderlin's contention that *"Leben ist Tod, und Tod ist auch ein Leben."*[55]

When occupying himself with the essence of poetry, especially with the poetry of Hölderlin, Heidegger attains not only the understanding of the crucial peril bound with the poetic vocation, but the overall revision of the ontological structure of being-there. The ontological project of being-there as adumbrated in *Erläuterungen zu Hölderlins Dichtung* makes it clear that to step out of the mediocre everydayness and its familiar world is not a step taken toward simple self-discovery and self-gain, but a setting out into the unknown where nothing is as certain as the fact that our existence can go astray and lose itself. It follows from the description of the poet's exposure to chaos that here the question concerns not so much one's own return from involvement with beings back to oneself as it concerns a dangerous movement in which the poet's individual being is permanently jeopardized and interfered with.

The temporal dis-unity of existence, which becomes urgent together with the coming of chaos, forces the poet not to completely throw himself at the mercy of chaos, to maintain at least a rudimentary relation to the present beings that can be of support for him, until a work comes into being, in which chaos shall be preserved via mediation without further jeopardizing the existential unity of the poet's individual being.

However, the poet's experience does not only bear witness to the temporal rupture in which the ontological unity of individual being splits, but also bespeaks a change in the understanding of the relation between being-there and the clearing of being: the clearing of being is no longer considered on the basis of the unity of a transcending existence, but being-there is thought on the ground of the temporal dis-unity in which the clearing of being gives and withholds itself. The temporal instability of being-there, and consequently also the instability of its individual being, is comprehensible only in the light of chaotic openness to which being-there essentially belongs.

Chaos, which opens up the space for the birth of a new law and order, is indeed virtually present in all beings, and yet it never shows itself as something present. In this sense, chaos pertains not only to human existence, but to all living and lifeless beings, although the possibility of observing the arising of order out of chaos, and thereby of attesting to its inclusion in nature, remains reserved for human being.

All this leads us to the conclusion that *Erläuterungen zu Hölderlins Dichtung* abandons the romantic arrangement of the ontological structure of being-there that was elaborated in *Sein und Zeit*.[56] Although, at first sight, the description of the

---

[55] Cf. Hölderlin's poem "In lieblicher Bläue blühet."

[56] Note: the word "romantic" is used here not in its common sense, but in the one it is attributed by Deleuze and Guattari in *Mille plateaux* where, "for lack of a better term," they distinguish between the classicist, romantic and modern arrangement. What is, according to them, characteristic of the romantic orientation is the motif of the hero who abandons the familiar home in order to face uncanniness in which he finds his own origin. However, there is no disintegration of individual being taking place in this process, which is how the romantic orientation differs from the modern one that challenges the foundational unity of thought.

poetic expatriation and repatriation seems marked by many romantic features, what occurs at its heart is a delicate yet momentous shift that brings it closer to the post-romantic strategy of thought. After all, Heidegger's advancement from the romantic to the post-romantic orientation does not consist in abnegation of all he has hitherto claimed; rather, it is a matter of a subtle shift of accent: instead of the temporal unity of the individual existence that relates to the clearing of being, the emphasis is on the clearing of being that gives itself and withholds itself in its temporal dis-unity, thus determining the way being-there relates to it.

It is no coincidence that this change occurs in the philosophical dialogue with Hölderlin, who is classed in *Mille plateaux*, together with Kleist, as a post-romantic author. Although often classified as belonging to the period of late Romanticism, Hölderlin remains for Deleuze and Guattari a poet of a tragically disintegrated individual being, a poet who sets out not from fundamental unity and constancy, but from the fundamental disjointedness of human existence, which puts him outside of the scope of the romantic thought.[57] And as De Man most pertinently observed, Hölderlin is also the only author whom Heidegger in his late period „cites as a believer cites Holy Writ".[58] Whereas Kant, Hegel, or even Kierkegaard and Nietzsche are not spared critical remarks, Hölderlin is for him the one who shows the way toward the clearing of being. Since the elucidation (*die Erläuterung*) of his poetic work is led by no other ambition than to make it resonate, this explication can function as a post-romantic turning point in which the existential analysis turns into a post-existential analysis, i.e. into such a mode of analysis that does not seek the principle of human existence in the autonomous and consistent individual being, but rather in one that is heteronomous and inconsistent.[59] As opposed to the existential analysis that connects transcendence from beings to being with the individuation and self-discovery of the lone being-there, the post-existential analysis demonstrates that being-there can fulfill its involvement in the clearing of being only at the cost of disintegration of its individual being. As long as some sort of individuation occurs in the chaotic openness of the clearing of being, it is only in the sense of an uncertain consolidation of the disintegrated individual being.

Unless one pays regard to this shift in the view on the ontological structure of being in disclosedness, the critique of Heidegger's philosophy cannot pay justice to it. Of course, one can state that what is underestimated within the framework of the existential analysis of being-there is the peril lurking in the abandonment of the inhabited familiar world and in the exposure to the uncanny openness of being. But unless one pays heed to the change in the ontological project of being-there that occurs in *Erläuterungen zu Hölderlins Dichtung*, it is too simple to point out that the thought of being betrays the deterritorialization, locating it in the difference between beings and being, and that it remains imprisoned in the categories of the Same and

---

[57] Deleuze, and Guattari. *Mille plateaux*, 328–9. Deleuze. *Différence et répétition*, 82, 118.

[58] De Man. Heidegger's Exegeses of Hölderlin. in *Blindness and Insight*, 250.

[59] See preface to the second edition of *Erläuterungen zu Hölderlins Dichtung*, 7–8. English edition: Heidegger. *Elucidations of Hölderlin's Poetry*, 31.

the One instead of revealing the essential non-sameness and dis-unity of individual being that issue from the way being-there relates to the clearing of being.

On the other hand, one must concede that Heidegger himself is incapable of maintaining the post-romantic position permanently, since he keeps coming back in his various thought-paths to the presupposition of a unified ontological constitution of being-there. The very shift of the perspective from which the relation of being-there and the clearing of being is viewed is far from sufficient for abandoning the idea of a unified ontological structure of sojourning in disclosedness, which is grounded upon the ecstatic unity of temporality. A document of this can be seen in *Zollikoner Seminare*, for instance, where the inseparable unity of the three temporal ecstasies, just as the ontological unity of individual being which is grounded upon it, present basic points of departure of the phenomenological approach to the questions of mental health and illness. Even though being-there is thought in that case from the viewpoint of the clearing of being in which it dwells, the unified ontological structure of its individual being is not in the least problematized. It becomes therefore clear that the crucial shift lies not in whether being-there is thought from the perspective of the clearing of being or vice versa, but in how this change in perspective is reflected in the project of the ontological structure of being-there.

Even if Heidegger attains the post-romantic orientation by explicating the clearing of being as gaping chaos, out of which arise law and order, this still does not necessarily mean that his conception of chaos tallies perfectly with the one of Deleuze and Guattari, in which chaos is thematized as an endlessly rapid changeability. The fact that the topic of chaos is on the very verge of what Heidegger is capable of thinking can also be tracked in his *Beiträge zur Philosophie* where the notion of chaos is explicitly denied. What gains prominence here instead of the arising of order out of chaos is the motif of the abysmal absence of ground (*der Ab-grund*) in which every substantiating ground is refused.[60] The openness of being is thus understood not as an opening (*das Aufklaffen*) of chaos, but as an empty abyss whose time-space is established in the receding and refusal of the substantiating ground. It is in this receding and refusal of the ground that the clearing of being clears itself, proving thereby that what belongs to it is not only unconcealment, but also concealment.

But even though the time-space of the abyss is thought positively, and not as some lack or unfulfilled wish, the polarity of concealment and unconcealment that polarizes itself therein still does have its limits that appear when we try to thematize psychopathological disorders on its "ground." The tension between the concealment and unconcealment precludes a subtle insight into the nature and structure of the variegated forms of madness by oscillating between two extremes that refer to each other only so that they oppose one another. The polarity between concealment and unconcealment erases the sense of perceiving the indiscernible states, which remain irreducible to any one of the two opposite extremes. What becomes blurred by the same token is the sense of perceiving gradual transitions or abrupt twists during

---

[60] Heidegger. *Beiträge zur Philosophie*, 381. English edition: Heidegger. *Contributions to Philosophy*, 266.

which health turns into suffering. Suffering itself in its psychosomatic structure cannot be accessed on the basis of concealment that belongs to the clearing of being.

On the other hand, the topic of the openness of chaos out of which arise law and order renders the entire spectrum of pathological phenomena and the inner logic of their evolution understandable; moreover, it allows us to better understand the question of the psychosomatic whole of human existence or the issue of old age and aging. All this shall be documented in the following chapter.

References

1. Alleman, Beda. 1954. *Hölderlin und Heidegger*. Zurich: Atlantis Verlag.
2. Deleuze, Gilles. 1968. *Différence et répétition*. Paris: PUF. English edition: Deleuze, Gilles. 1995. *Difference and Repetition*. Trans. Paul Patton. New York: Columbia University Press.
3. Deleuze, Gilles, and Félix Guattari. 1980. *Mille plateaux: Capitalisme et schizophrénie*. Paris: Minuit. English edition: Deleuze, Gilles, and Félix Guattari. 1987. *Thousand Plateaus*. Trans. Brian Massumi. Minneapolis: Minnesota University Press.
4. Deleuze, Gilles, and Félix Guattari. 1991. *Qu'est- ce que la philosophie?* Paris: Minuit. English edition: Deleuze, Gilles, and Félix Guattari. 1994. *What is Philosophy?* Trans. Hugh Tomlison and Graham Burchill. New York: Columbia University Press.
5. De Man, Paul. 1983. *Blindness and insight. Essays in the rhetoric of contemporary criticism*. Minneapolis: University of Minnesota Press.
6. Gosetti-Ferencei, Jennifer Anna. 2004. *Heidegger and the subject of poetic language. Toward a new poetics of Dasein*. New York: Fordham University Press.
7. Heidegger, Martin. 1951. *Erläuterungen zu Hölderlins Dichtung*. Frankfurt am Main: Vittorio Klostermann. English edition: Heidegger, Martin. 2000. *Elucidations of Hölderlin's Poetry*. Trans. Keith Hoeller. New York: Humanity Books.
8. Heidegger, Martin. 1987. *Zollikoner Seminare. Protokolle, Gespräche, Briefe*. ed. Medard Boss. Frankfurt am Main: Vittorio Klostermann. English edition: Heidegger, Martin. 2001. *Zollikon Seminars*. Trans. Franz Mayr and Richard Askay. Evanston: Northwestern University Press.
9. Heidegger, Martin. 1989. *Beiträge zur Philosophie (vom Ereignis)*. Frankfurt am Mein: Vittorio Klostermann. English edition: Heidegger, Martin. 1999. *Contributions to Philosophy (From Enowning)*. Trans. Parvis Emad and Kenneth Maly. Bloomington: Indiana University Press.
10. Heidegger, Martin. 1993. *Sein und Zeit*, 17th ed. Tübingen: Niemeyer. English edition: Heidegger, Martin. 1996. *Being and Time*. Trans. Joan Stambaugh. Albany: SUNY Press.
11. Lacue-Labarthe, Phillippe. 2007. *Heidegger and the Politics of Poetry*. Trans. Jeff Fort. Urbana/Chicago: University of Illinois Press.
12. Richardson, William J. 1963. *Heidegger: Through phenomenology to thought*. The Hague: Martinus Nijhoff.
13. Torno, Timothy. 1995. *Finding time. Reading for temporality in Hölderlin and Heidegger*. New York: Peter Lang.

Chapter 7
Psychopathological Consequences

While the preceding chapter has pointed out new thematic possibilities of the ontological analysis of human existence, the aim of the following chapter is to make use of these possibilities in the area of psychopathology. Suffering conditioned by the temporal disintegration of the self and accompanied by the collapse of the order of experience needs to be illustrated on concrete clinical studies. For the sake of such exemplification, some case studies presented by Binswanger, Blankenburg and Laing are here analyzed; they provide a material that is to be reinterpreted by the post-existential analysis. In this way we arrive at a new understanding of hebephrenic schizophrenia, paranoid delusions, as well as schizoid structure of personality. All these pathological states are understood not as privative forms of existence related to some normative ideal, but as positive phenomena which have their own logic. Yet, this is not to say that they are advantageous or enviable. On the contrary, the suffering that speaks through the psychopathological phenomena is even more terrible if seen in its own light, and not from the perspective of some normative ideal. Since suffering is connected with the very finitude of human existence, it cannot be simply eradicated from human life. It can be only alleviated, but the temporal rupture from which human existence suffers can never be healed. And it is precisely this rupture that ontologically enables mental disorder as well as oldness that inseparably belongs to the finitude of human existence, even though Heidegger does not pay any attention to this phenomenon.

We have already seen that the ontological project of being-there as adumbrated in *Erläuterungen zu Hölderlins Dichtung* is not grounded on the idea of an *a priori* unity of the three temporal ecstasies. The ecstatic unity of the having-been, the future and the present that joins and unites the ontological structure of being in disclosedness is here replaced with the abysmal disunity of the having-been and the future in which the gaping openness of chaos heralds itself. In its light, one's own belonging to the gaping chaos appears neither integral nor unified; one's own existence is not unified by the ecstatic unity of temporality, but on the contrary falls apart in the tension between the having-been and the future. In its deepest foundation, being-there is disunited and disintegrated, since it is disturbed by the temporal

© Springer International Publishing Switzerland 2015
P. Kouba, *The Phenomenon of Mental Disorder*, Contributions
to Phenomenology 75, DOI 10.1007/978-3-319-10323-5_7

rupture that must be incessantly reintegrated, an action which being-there performs by anchoring itself in the present. By virtue of its sense of the present that binds it to things of concern, being-there can maintain its individual being in integral unity. However, our existence can corroborate its belonging to openness, which opens itself as chaos, only by accepting the essential disunity in which its individual structure is torn between having-been and the future. Thus, our temporal disjointedness appears as the source of the deepest suffering. However much we can alleviate or cover up the suffering by clinging to the seemingly unshakeable reality of the everyday world, we can never fully rid ourselves of it.

As long as we are to thematize the phenomenon of mental disorder, we must take into account suffering, which consists in our vulnerability to the bottomless abyss of chaos and turn it into a point of departure of our meditations. Understanding mental disorder on the basis of suffering from chaos does not imply a return to interpretations that explain it as an organic disorder of the brain or as a disorder in the functioning of the psychic apparatus. Rather, this approach is much closer to the view of mental disorder offered by John Caputo, who in his *More Radical Hermeneutics* claims madness to be a "disturbance" in a twofold sense of the word.[1]

Madness is firstly that which disturbs us, the "normal" ones, from the established order of the everyday being-in-the-world by reminding us of what we would rather know nothing about. It is a mirror that lets us peer inside the deep rupture in human existence, telling us who we are. When facing madness, we have to realize that our perfectly organized, conventional existence is a mere cloak of a deep dissonance that resounds from within the heart of our being. The madman who tells of this dissonance by his whole being coerces us to encounter what we suppress inside ourselves in order to exist "normally", even though it can never be suppressed completely.

The madman, however, can bear witness to the irrevocable rupture in human existence only at the cost of his own suffering. Thus, what unveils itself in the madman's suffering is the other meaning of disturbance Caputo speaks of. In this respect, Heidegger's explication of the essence of suffering implies a disturbance in the sense of a rupture in the ecstatic unity of temporality, thanks to which we, the "healthy," are capable of finding the proper place and sense of our existence in that with which we occupy ourselves, i.e., not only in our work, but also in our interests and hobbies, in which we become naturally bound with those around us. The madman, on the contrary, finds the primary sense not in his occupations, but in his suffering; his behavior is led not so much by practical interest as by the need to escape suffering that follows from the temporal rupture in his existence. His experience is permeated by suffering that we others sense only indistinctly beyond the dark horizon of our world.

Let us not therefore be deceived. There is no idealized figure of the madman who knows more than all wise men here. What the madman gives us to understand in his suffering, what we can learn from him, is nothing but the tidings of the radical

---

[1] Caputo, John D. 2000. *More Radical Hermeneutics, On Not Knowing Who We Are*. Bloomington and Indianapolis: Indiana University Press, 36–8.

finitude of our being. As long as we want to hear and truly understand these tidings, we must bracket all scientific knowledge which gives us the false impression that we know what mental disorder is when we are able to explain its causes or reveal the correlative changes in the functioning of brain centers; instead, we must regard mental disorder as the expression of our finitude consisting in our belonging to chaos.

Mental disorder is to be viewed from the perspective of chaos in whose openness the sense, order and cohesion of experience dissolve. Suffering which permeates mental disorder is essentially the suffering from chaos in whose abyss the temporal unity of the individual existence disintegrate. To approach the essence of psycho-pathological disorders is therefore possible only when we conceive of them on the basis of suffering, which in itself is nothing but the suffering from the disintegration of the individual being. This is not to say that the suffering patient must be under-stood directly as impersonal chaos; rather, it is necessary to understand him/her from what he/she has to face, i.e., from the imminent threat of the disintegration of his/her individual being. Only thus is it possible to thematize psychopathological disorders in a non-normative way.

The concept of psychopathological disorder that puts the primary focus on the suffering from chaos cannot be normative already because, instead of the standpoint of normality or adequacy to norm, it chooses a standpoint of the extreme. From the perspective of chaos, mental disorder appears as neither a deficiency of openness, nor a privation of the ontological unity of individual existence. In comparison with the normal, socialized mode of existence, mental disorder does indeed display many deficient features, but their mere enumeration does not help us to attain an under-standing of its inner logic. Even though it does entail the loss of many possibilities, mental disorder is no mere relative disability, since it opens way for new modes of behavior that respond to the terrifying nearness of chaos. Even a disorder as severe as schizophrenia cannot be sufficiently understood merely in negative terms. The suffering of the schizophrenic manifests itself not only in the derealization and depersonalization, but mostly in a multitude of defense mechanisms that are to fore-stall the frightful onslaughts of chaos. Already the first attack of schizophrenia with its delusions and hallucinations encompasses the effort to consolidate individual being, re-establish order of experience and reconstruct a world in which one could exist. Nothing can be changed about it even in the case of paranoid schizophrenia where the individual being becomes a desperate outcast in a world full of omnipresent intrigues and threats which reflect the bottomless awesomeness of chaos. Since the familiarity with the intrigues of the pursuers and enemies that people the schizophrenic's world is merely a different expression of the awesomeness of chaos, its original sense can emerge only against the background of the uncanny awesomeness to which human existence is essentially exposed. The example of schizophrenia, more than any other, corroborates that the uncanny awesomeness of chaos allows suffering to be seen as an original phenomenon, and not merely as a privation of health.

What necessarily changes together with the image of suffering is also the image of health. Since the gaping openness of chaos makes it possible to understand that health does not mean a total absence of suffering, but is rather substantially related to it, the relation between health and suffering gains a completely new dimension. It is obvious that the effort to do away completely with suffering would, having attained its fulfillment, necessarily lead to the elimination of health, for it would create a human being who wouldn't be confronted with chaos at all, thus remaining imprisoned in one situation whose order could be neither changed, nor abandoned. However, since health proves itself not only in the tranquil and easy existence within a firmly given order, but especially in situations where the old order disintegrates, succeeded by a new one, suffering must be inseparably connected with it.

Health understood as absence of suffering or indubitable awareness of the world order is a mere caricature of health. Such a caricature can be found within the framework of Boss's psychiatric conception, where health is presented as maximal ability to respond to the significative givens of the world combined with the "bovine peace of mind," as Nietzsche would say. Since by choosing some possibilities we necessarily lose others, one cannot even say that health would be given by maximum amount of possibilities accessible for the individual.

Conceived of in the light of chaos, health appears rather as the ability to lose sense, to face non-sense, the absurdity of the world and the contingency of our existence. It is the ability to bear chaos out of which arise a new sense and order, the ability to undergo the disintegration of one's own self and reintegrate it again. To be healthy means to be able to die and be born again in the chaotic field of individuation. It is clear that health thus understood is not only permeated by suffering, but also harbors a whole plethora of traps that can turn it into unbearable suffering at any moment. The moment when the heady desire to abandon the given circumstances and one's own self turns into a total ruin of the world and self is difficult to predict and can be determined with certainty only when it is only too late.

Knowing this, it is all the more necessary to remember the rift dividing the healthy development, in which the accepted and habitual forms of thought, perception and action are destroyed, from the pathological breakdown that leads to schizophrenic derangement out of the familiar sphere of relevance and significance. Even though the schizophrenic derangement out of the sphere of meaningfulness, and thus also of a certain restraining obligation, can at first appear very inconspicuously, it still presents an essential change in the way in which human existence exposes itself to chaos. In the case of a healthy development the disruption of the established order of the world is a mere transitional phenomenon followed by the re-consolidation of the sphere of relevance and significance, whereas what occurs in the case of schizophrenic alienation is an interruption of this development.

This is why Wolfgang Blankenburg, who focused in his clinical studies especially on various forms of disorganized schizophrenia, speaks in connection with schizophrenic alienation of the loss of "natural self-evidence" (*die natürliche Selbstverständlichkeit*), in whose atmosphere the everyday being-in-the-world goes on.[2] In his opinion, "hebephrenic" patients lose the feeling of security and safety

---

[2] Blankenburg, Wolfgang. 1971. *Der Verlust der natürlichen Selbstverständlichkeit. Ein Beitrag zur Psychopatologie Symptomarmer Schizophrenien.* Stuttgart: Ferdinand Enke Verlag, 79–81.

provided by the anchoredness in the significative and referential context of the everyday world, and they behave accordingly. Restlessness and inattention, so typical of these patients, result from the disturbance of the self-evident certainty with which individual existence relates to the surrounding beings and to its close ones. The surrounding beings and people don't vanish, but rather appear in their peculiar strangeness that hampers any meaningful activity. The loss of natural self-evidence thus becomes manifest as a loss of the sense of reality, or more precisely, as a primary disturbance in concerned being-together-with beings. The total loss of being-together-with beings, however, is opposed by the effort to amend the disintegration of the significative and referential context of the everyday world by means of persistent control over every situation in which the schizophrenic finds himself/herself. The immoderate meticulousness and "neatness" which can be noticed in many schizophrenic patients are expressions of a desperate need to avoid all unexpected surprises which could evoke the invasion of chaos into the preordained order. The fact that these patients must, so to speak, pre-prepare every situation in which they find themselves, nevertheless, attests to the fragility of the provisory order of their world: this order is not something self-evident and immediately given, but something which is to be constantly re-built and defended. The referential and significative connections on which this order relies result from an intentional act which requires an enormous effort, whereas a healthy individual finds a whole order of the referential and significative connections without having to think about it explicitly.

Another risk is hidden in a self-destructive strategy of people in situations where they have no way out, where they find themselves in checkmate, as they are bound by mutually contradictory requirements. Schizophrenia then appears as a specific strategy which the individual puts into effect in a situation that cannot be endured, nor abandoned. This strategy consists in the interiorization of mutually contradictory requirements, which nevertheless leads in the end not to the overcoming of the pathogenic situation, but merely to its shift from the interpersonal to the personal level. Such a strategy can be observed in the behavior of Binswanger's patient Ilsa, who oscillates between a raving love, an almost venerating respect for her father and deep disapproval of his tyrannous way of dealing with his wife and children.[3] Since this discrepancy can be solved neither by redressing the father's behavior, nor by his abandoning the family, it becomes the discrepancy between Ilsa's mood and understanding. For her, the dissonance between understanding and mood is the fundamental existential rupture that cannot be overcome even by a desperate gesture of sacrifice (burning of arm), and thus brings about her psychotic breakdown.

Although the dissonance between mood through which the individual is thrown into the world and the understanding through which individual existence projects itself to its possibilities is felt to some extent by everyone, for it reflects our ambiguous position in the world, this discrepancy also harbors the possibility of a psychotic breakdown, which can best be explained on the temporal level of being-there where it becomes clear that the existential project involves openness to the future, whereas

[3] Binswanger. *Schizophrenie*, 3–4.

thrownness falls back into the past. The discrepancy between thrownness and existential project is thus essentially a temporal rupture, and unless individual existence overcomes it in its relation to the people around it and to beings that address it in the dimension of the present, it can precipitate even a schizophrenic disintegration of its being.

The outbreak of schizophrenia has a rather different course in the case of Binswanger's patient Suzanne Urban, whose mental collapse occurs upon her hearing about her husband's cancer. The news of her husband's incurable disease evokes in her a paranoid fear of police conspiracy and the persecution of her family. This, however, could not happen unless this woman had already been jeopardized by the uncanny awesomeness. Paranoid delusions are mere concretizations of the awesome abyss over which Suzanne Urban has insecurely balanced her whole life. If we reinterpret Binswanger's description of her life history against the background of the gaping openness of chaos, we can find the fundamental theme of this pathogenesis: it is the vulnerability to the uncanny awesomeness of chaos in which the integrity of the patient's individual being as well as the overall order of her world disintegrate. Chaos as such, however, is not the cause of this mental disorder, but rather its enabling condition. The immediate impulse that precipitated the change of Suzanne Urban's life into the "awesome stage" of madness was her husband's disease and the ensuing disintegration of the whole system of safety guarantees that were to protect her against the horrible onslaught of chaos.[4] One could say that the deadly disease of her husband shattered her hitherto considerably neurotic model of experience, which then had to be superseded by the martyrdom of paranoid schizophrenia where the awesome abyss of chaos substantiated itself.

Another example of psychotic breakdown is the fate of the 14-year-old Phillip mentioned by R. D. Laing in *Wisdom, Madness and Folly*.[5] His psychosis broke out after he had lost both his parents within a brief period of time: first, he found his mother lying in a pool of blood (she had suffered from lung tuberculosis and choked on her own blood), and 2 months later he found his father hanged, for he had not come to terms with her death. Prior to his suicide, however, he had managed persistently and repeatedly to blame his son for his mother's death, for having exhausted her during pregnancy, childbirth and throughout his whole life. This resulted in Phillip's psychotic breakdown marked by "autistic" behavior and "catatonic" stupor, at times replaced by hectic, uncoordinated motion. Phillip "was broken up, shattered to pieces by what had happened. He was staggering. He had been through a literally *staggering* experience. He was *staggered*. He had been struck – not quite *dumb*. He could utter sounds, but nothing coherent came out of his mouth. Just scraps, shreds, drivel, a sudden bellow, a moan, a laugh."[6] All this was accompanied by utter inertia to the surrounding world and permanent reek (the patient suffered also from the incontinence of urine and excrement) that escalated the

---

[4] Binswanger. *Schizophrenie*, 416–7.

[5] Laing, Ronald D. 1998. *Wisdom, Madness and Folly. The Making of a Psychiatrist 1927–57.* Edinburgh: Canongate Classics, 148–53.

[6] Laing. *Wisdom, Madness and Folly*, 150.

impression of total ruin and decline. The boy's acute psychosis had reached a degree at which the presence of the surrounding beings no longer concerned him; he himself remained utterly outside reality, whereas his body was just "a smelling reminder of his own story."

Of course, Laing concedes, it was a reactive psychosis that probably wouldn't have broken out had there not been the drastic life experience, under whose onslaught Phillip's world broke apart. Not everyone must react to a catastrophic loss by psychotic collapse. But therein lies the rub: we never know in advance where the threshold of our resistance is, how far we can go and how much we can bear. That something is beyond our strength we learn usually when it is all too late.

Yet, Phillip's case is interesting also for another reason – its happy denouement. Despite his grave diagnosis, since both his parents were probably psychotic and the boy himself was weakened so much that one could only predict chronic schizophrenic, the worst case scenario did not occur. What was to be given credit here wasn't the appropriately chosen medication, insulin or electric shocks, but the proximity of another human being despite the boy's repulsive condition. In spite of evoking the feeling of primary, pre-reflexive revulsion that distanced from him even those who wanted to take pity on him, Phillip's state was first and foremost a call for the proximity of someone else. Not for compassion, but for real proximity. Without it, Phillip could never have extricated himself from his "isolation" and gradually have attained a normal, stabilized state, which he eventually managed to do.

The very first couple of sessions in Laing's consulting room allowed the patient to re-establish after many months the contact with his surroundings and turned him into a person who quietly related his visions, hallucinations and the mysterious hyperspace in which he found himself most of the time. As Laing remarks, had this effect been achieved by means of medication without any undesirable side effects, it would present a momentous breakthrough in medical psychiatry, and the discoverer of such a drug could right away be nominated for Nobel prize. Even if it were to be discovered one day, and this day may not be too far, such a drug could never substitute for the help that a madman can be provided with by the proximity of another human being.

This is why it is of essence to consider the way in which the encounter between the mentally deranged and the therapist takes place. What is the condition and precondition of such an encounter? At the beginning there is always the doctor's confrontation with a human being displaying certain features of behavior that are perceived in the common, everyday world as unreasonable and nonsensical. In order to understand nonsensical behavior, however, it is by no means enough to take these behavioral features for pathological symptoms that refer to this or that category of the nosological system. As long as the encounter between the doctor and the patient (perceived not as an object of a therapeutic treatment, but as someone in suffering) is to take place at all, the therapist must be able to see in the mental disorder a possibility that has bearing also on himself. The therapist must be aware that what has happened to the patient can happen to anyone, for what is at work here is not some external danger, but a fundamental jeopardy that establishes and determines the character of human existence. As Caputo says, what is at stake is not to regard mental disorder as an objective process that does not pertain to us, but to understand it as a principal possibility of human existence of which the suffering patient "knows" more than the whole medical science. If the therapist really wants to approach the patient, he/she cannot do this solely with a professional erudition – what he/she needs most of all is the capacity for listening *sym-pathy* that enables him/her to discern in the psychopathological disorder the expression of the unstableness and insecurity of human existence as such. This art of sympathy needs to be distinguished from sentimental pity for the madman which does not surpass the barrier of his primordial otherness, and thus can never lead to a real proximity.

Quite special claims are made on the therapist by the care for the schizophrenic patients who don't remain within the one commonly shared world and whose behavior often gives the impression that there is no one behind it any more. These patients can be approached only if the therapist temporarily forsakes his/her own judgments about what is real or unreal, trying to transport himself/herself into the order of their experience. In claiming to have been long dead, to be unreal or threatened by hostile alien forces, the psychotic need not be wrong, but can be absolutely right, and not only in the metaphorical sense. To understand similar statements, however, it is necessary to leave the significative order of the everyday world and learn to orientate oneself within the significative structures of the schizophrenic experience. The capacity for such de- and re-orientation is, as Laing claims in his *The Divided Self*, a prerequisite indispensable for therapeutic work with psychotics.[7] Without it, all theoretical knowledge about schizophrenia as a specific illness is utterly worthless, since it does not suffice for breaking through the wall of isolation behind which the schizophrenic dwells. If, on the contrary, one manages to surmount the barrier of misunderstanding, which the schizophrenics oftentimes build for themselves in order not to jeopardize their own integrity by an open conversation with another human being, the first step toward successful cure has been taken. Similarly to Jung, Laing believes that the schizophrenics are able to consolidate and integrate their being once they have the feeling that they have encountered someone who understands their suffering. But as long he/she is to approach the schizophrenic's situation, the therapist must "draw on [his/her] own psychotic possibilities."[8]

In other words, the prerequisite for the therapist's encounter with a psychotic patient is his/her own experience with the ungraspable and uncontrollable chaos that gives him/her the opportunity to understand the behavior which appears bizarre and nonsensical in the common everyday world. Chaos is the shaky ground which eventually enables the encounter between the doctor and the patient: without having experience with chaos, the therapist couldn't approach the suffering of another human being, since he/she would lack elementary knowledge of what imbues all pathological forms of behavior with their content. This is confirmed both in the case of paranoid delusions whose structure substantially diverge from the significative context of the common world of everyday existence, as well as in the cases of "hypochondria" or pathological jealousy. Without a primary insight into the

---

[7] Laing, Ronald D. 1960. *The Divided Self*. London: Tavistock Publications.
[8] Laing. *The Divided Self*, 34.

awesome character of chaos, all these forms of experience could easily seem certain variants of fallacious understanding or error. The vulnerability to chaos in its abysmal immensity enables the realization that "hypochondria", pathological jealousy or "paranoia" have their own logic that has nothing to do with the categories of fallacy or error. The therapist himself should therefore at least once go through the disintegration of the structure of being-there that would lead him/her away from the common everyday experience to the possibility of a delirious experience, thus enabling him/her to recognize the awesomeness from which the madman strives to escape as the essential possibility of his/her own being.

But unlike the madman, the therapist must be capable of reverting from this journey back into the significative context of the everyday world, and not to repeat it hopelessly in the fear of enemies, abandonment or illness. In this respect, the therapeutic role is akin to the role of the poet who exposes himself to chaos in order to return from it to the familiarity of home. Both the poet and the therapist must set out for an unknown terrain where a new order arises out of chaos. Whereas the former does this in order to bring about a work out of chaos which shall put familiar things in an utterly new light, the latter does so in order to lead his/her neighbor out of chaos.

The similarity between the poet and the therapist that lies in the necessity to advance beyond the boundaries of the familiar world and to experience the excess of awesomeness did not remain hidden to Binswanger, although he did not manage to grasp the openness of chaos as such. He was also well aware of the significance that the knowledge of the Awesome and the Annihilating to which the madman is exposed in his/her whole existence has within the field of psychotherapeutic communication.[9] As long as we renounce the idea of the principal ontological unity of individual being borne by the unity of the three temporal ecstasies, not speaking of the concept of the infinite moment of being-beyond-the-world, we can thus use a certain part of Binswanger's clinical observations as documentary material.

What is clear from Binswanger's description of paranoid schizophrenia is that paranoid systems of delusions cannot be sufficiently explained as mere products of lively unrestricted fantasy, but rather must be perceived against the background of that to which the schizophrenic is exposed, that is, the awesome and annihilating chaos. The pathological nature of the fear of omnipresent chasers lies not so much in its exorbitance or inappropriateness to the real circumstances as in the overall atmosphere of jeopardy and danger that ensue from the awesomeness of chaos. Conspiracy, persecution and sadistic orgies prepared by one's enemies are not primary in their essence; the irrefutable certainty with which the schizophrenics expound on their theories of conspiracy and persecution is merely a secondary moment of the disruption and disintegration of the order of their experience. The role of paranoid delusions consists in covering and filling up the holes that arise once the order of experience has fallen into chaos. The need to reintegrate the disintegrating order of experience leads the schizophrenic to constructions by means of which the uncanny awesomeness of chaos changes into the impending presence of

---

[9] Binswanger. *Schizophrenie*, 435–6. Binswanger. *Der Mensch in der Psychiatrie*, 32–3.

the Enemy. What follows in lieu of the indefinably and unutterably awesome are the "well known" intentions of thieves and murderers. In this way, the inconsistency of experience turns into the absolute consistency of a delusion.

However, since the disintegration of the order of experience is accompanied not only by the collapse of the significative structure of the world, but also by the breakup of individual being, it is at least inaccurate to speak here of some individual who would construe paranoid systems of delusions. The paranoid "I" itself is rather the product of the integration of chaos, and thus one can in such cases speak not of an individual, but only of an experience of the disintegration of the world and individual being from which the attempts to reconstruct the world and reintegrate individual being set out. Nevertheless, even if the overall order of the world has been at least partially reconstructed and individual being reintegrated within the frame of the paranoid system of delusions, the schizophrenic still cannot escape the uncanny awesomeness of chaos in this way. A world in which one must constantly be on guard against the murderous designs of enemies, a world where no one can be trusted, cannot be a safe home. Despite the alleviation of the suffering and the relative stabilization incurred by the paranoid phase of madness, the schizophrenic experience is reminiscent of a barge that can at any time sink in the endless sea of chaos. Such is the case of Binswanger's patient Lola Voss who suffered not only from "paranoia", but also from superstition and fear of changing clothes: since her existence was shaken and disrupted to its very ground, she had to seek support in her clothing that could at least provide her with a semblance of stability and constancy. Any change of clothes, on the other hand, presented to her a threat of the annihilating onslaught of chaos in which both the order of her world and her individual being would perish.[10]

How far can a description of a pathological experience go, which departs from the abysmal openness of chaos where attempts at reconstructing the world and individual being take place, can be illustrated by the last stages of schizophrenia. In such cases human existence capitulates to the annihilating force of chaos that shatters the significative structure of the world and the integral constitution of individual being. The desperate attempts at escaping chaos, during which the schizophrenic becomes the more fatigued the more he/she strives for maintaining at least a sham order, end in a total exhaustion. Afterward, there is nothing to prevent the end of the world and the disintegration of individual being, since the schizophrenic loses any relation to the present reality and the temporal unity of his/her existence breaks apart in the non-connectible having-been and future. The essence of these forms of schizophrenia thus lies not only in the loss of the sense of reality, but rather in the overall disintegration of the ecstatic unity of temporality. A resignation to maintain the integral unity of the three temporal ecstasies also stands in the background of the decomposition of individual being, referred to in the clinical jargon as "personality dissociation".

Once the overall disintegration of the ecstatic unity of temporality has occurred, it has little sense to refer to the difference between authentic and inauthentic

---

[10] Binswanger. *Schizophrenie*, 323.

existence as thematized in *Sein und Zeit*. Both authentic and inauthentic existence present merely two different modes of temporalization of the ecstatic unity of temporality; however, a schizophrenic breakdown of individual being which becomes consummated in the emptying out of existence or in the catatonic torpor cannot be thematized on the basis of the indivisible temporal unity of being-there, unless we don't want to settle for "explaining" it as a privative form of the original unity of individual existence.

As long as the schizophrenic undergoes the disintegration of the ecstatic unity of temporality, it still does not mean that his/her being-there changes definitively into no-longer-being-there. One must rather understand that even the schizophrenic existence, whose temporal unity has completely fallen apart, can still integrate its individual being and re-unite the order of its experience. In order to conceive of that, it is necessary to undertake a re-description of the openness of being to which human existence essentially belongs, and to describe it as the gaping openness of chaos.

The adumbrated re-description of being in openness requires, among other things, a change in the understanding of the finitude of being-there. As long as the clearing of being is thematized as the gaping openness of chaos, one can abandon the conception of finitude that ties death with the final exit into the all-negating concealment and conceive of the finitude of being-there as vulnerability to chaos in which both the temporal unity of individual being and the structured order of experience fall apart.

Not until the finitude of human existence is seen in its essential belonging to chaos is it possible to explain why even a totally burnt-out schizophrenic can temporarily or even permanently unify his/her disintegrated individual being and reorganize the order of his/her experience so as to render it accessible to other people as well. Such a return from the "realm of the dead" proves that death is not only the extreme, not-to-be-bypassed possibility to which we relate with understanding. Insofar as the individual existence is becoming dead whenever its individuality disintegrates and the structured order of its experience breaks down, death has not a singular, but rather a plural character. In its belonging to chaos, the human existence is becoming dead, time and again. Its becoming-dead – which is not the same as being dead – is therefore to be sharply distinguished from dying, which is thematized on the basis of the temporal unity of being-there, as is the case in *Sein und Zeit* where Heidegger understands dying in the light of the phenomenological structure of care.

Unlike the existential analysis which displays dying on the ground of the indivisible ontological constitution of care, the post-existential analysis combines the process of becoming-dead with the gradual disintegration of this ontological constitution. The relation to death is thus no longer subjected to the ontological structure of being-there, but rather this ontological structure is subjected to death understood as the breakdown of the ecstatic unity of temporality. From the viewpoint of the post-existential analysis, an individual who is dying is not *the one who understands* death as his/her very own possibility. A dying man does not relate to death as an existing individual relating to his extreme and ultimate possibility, but rather is absorbed by it without the slightest distance. Of course this does not mean that he wouldn't know about it; his understanding, however, is part of an overall disintegration of experience that occurs in the framework of the process of dying.

This shift in the understanding of dying and death must also be felt in the new conception of the process of individuation. Its vanishing point can no longer be death understood as one's very own and ultimate possibility of individual existence, but chaos, in which human existence repeatedly encounters death. As the fundamental constant that determines human existence not only in its pathological states, but also in the moment of creative and intellectual search, chaos can be defined as a "field of individuation." Individuation, which occurs in the boundless and ungraspable chaos, is not a moment of a constant individual being that finds the way out of the public space of the everyday world back to itself, but on the contrary a moment of the disintegrated individual being torn between the having-been and the future, having to cling to something present in order to consolidate itself. Inasmuch as individuation is to be something more than a mere turning-away from the familiar beings and a return to one's own being, individuation must contain a moment of disintegration and the subsequent reintegration of individual being.

Individuation thus understood harbors not only the risk of utter self-destruction, but also the hope of salvation for those who have lost their individual being and their familiar home. This applies, among others, to schizophrenics who are suddenly brought out of their closedness and regress into it after a while of common coexistence with others. In his *Wisdom, Madness and Folly*, Laing thus describes unapproachable, catatonic schizophrenics who interrupt their motionless lethargy once a year in order to wish each other a happy new year and return to their original state.[11]

This extreme case alone suggests the importance of the role of another human being in the process of individuation. It is the other who can be the decisive factor in enabling the mentally ill to regain the relation to the temporal dimension of the present, and thus to re-consolidate his/her disrupted or shaken individual being. The other is not only a part of the existential being-with others that links being-there to people by the bond of mutual solicitude, but also the one who opens for being-there the dimension of the present and together with it the way to its own individual being. This is confirmed both by the story of Phillip, whom the presence of the other helped to wake up from a total psychotic breakdown, and by the case of another one of Laing's patients whose individual being was secured only when she felt the presence of someone who cared about her. Without it, she relapsed into abysmal anxiety in which her insecurely constituted individual being was jeopardized by the deepening depersonalization.[12] In general, one can say that something similar applies also to small children whose individual being has not been firmly constituted quite yet and who need the presence of another human being in order to create it. One need not specify that the other *par excellence* in this connection is the mother. As Laing observes:

---

[11] Laing. *Wisdom, Madness and Folly*, 31–2.
[12] Laing. *The Divided Self*, 54–8, 119.

It seems that loss of the mother, at a certain stage, threatens the individual with loss of his self. The mother, however, is not simply a *thing* which the child can see, but a *person* who sees the child. Therefore, we suggest that a necessary component in the development of the self is the experience of oneself as a person under the loving eye of the mother.[13]

Just as the other – whether the mother or the father – is a prerequisite of the child's individuation, the other is also the one who mediates for the child the world by bring an elementary order into the chaotic experience.

The mother and father greatly simplify the world for the young child, and as his capacity grows to make sense, to inform chaos with pattern, to grasp distinctions and connexions of greater and greater complexity, so, as Buber puts it, he is led out into 'a feasible world.'[14]

What is at stake in connection with the gradual modulation of the small child's experience is not only the factual presence of mother and father, but rather the 'family' as a whole structure of interpersonal relations that form in a certain way our being-with others. The 'family', as Laing shows in his *The Politics of the Family*, is not only a community of a few relatives, but rather a formal structure of being-with others that determines the very foundations of existence of every single one of its members.[15] Family thus understood is accordingly not abandoned by an individual even if he/she becomes physically remote from his/her relatives. In moments of physical absence of others, the fundamental structure of the familial being-with others can actually manifest itself to being-there much more clearly than ever before, or the individual can further reproduce it without becoming explicitly aware of it.

Yet, even this structure of being-with others can be abandoned, although not simply by leaving the parent's house and beginning to live on one's own. To gain independence, it is necessary in the first place to break through the virtual structure of coexistence with others presented by the 'family'. This step, however, is quite risky, since outside of the family there is no solitary being-in-the-world to which being-there could simply return in order to find the source of the original uniqueness of its own individual being. What is rather the case is that individual being is possible only within the frame of being-with others, whether it takes form of the family in the narrow sense of the word or of a family such as the Church, a political party or other community. One can say of all these forms of coexistence what Laing says of 'family', i.e. that "the preservation of the 'family' is equated with the preservation of self and world and the dissolution of the 'family' inside *another* is equated with death of self and world-collapse."[16] To step out of the binding structures of 'family' or to transform them into some looser form is thus possible only by transcending oneself, by disrupting the overall unity of individual being and the structured order of one's own world. As long as the familial constellation of being-with others determines who being-there is in its individual being and what is the order of its

---

[13] Laing. *The Divided Self*, 116.

[14] Laing. *The Divided Self*, 189.

[15] Laing, Ronald D. 1971. *The Politics of Experience*. Harmondsworth: Penguin Books, 4–5.

[16] Laing. *The Politics of Experience*, 14.

world, the abandonment of 'family' precipitates the disruption in the integral individual being and the annihilation of the integrated order of the world.

What is also clear here is that such a disruption affects not only the one who leaves the established familial structures of being-with others, but all others who participate in these structures. It is also their own being and the order of their experience that are shaken by this disruption, and unless they are to totally break down they must undergo a momentous transformation.

The renovation of the lost integrity of individual being and a new arrangement of the disintegrated world order are all the more necessary for someone who has set out outside of the frame of familial coexistence. Lest the abandonment of 'family' should turn into utter self-destruction, being-there must reintegrate its individual being and create a new order of world, which is only possible through the discovery of a new form of being-with others. A primary example of a process in which all this happens at once is pubescence, and it is no coincidence that a vast amount of schizophrenic cases occur precisely in this complicated life period.

What consequences there are to the disruption or blockage of the process in which being-there strives to break free from the familial structures of being-with others, from the established order of the world, and from its old self in order to find it all in a new form, can best be illustrated by the casuistry of a 26-year-old schizophrenic Julia, characterized in *The Divided Self* as a chronic schizophrenic of the catatonic-hebephrenic type.[17] Since this girl did not manage to break free from the binding family patterns, nor was she able to bear their suffocating weight any more, a collapse occurred in which both the structure of her being-with others and the overall order of her experience perished along with the integral structure of her individual being.

When Laing meets Julia, her individual being has already disintegrated so much as to give the impression that there is "no one behind" her bizarre behavior and incomprehensible statements, that there is nothing that would provide them with an intentional unity and personal integrity. Her ways of speech, intonation and gesticulation change at any time without the slightest possibility of unveiling what it is that mutually links the incongruous pieces of speech, gestures and attitudes. It seems rather that what is at work in them instead of one individual being is several fragmentary, mutually independent "personas" distinguished by diction, intonation and behavior. As Laing observes, to communicate with Julia is similar to doing "group therapy with the one patient." In her behavior and expression, several quasi-autonomous systems of experience are palpable, with each of them having its own focus and its own "self." What develops here in lieu of one integrated individual being are a number of fragmentary foci of experience, each of which perceives itself as a "self" and others as "non-self." A set of these fragmentary "selves" creates a conglomerate of heterogeneous systems of experience that enter into a mutual, oftentimes agonistic interaction. The mutual interaction of partial systems of experience has no higher unity: although one fragmentary "self" can relate to another one, it can never permeate the system of its experience and become aware of what

---

[17] Laing. *The Divided Self*, 178–205.

the other "self" experiences. In its essence, the inner relation between two partial systems of experience is disjunctive.

According to Laing, what occurs in Julia apart from the "molar" fission of the unity of being within whose framework Julia's individual being dissipates into a multitude of fragmentary "personas" is also the "molecular" cleavage that disrupts every continuous succession of perceptions, actions and even breaks apart the grammatical coherence of words. Even though some of the many partial personas can express themselves in a relatively coherent and prudent way, they all eventually fall apart into utterly inconsistent, chaotic utterances. All this approaches the state which Laing, referring to William Blake, describes as "chaotic nonentity." This chaotic state, in his opinion, is marked by a total disintegration of individual being, in which there is no trace of unity or constancy.

> In its final form, such complete disintegration is a hypothetical state which has no verbal equivalents. We feel justified, however, in postulating such a hypothetical condition. In its most extreme form it is perhaps not compatible with life. The thoroughly dilapidated, chronic catatonic-hebephrenic is presumably the person in whom this process has gone on to the most extreme degree in one who remains biologically viable.[18]

It can thus be said of Julia that her state approximates "chaotic nonentity." Just as other schizophrenics of the hebephrenic-catatonic type, she reaches the phase of existential death where nothing happens, where there is no graspable possibility, no present. Unlike paranoid schizophrenics in whom the elementary integrity of individual being still persists, the schizophrenics of the hebephrenic-catatonic type "find" themselves in a stage described by Laing as "death-in-life."

Not even the state of total disintegration, however, must necessarily be once and for all irreversible and fossilized. Even Julia, as if by a miracle, can sometimes "pull herself together" and consolidate her individual being, even though she fears doing so, for the repeated disintegration means for her an unspeakably terrible experience. Rather than the repeated attempts at reintegrating her individual being, what is more bearable for "her" is the state of existential death, of unreality and disintegration in which she survives only within the framework of interaction of mutually disparate systems of experience.

Each of these systems has "within it its own focus or centre of awareness; it [has] its own very limited memory schemata and limited ways of structuring percepts; its own quasi-autonomous drives or component drives; its own tendency to preserve its autonomy, and special dangers which [threaten] its autonomy."[19] What, on the other hand, Julia lacks is a reflexive self-awareness and long-term memory, i.e. all the functions that depend on the overall unity of individual being. The impossibility of reflexive relation to one's being as well as the correlated impossibility of relation to one's having-been are also reflected in the very vague consciousness of one's own limits. Insofar as it has no relation to its own being, being-there is permanently threatened by the possibility of confusing itself with what it relates to at the moment.

---

[18] Laing. *The Divided Self*, 162–3.
[19] Laing. *The Divided Self*, 198.

Not clearly defined against her surrounding and freely identifying herself with the perceived objects and other people, Julia can be virtually whatever or whoever. Her existence cannot therefore have a singular character. As she states herself: "I'm thousands. I'm an in divide you all. I'm a no un." [20]

Such a plural mode of existence won't be comprehended, as long as we regard it as some privation of one integral individual being. The "split states of being," on the contrary, must be seen in and out of themselves, i.e. in their specific multiplicity that only makes it possible to penetrate into the logic of partial systems of experience, into their autonomous functioning and mutual relations. These autonomous systems of experience, each of which has its own focus and center of awareness, create an incessant conglomerate of relations whose only external boundary is chaos that dissolves all consistency. The relative stability of partial systems of experience and unsteady balance of their mutual relations are related not to some atomic or implicit individual being, but to the all-shaking chaos. As long as partial systems of experience establish at least an elementary order, it is only at the cost of an unremitting confrontation with chaos.

Therefore, we must go even further than Laing who still regards the schizophrenic experience from the perspective of an integral, independent individual being instead of thematizing it against the background of that "chaotic nonentity" in which all sense and order disintegrate and get reborn. Even he is not yet able to explicate the schizophrenic experience in the light of a total disintegration of individual being, constantly reverting to the individualistic conception of unity which schizophrenics fail to realize. Despite the exact description of partial systems and fragmentary foci of experience as presented in *The Divided Self*, the existential approach to mental disorder is still at work here, which is why chaotic nonentity is accepted merely as a hypothetical limit, and not as the ontological ground and the enabling condition of a schizophrenic disintegration of individual being. The post-existential analysis of being-there, on the contrary, leads to the realization that chaos in which all unity and integrity of individual being vanish is the condition enabling the breakout not only of disorganized schizophrenia, but also of all other forms of this illness.

This is in a way corroborated also by Blankenburg's clinical studies in which, apart from the disorganized form of schizophrenia, the focus is the so-called *schizophrenia simplex*, i.e. a disorder in which no paranoid systems of delusions but merely the derangement from the order of the everyday being-in-the-world and the lapse of its natural self-evidence occur. Unlike paranoid schizophrenia, *schizophrenia simplex* is marked by the fact that although it disrupts one's own rootedness in the significative context of the everyday world, this disruption is not covered by means of the rigid structure of delusions, but rather revealed in its naked form. This "pre-paranoid" alienation thus opens up a way toward understanding the very foundations of schizophrenic illness. Although it is a relatively rare form of schizophrenic alienation, Blankenburg sees in it the matrix and enabling condition for schizophrenia as such. It is only in its light that one can, in his opinion, adequately

---

[20] Laing. *The Divided Self*, 204.

elucidate both the creation of paranoid delusions and the origin of schizophrenic detachment from the world.

The "loss" of natural self-evidence that lies in the heart of schizophrenic alienation, however, does not mean any deprivation in the sense of privation. As Blankenburg never fails to emphasize, the non-self-evidence of being-in-the-world is not opposed to the natural self-evidence as its deficiency.[21] Its non-self-evidence and insecurity are as constitutive of being-in-the-world as the self-evidence and security of the order in which being-there safely orientates itself.[22]

From the viewpoint of post-existential analysis, the same is true also for the disintegration of individual being tied to the loss of natural self-evidence of being-in-the-world: whereas the firm order of the everyday being-in-the-world provides the individual being with support, a breach in this order disrupts the unity of individual being and ruins its integrity. Hence, every imperilment of the familiar order of the world entails also the threat to the integrity and constancy of individual being, of which all mentally ill individuals are more or less aware. This implies that the loss of natural self-evidence in whose atmosphere being-there becomes familiar with the referential and significative order of its world ontologically enables not only schizophrenia, but a whole range of other psychopathological disorders.

That this is the case can be illustrated by the example of individuals with the schizoid personality disorder whose behavior is described in Laing's *The Divided Self*. Even though in these cases the loss of natural self-evidence does not reach the same degree as in schizophrenic alienation, they are still marked by the feeling that the individual existence is not sufficiently settled in the world and is not "at home" there. Despite not being exposed to the immediate breakup of individual being, the schizoid individuals experience an incessant jeopardy of their being. Neither the surrounding world nor their close ones evoke in them the feeling of primary safety and security, but on the contrary expose their individual being to the threat of being devoured and dissolved in the chaotic nonentity. In a world they share together with others lurks the fear of the fall into chaos and of the loss of the individual being.

What characterizes the schizoid personality disorder is "ontological insecurity" in which the post-existential analysis detects the vulnerability to chaos full of suffering. This ontological insecurity forces being-there to take various safety measures that are to protect its individual being from the fall into chaos. The schizoid personality strives to evade anything that could deepen the state of primary ontological insecurity. This pertains especially to the relation with other people from which the schizoid personality withdraws into itself, dealing with mere unsubstantial specters and phantasmal illusions rather than with their real presence, for they are the only ones it lets in through the ramparts of its fortress. Nevertheless, not even the voluntary isolation into which the schizoid person closes itself off can save the individual being in the state of ontological insecurity. Even though he/she is ready to renounce all but his/her individual being, it is a tragic paradox that the schizoid person destroys more of his/her individual being the more he/she distances himself/herslef

---

[21] Blankenburg. *Der Verlust der Natürlichen Selbstverständlichkeit*, 58.

[22] Blankenburg. *Der Verlust der Natürlichen Selbstverständlichkeit*, 58.

from those around him/her and their shared world. For without a real relation to others and the world, individual being gradually disintegrates, eventually reaching the point of a complete schizophrenic breakdown.

When analyzing the way the schizoid person gradually approaches the schizophrenic state, Laing notices various defense mechanisms that are meant to protect the imperiled individual being, while actually devastating it the most. In the relation to other people, it is especially the above-mentioned withdrawal into isolation opted for by the individual in the state of ontological insecurity in order not to become wholly devoured by the claims and feelings of others.[23] The fear of becoming wholly absorbed by others coerces schizoid personality to pull away from them and remain in total solitude. The same effect is that of a fear of implosion, i.e. of others devouring the schizoid person like gas filling the vacuum. Apart from recoiling into isolation, an individual suffering from such fears can also use the so-called petrifaction strategy. It is based on the decision to regard the other as a mere thing, as some "it," and treat it accordingly. It is a means to rid oneself of the disturbing presence of the other and of the responsibility for the other's feelings. This depersonalization and reification of the other is to prevent the other from doing the same: afraid of becoming devoid of his/her personal sovereignty, the schizoid person must neutralize others before they neutralize him/her. In order not to become a thing for the other, he/she must rid the other of all personal status and change the other into a thing. However, this strategy results in a situation in which there is no one left who could confirm the fact of the schizoid's existence by acknowledging his/her unique personality. Since being-there cannot maintain its individual being without relating to those around it who respect it as a unique and independent person, the schizoid person loses even the much sought-after certainty of himself/herself. In the absolute solitude, he/she cannot at all preserve the integrity of his/her own individual being.

Pathogenesis, within which human existence advances from the schizoid position to the schizophrenic disintegration of individual being, also encompasses the construction of a false "self" that the schizoid person shows others as a mask hiding his/her true face. To remain unrecognized is for him/her to remain safe. That is the reason why he/she creates a false "self" which he/she allows to perceive and act, while remaining an unaffected observer. His/her own individual being remains aloof and untouchable, for there is nothing "out there" that concerns him/her. The schizoid person holds everything at a distance. Instead of perceiving and acting spontaneously in a world shared together with others, the schizoid person becomes enclosed in himself/herself, which allows him/her to gain absolute control over himself/herself and to indulge imperturbably in his/her own fantasies.

As he/she withdraws his/her individual being from the world and leaving all action up to the false "self," his/her individual being becomes gradually derealized. As long as his/her only activity lies in aloof observation connected with fantasy, the schizoid person cannot preserve a living relation with the real present, since he/she never really encounters it. The schizoid individual being relates to the world merely by means of a false "self" which it has created so that it may live instead of it in the

---

[23] Laing. *The Divided Self*, 43–9.

real presence of things and others. Without a direct relation to things and people, however, even the integrity of individual being cannot last for long. Even though individual being, in its detachment from the real present, enjoys a seemingly boundless freedom, it is merely an empty powerlessness in which it has nothing to hold on to, and thus inevitably disintegrates. In the end, the schizoid person cannot preserve even the uncertain integrity of individual being which he/she has striven to save from dissolution in the chaotic nonentity. Hence, the only possible way of evading a schizophrenic breakdown is to enter directly into the world shared with others, even though it means to accept the ontological insecurity that reflects the contingency and finitude of human existence.

In this connection, it must be noted that ontological insecurity is not only something pathological. The state of ontological insecurity as reflected in the consciousness of the ambiguity, inconsistency and disarray of our world and of our position therein, does not mean only the pathological disturbance in the unshakeable ontological certainty, as Laing sometimes implies.[24] Ambiguity, inconsistency and disarray belong to being-in-the-world as fundamental expressions of its insecurity and unanchoredness. Ontological insecurity that unveils our vulnerability to chaos has its irreplaceable place wherever a fundamental problematization of individual existence occurs, with its decontextualization and consequent re-contextualization, with the creative search for the meaning of being, albeit at the cost of the threat of one's own ruin.

What is definitely not at stake here is to exclude every vestige of chaos out of the world and render it a place of perfect order. That would merely attest to the neurotic effort to attain absolute safety, peace and harmony. Real health lies rather in the ability to bear danger, suffering and disharmony that form an irreplaceable part of human existence.

Whereas true health always encompasses the possibility of abnormal behavior whose sense escapes not only others, but the acting agent himself, the schizoid individual can behave in an utterly normal, socialized way. His/her semblance of health is concentrated around the system of the false "self" that expresses itself as one is expected to behave in a given situation. As Laing says: "We see a model child, an ideal husband, an industrious clerk."[25] What lies behind this façade, however, is a schizoid personality who secretly hates the false "self" with all its social adaptability. Once the hate for the false "self" has surfaced, its outburst that destroys the system of the false "self" often involves accusing people, to whom the schizoid person has subjected himself/herself for many years in his/her outward behavior, of trying to kill him/her, of intending to steal his/her soul or brain. In such cases, one speaks of a sudden outbreak of psychosis, inexplicable by the external circumstances.

There is also the possibility of a long latent stage of mental disorder during which the schizoid individual remains seemingly healthy, although his/her behavior becomes increasingly stereotypical. The normality of behavior is paid for by

---

[24] Laing. *The Divided Self*, 39, 42.

[25] Laing. *The Divided Self*, 99.

permanent hypocrisy in which individual being hides behind the action of the false "self" without identifying with it. One of Laing's patients who seemed to live quite an ordinary life reached in his schizoid state the point where he wasn't able to have intercourse with his wife, but only with his idea of her: when making love with her, his hidden individual being merely watched what he was doing or imagined having sex with his wife as the object of his imagination.[26] Not even in the moment of greatest physical proximity and intimacy was this patient able to bring his individual being out of isolation. Without her having the slightest idea about it, his wife was a mere object of imagination for him to which he wasn't connected by any real bond.

The problem of Laing's patient also points to another important aspect of the schizoid personality disorder, namely the bodily experience. When withdrawing from the world, the schizoid person adopts also a distanced attitude to his/her own body. One's own body is no longer the point of departure of one's experience. The individual being does not participate in any physical activities, reserving for itself the purely spiritual sphere in which it can exist without any restriction that follows from the human corporeality. All bodily functions, whether perception- or action-based, are left over to the false "self" which takes responsibility for them. Whereas the false "self" realizes itself in connection with the body, one's own individual being remains bodiless. Not incarnated, the schizoid individual perceives his/her body as that which does not belong to him/her, or he/she perceives it only in an arbitrary way. As Laing notes in this connection, "the body is felt more as one object among other objects in the world than as the core of the individual's own being."[27] What thus occurs is the depersonalization which can lead as far as to make one consider one's own body a mechanic object or a pre-programmed automaton. The depersonalization of the body is the inevitable result that arises from a process in which the disembodied spiritual self is placed on the one side and the corporeality maintained by the system of the false "self" on the other.

In this respect, it remains a question whether the depersonalization of one's own body experienced by the schizoid person can be interpreted as a pathological phenomenon as long as one uses a theory relying on the model of the somatic apparatus and conceiving of the human body as a complex machine. Laing summarizes this dilemma very concisely: "A man who says that men are machines may be a great scientist. A man who says he *is* a machine is 'depersonalized' in psychiatric jargon."[28] But how more insane is he who severs his spiritual self from his body, from the community with others and from the world, than a conception that divides the soul from the body, from the community with others and from the commonly shared world, in order to regard it a subject against a sphere of objects? Is not the Cartesian view of human existence actually the expression of the schizoid position of thought? In any case, the Cartesian division of the body and the soul can barely contribute to an understanding of the schizoid dissociation of body and self, since it offers nothing that would show its inner disputability and existential untenability.

---

[26] Laing. *The Divided Self*, 86.
[27] Laing. *The Divided Self*, 69.
[28] Laing. *The Divided Self*, 12.

An adequate explication of the schizoid position requires the thematization of the complex connection of the bodily being and individual being. For even the catatonic schizophrenic is not reduced to a mere corporeal thing (*der Körper*), but rather undergoes an extreme change in his/her lived body that belongs to his being-in-the-world.

Although the phenomenological thematization of the lived body (*der Leib*) offers in this respect a much better way of understanding than the Cartesian schism of *res extensa* and *res cogitans*, it still cannot be quite sufficient as long as it restricts the bodily being to the realm of sensory perceptions and turns the understanding of being into a matter of pure contemplation. As Heidegger states in *Zollikoner Seminare*, the lived body does not participate in the understanding of being, for that is only a matter of pure thought. Once, however, the performance of the lived body is reduced only to the realm of the everyday being-in-the-world and to the relation to what appears within the context of its familiar order, it is practically impossible to understand such phenomena such as hallucinations, which present an important factor of a schizophrenic breakdown.

Hallucinations and delusions which pervade the schizophrenic experience cannot be judged by the categories of fallacy or illusion, nor is it sufficient to understand them as expressions of a deficient openness to the sensual givens of the everyday world. The hallucinating schizophrenic is transposed out of the significative context of the everyday world and at the same time extremely desocialized, which prevents him/her from correcting his/her own experience according to the experience of others. This leads to the disintegration of the structured order of experience, to the shattering of the arranged existential space, where what is nearby is distinguished from what is remote, what is present from what is absent, what is large from what is small. Instead of the delimited world governed by direct lines and distinct proportions, the schizophrenic lands in a boundless space, where the lines freely cross each other, things suddenly change their position and sounds come out of nowhere. All that is permeated by the atmosphere of unidentifiable peril and uncanny awesomeness, which supplant familiarity with the firm order of the everyday world. In sum, the derailment from the significative context of the everyday world and the correlated desocialization throw experience into chaos where even the most elementary certainties cease to be valid. The deeper the world falls into the uncanny awesomeness of chaos, the more desperately the schizophrenic strives to hold on to anything offered to him/her, regardless of whether it is perceived by others, or not. Thus, hallucinations originate neither in fallacious sensory perception, nor in falling prey to the appearing givens of the world, but spring from the openness of chaos to which the schizophrenic is exposed.

Hallucinations are at the same time a clear proof of the fact that chaos has both a mental and a physical "reality" (as long as we comprehend it in the sense of φύσις). Even though chaos is not given as something present, it is never only the pure thought, but also sensuality that is influenced by it. Chaos as such cannot be seen or heard, but it still affects our senses through beings that lose their sense, shape and consistency. A confrontation with chaos therefore necessarily evolves upon the "psychosomatic" level. As long as chaos dissolves all cohesion, it must be there that the disintegration of thought as well as the disintegration of the lived body take place. The bodily disintegration is reflected in the breakdown of the overall unity of sensual spheres, which is grounded in the ecstatic unity of temporality. We know that the open unity of sensual spheres, in which the performance of the lived body is realized, is borne by the temporal unity of being in openness. Whereas under normal circumstances, the overall unity of sensual spheres is guaranteed by the ecstatic unity of temporality, outside of the frame of common everydayness this is no longer the case, since the integral unity of temporality is here exposed to chaos in which it disintegrates. Since chaos opens itself as a bottomless abyss of the having-been and the future, the ecstatic unity of temporality falls apart therein and the sensual unity of experience disintegrates. This is not only the enabling condition of schizophrenic hallucinations, but also the very substance of suffering to which the lived body is essentially exposed. Therefore one can say together with Laing that in fact we are all 2 or 3° C away from the psychotic type of experience: "Even a slight fever, and the whole world can begin to take on a persecutory, impinging aspect."[29]

How deeply the lived body is imbued with suffering that disintegrates its sensual unity is also confirmed by the phenomena of panic and vertigo, which in themselves need not be of a pathological character. If in panic we are seized by chaos, then in vertigo we look straight into the abysmal depth of the having-been and the future that gapes underneath us. What appears within the frame of disintegration of the lived body are, nonetheless, also the phenomena of ecstasy and physical pleasure. The disintegrated unity of the lived body is a field of not only suffering, but also of passion and ecstasy that transport our existence out of common everydayness. Related to this rapture is the process of desocialization in which the our existence abandons its learned roles and its normalized being-with others. Nevertheless, desocialization is certainly not a path toward a lone being of an individualized existence, for what occurs in its course is not only the disintegration of the lived body, but also the decomposition of integral individual being. Already for this reason it is necessary that the destabilization of the lived body should be followed by a phase of reconsolidation. Unless the disintegration of the lived body is to degenerate into a self-destructive fall into the gaping chaos, a germ of a new reintegration must be included therein from the start. The peril of too radical or too sudden disintegration that may throw the lived body into the all-destroying chaos is nevertheless still actual.

All these phenomena remain necessarily veiled as long as Heidegger sets aside the lived body from the immediate relation to the clearing of being. While he holds the opinion in *Zollikoner Seminare* that the understanding of being does not have its correlate in the lived body, and thus renews the Cartesian schism of sensuality and pure contemplation, the theme of chaos makes it possible to definitively overcome the difference between the body and the soul, and at the same time to understand how our belonging to the openness of being bears upon the schema of the lived body. The gaping openness of chaos is a field where the disintegration and ensuing

---

[29] Laing. *The Divided Self*, 46.

reintegration of the unity of sensual spheres forming the lived body take place. As such, chaos is the source of both extreme suffering and extremely cheerful ecstasy.

Only with chaos explicated as a gaping openness to which our existence essentially belongs can *Leiblichkeit* be seen in its contingency and finitude, in its vulnerability and mortality. It is also in this phenomenal sphere that the sense of such phenomena as old age and aging is to be sought.

Despite having written numerous pages of meditations on the finitude of human existence that manifests itself as being-toward-death, Heidegger has unfortunately left the phenomena of aging and old age practically without mention. What sense, however, does it have to speak of being-toward-death, if old age and fatigue from existence are not tied to it? Unless being-toward-death is to remain a merely formal determinative of our existence, one must add to it the understanding of how the performance of this existence is burdened by the vulnerability to chaos. Aging is not only a question of irreversible physiological changes in the organism; it is much rather a certain relation to the openness of chaos to which human existence essentially belongs.

This uncertain and unstable relation to chaos is described by Deleuze and Guattari in their *Qu'est-ce que la philosophie?*, where they argue that old age can take two forms: either a fall into a mental and sensual chaos, or a fossilization in the ready-made opinions, attitudes and habits, in which fatigued thought seeks shelter from chaos.[30] This is to say that old age is simply not given by many years of living, but that it follows from fatigue, marked either by a fossilization of opinion and clinging to established habits, or by senile dementia as a gradual breakup of the integrity of individual being. Both these possibilities don't pertain to only people advanced in age, but relate also to the young to whom fatigue shows the limits of their capacities. That is why Kraepelin could with some justification label schizophrenia as *dementia praecox*. However, just as in the case of psychopathological disorders, old age is not only a deficient form of youth. The true sense and meaning of old age can be understood once we have ceased to consider it as a privation of youth, regarding it instead on the background of chaos, in which our being and thought come to their end.

References

1. Binswanger, Ludwig. 1957. *Schizophrenie*. Pfullingen: Neske.
2. Binswanger, Ludwig. 1957. *Der Mensch in der Psychiatrie*. Pfullingen: Neske.
3. Blankenburg, Wolfgang. 1971. *Der Verlust der natürlichen Selbstverständlichkeit. Ein Beitrag zur Psychopatologie symptomarmer Schizophrenien*. Stuttgart: Ferdinand Enke Verlag.
4. Caputo, John D. 2000. *More radical hermeneutics: On not knowing who we are*. Bloomington/Indianapolis: Indiana University Press.

---

[30] Deleuze, and Guattari. *Qu'est-ce que la philosophie?*, 187.

 5. Deleuze, Gilles, and Félix Guattari. 1991. *Qu'est- ce que la philosophie?* Paris: Minuit. English edition: Deleuze, Gilles, and Félix Guattari. 1994. *What is Philosophy?* Trans. Hugh Tomlison and Graham Burchill. New York: Columbia University Press.
 6. Heidegger, Martin. 1951. *Erläuterungen zu Hölderlins Dichtung.* Frankfurt am Main: Vittorio Klostermann. English edition: Heidegger, Martin. 2000. *Elucidations of Hölderlin's Poetry.* Trans. Keith Hoeller. New York: Humanity Books.
 7. Heidegger, Martin. 1987. *Zollikoner Seminare. Protokolle, Gespräche, Briefe.* ed. Medard Boss. Frankfurt am Main: Vittorio Klostermann. English edition: Heidegger, Martin. 2001. *Zollikon Seminars.* Trans. Franz Mayr and Richard Askay. Evanston: Northwestern University Press.
 8. Heidegger, Martin. 1993. *Sein und Zeit*, 17th ed. Tübingen: Niemeyer. English edition: Heidegger, Martin. 1996. *Being and Time.* Trans. Joan Stambaugh. Albany: SUNY Press.
 9. Laing, Ronald D. 1960. *The divided self.* London: Tavistock Publications.
10. Laing, Ronald D. 1971. *The politics of experience.* Harmondsworth: Penguin.
11. Laing, Ronald D. 1998. *Wisdom, madness and folly. The making of a psychiatrist 1927–57.* Edinburgh: Canongate Classics.

Chapter 8
Conclusion

In conclusion, the new notion of mental illness and health can be summarized as follows. Since the revision of the daseinsanalytical approach to mental health and illness sheds new light on the overall ontological structure of human existence, it is also necessary to spell out how the post-existential analysis changes the character and the mutual relation of the authentic and inauthentic existence. One can say that the appropriate approach to suffering also changes the view of the inauthentic existence that ceases to be a mere privative modification of the authentic existence and becomes its necessary counterpart which balances the disruptive power of the openness of being. Without the inauthentic existence, being-there would immediately dissipate in the chaotic openness of being. In order to exist, being-there must thus maintain a balance between the authentic and inauthentic way of being. This labile balance can be compared to the way Deleuze and Guattari describe the oscillation between the schizophrenic and paranoid tendency of life. Although one should not confuse the ontological analysis with schizoanalysis, their comparison may prevent the normative usage of the authentic existence and the underestimation of all the risks connected with it.

We have tried to demonstrate that the precondition of a non-normative view of mental disorder, i.e., one which wouldn't regard it as a mere privation of a normal state but would reveal it as an original phenomenon, is the interpretation of the clearing of being as chaotic openness in which the order of our experience arises and perishes. What appears against the background of the chaotic openness, in which our existence dwells in that it initially and for the most part turns away from it, is that mental disorder is determined by the way in which one relates to order and chaos. Unlike the socialized existence in the world of common everydayness where order prevails over chaos, the mentally disturbed existence is marked by an extreme sensitivity to the urgency of the all-devouring chaos. However, it is precisely the heightened sensitivity for the openness of chaos in which countless possibilities arise and perish that prevents us from branding mental disorder as a mere deficiency of normality. The normative approach to mental disorder is unacceptable also given that the fixation to the firmly given order of world that marks the everyday mode of

P. Kouba, *The Phenomenon of Mental Disorder*, Contributions to Phenomenology 75, DOI 10.1007/978-3-319-10323-5_8

existence is far removed from real health. The thesis that mental disorder is an utterly original, irreducible way of being does not of course mean that there is no difference between health and illness. Rather, the opposition between health and illness shouldn't be viewed solely from the perspective of health, from which mental disorder does appear a certain negation. Just as illness can be perceived from the viewpoint of health, health can be viewed from the perspective of illness which – as if through a magnifying glass – shows what is always already hidden in health, albeit in the form of an unclearly divined threat. In its primary otherness that distinguishes it from health, illness not only makes it possible to understand better what it is to be healthy, but also opens a new, more penetrative way of looking at human existence as such. As Nietzsche says, "being ill is instructive, we don't doubt, more instructive than being well."[1]

Let us therefore repeat one more time how illness differs from health. The difference between health and illness lies not only in the contradiction between order and chaos; the ill is not simply one whose experience disintegrates in chaos, just as the healthy is not one who maintains a perfect order of experience. Since our existence essentially stands *between* order and chaos, the difference between health and illness rather depends on the mode in which order and chaos relate to one another. It depends on whether the dynamic connection in which order and chaos provoke and potentialize each other is preserved, or whether the relation between order and chaos is purely negative. One can speak of true health only when human existence stands between order and chaos in that it preserves their dynamic tension and develops it further. Our belonging to both order and chaos is best attested to when we abandon the established order of the world and expose ourselves to the gaping openness of chaos, out of which new order and sense arise. On the other hand, mental disorder occurs when the polarity of the firm order and annihilating chaos is experienced as an insoluble dilemma. Instead of a dynamic connection of order and chaos, it is their separation and absolutization that takes place here. Chaos and order manifest themselves no longer as two constitutive areas in which human existence dwells, but as two inconsolable spheres between which human existence is cleft. Where a healthy human being experiences a dynamic connectedness of order and chaos, the ill person feels a painful cleavage that coerces him/her to seek shelter from the devastating effect of chaos in the rigid order. While health allows us to undergo the breakup of the order of experience and partake in the birth of a new order out of the infinite chaos of possibilities, mental disorder compels us to cling desperately to the frail order of experience unless we want to drown in the sea of chaos. Every single drop, every vestige of chaos can become fatal. The need to maintain the uncertain order of experience can bring a mentally ill person so far that he/she is practically unable to change opinion. As one of Laing's patients says: "You are arguing in order to have pleasure of triumphing over me. At best you win an argument. At worst you lose an argument. *I am arguing in order to preserve my*

---

[1] Nietzsche, Friedrich. 1994. *On the Genealogy of Morality* (trans. Diethe, Carol). London: Cambridge University Press, III, section 9.

existence."[2] Unless compelled by the desperate need to protect itself, human being can change its perspective on the world and its role in it even if the cost is the disintegration of the whole order of its experience and breakdown of the integral constitution of its individual being. The possibility of such a change, which in no way precludes the capacity for keeping one's conviction unless it is proven wrong, is unbearable for the mentally ill, however. His/her misery lies in the fact that he/she is situated in an either-or situation: either the existence in the integrated order of experience, or the fall into chaos. Either life, or death.

Yet, it would be too simple to regard this state as a pathological defect and to restrict oneself to a mere enumeration of the possibilities of which human existence deprives itself by either becoming hermetically closed in a fixed order, or falling hopelessly into chaos. Rather than to explicate the peculiar sharpening of the polarity between order and chaos in the notions of deficiency, it is much more pertinent to understand it as a certain modification of the relation between order and chaos.

Order keeps incessantly emerging out of chaos and dissolving therein again. The stable order, order with clearly defined contours, comes into being only when it is separated from chaos by a horizon which protects it from the annihilating forces of chaos. This horizon can be more or less impenetrable, and the degree of its impenetrability is precisely what decides whether the relation between order and chaos is conjunctive or disjunctive. Whereas in the first case the relation between order and chaos is modulated by means of a process during which order opens itself to chaos, lets itself be penetrated by it or dissolves in it in order to give way to a new order that takes its place, in the other case order and chaos merely contradict each other. As long as one can speak of "mental disturbance" here, then only in the sense of a disturbance in the dynamic connection between order and chaos, in which the door of the possible keeps opening and closing itself.

But who can ever say about himself/herself that he/she fully stands the ground of the chaotic openness in which the order of experience arises and perishes? Who does not restrict the dynamic connection of order with chaos for the sake of at least somewhat peaceful and balanced existence? Is it not the case, in the end, that most of us are neither really healthy, nor really ill? Do we not find ourselves mostly between health and illness, in the state of being somewhat healthy and somewhat ill? That perfect health is hardly attainable is attested to by the fact that free vulnerability to chaos, in which not only the order of experience, but also the unity of individual being disintegrates, is connected with suffering.

If we still reserve the right to speak of mental disorder, it is mainly because the confrontation with chaos is experienced in pathological states not as a moment of ecstasy or rapture, but as a state of immense suffering. Not even the bipolar affective disorder is in its manic phase an expression of a joyful ecstasy, but rather a headlong escape from suffering. The state in which this suffering appears in its extreme form is the schizophrenic collapse in which chaos fully breaks out.

---

[2] Laing. *The Divided Self*, 43.

Facing the extreme danger to which the weakened schizophrenic is exposed, psychiatry must not remain inactive. Its duty is to alleviate the patient's suffering, for which purpose it can avail itself of medication, which narrows down the frame of personal experience, thus enabling the patient to come to terms with the disintegrative effect of chaos, and it can also use the protected environment of the psychiatric asylum, where a certain daily order is observed. By virtue of all these measures, the schizophrenic can manage to reintegrate the disintegrated order of experience and consolidate the shaken individual being. Thus, the patient can reach a relatively stabilized state and regain control over himself/herself.

Real cure, however, lies not in stabilization reached by means of greater or lesser restriction of the patient's world, but rather in the gradual reduction of the barriers which prevent human existence from freely exposing itself to the disintegration of experience and participating in its renewed birth from out of the wild chaos. The objective of therapeutic help is therefore not to remove the patient's suffering altogether, but to help him/her accept it as an integral part of his/her existence, i.e., to learn to live with it as something from which he/she need not desperately flee or to which he/she must hopelessly succumb.

Especially nowadays, when suffering is understood as the opposite to health, and consequently repressed with the help of all possible means from the human life, it is increasingly necessary to point out the fact that we must not only remove suffering, but also learn to accept it to a certain degree.[3] Against the tendency to identify health with the absence of suffering whose excess is heralded in illness we should adopt the view that suffering forms an inseparable part of human existence understood as dwelling in the gaping openness of chaos. To remove from human existence the suffering from disintegration of its individual being and from the breakdown of the order of its experience would mean to eliminate from within it all possible ways of breaking through the everyday being-in-the-world. Without suffering, our existence would be impoverished of not only the possibility of joyful rapture and ecstasy, but also of the possibility of leaving the firmly established order of one's world and searching a new order and sense. For suffering is the price we pay for our freedom.

What is offered here is actually a perspective on suffering: suffering that springs from our vulnerability to the gaping openness of chaos is not something *per se* that is to be detected and removed. Suffering and health are correlative notions because they mutually condition and supplement one another. Every health has an ingredient of suffering, and *vice versa*. One could of course doubt whether the ultimate form of suffering, such as the schizophrenic disintegration of personality, still encompasses some traces of health. But it is precisely here, in this limit of our experience, that what eludes us in the everyday, socialized mode of existence is brought to light; that is, that suffering forms the dark side of health understood as the ability to expose oneself to the openness of chaos, in which all order arises and perishes.

[3] The tendency to understand health as total absence of suffering is affirmed and consecrated by the World Health Organization, according to which "Health is a state of complete physical, mental and social well-being and not merely the absence of disease or infirmity." [http://www.who.int/about/definition/en/]

What is at stake is of course not only suffering itself, but also such phenomena as fatigue or old age. Although we sense that suffering, fatigue and old age somehow relate to the finitude of human existence, this connection remains unclear until the above-mentioned phenomena are seen against the background of chaos, in which the order of our experience arises and perishes. It is only our belonging to chaos that allows us to understand the real burden of human existence; it is only this belonging that displays its instability and fragility in full light. The fact that human existence is exposed to chaos, in which its individuality disintegrates and vanishes, casts light on the abysmal dimension of its finitude. The essential unanchoredness and inconstancy of human existence is reflected in its incessant oscillation between order and chaos. By understanding such phenomena as suffering or fatigue and old age, we attain a new view of human existence as such. Yet, the overall picture of existence we thus obtain does not result from a mere application of certain "ontic" pieces of knowledge, but follows from an "ontological" meditation about being-there which experiences its finitude in the unremitting repetition of its end.

If human existence is to be thematized on the basis of its belonging to chaos, in which both individual being and the overall order of experience disintegrate, its picture must be substantially different from the project of being in disclosedness whose ontological structure is adumbrated in *Sein und Zeit*. Contrary to the existential analysis of being-there, in the post-existential analysis, one cannot speak of a binary opposition of authentic and inauthentic existence, especially not in the sense that the inauthentic mode of existence would be a privation of the authentic one. Existence which clings to the inhabited familiar world of common everydayness and to the conventionalized coexistence with others cannot be some privative form of a mode of being in which the lonely being-there sets out to face uncanniness, but rather must appear as an equally original modus of existence. Instead of the polarity of the authentic and inauthentic existence which oppose each other as two different modes of being between which one chooses, a much more subtle differentiation must be introduced, which would leave room for delicate oscillation, gradual alternations, prevalence and intermingling of various forms of existence, taking into account also the zones of their indiscriminability and indistinctness.

Even in *Sein und Zeit* one can find passages implying a scale of various degrees of inauthenticity, but this scale does not pertain to the fundamental difference between the authentic and inauthentic modes of existence.[4] Even though Heidegger does admit that one's absorption in the surrounding world can reach various degrees depending on how far being-there alienates from its very own potentiality-of-being, a re-appropriation of one's own being in disclosedness, according to him, is possible only by means of a crucial change in the overall mode of existence. In this way he opens up a path for Boss who consequently claims that mental disorder is essentially nothing but inauthenticity escalated to the extreme. Whereas the inauthentic existence can then serve as a model of illness, the authentic existence, with the special focus on its autonomy, constancy and integrity, becomes the ideal of health.

---

[4] Martin Heidegger. *Sein und Zeit*, 347.

The primary trouble with this view of authentic and inauthentic existence, however, lies not only in the psychiatric application of the two fundamental modes of existence, but mostly in the omission of the fact that authenticity has not only a positive value that consists in breaking free from the yoke of the existential routine, conventions and accepted opinions, but also its dangers and risks. By the same token, one must not forget that inauthenticity presents not only the threat of stagnation, self-alienation and self-oblivion, but that it also has a positive sense for us, providing us with the support of the familiar world and allowing us to lead an undisturbed, balanced existence. This must be kept in mind if we are to evade any normative use of the phenomenal structures of authentic and inauthentic existence.

In this respect *Erläuterungen zu Hölderlins Dichtung* presents an undeniable advancement beyond *Sein und Zeit* by clearly depicting the peril connected with the abandonment of the familiar inhabited world and the exposure to the chaotic openness of being. What becomes apparent here, apart from the recognition of the threat hidden in the self-destructive fall into the gaping openness of chaos, is that remaining in the familiar world of common everydayness and in the conventionalized coexistence with others is not only an expression of the existential decay, but also a pre-requisite of the preservation of the constant individual being and the overall order of experience. The mode of being which is understood in *Sein und Zeit* as inauthentic has its positive sense in that it is a guarantee of an integrated order of experience and of ones' own individual integrity; as such, it is an indispensable counterbalance equalizing the disintegration of experience and the collapse of individual being that occur in the *ecstatic* exposure to the chaotic openness of being. Were it not due to the so-called inauthentic mode of existence, we could maintain neither a firm order of experience, nor a constant unity of our individual being.

This, however, is not in the least to say that the inauthentic mode of existence should occupy the place hitherto reserved for the authentic existence. The point is that a full comprehension of the process in which being-there throws itself at the mercy of the chaotic openness of being enables us to appropriately appreciate also the undisturbed, ordered existence in the familiar world of everyday matters and the socialized coexistence with others.

Our balancing between the "authentic" and "inauthentic" modes of existence thus achieves a totally different dimension from the one it is attributed by the existential analysis of being-there undertaken in *Sein und Zeit*. On the one hand there is the firm order of everyday co-existence with others, which does provide us with support, and yet may become a bond that condemns us to unoriginality by hindering our free invention, and on the other hand there is the chaotic openness of being that makes it possible to escape from the captivity of old habits and accepted opinions, albeit at the cost of a breakup of the order of experience and of the integral unity of individual being.

The possibility of sudden twists, gradual shifts and subtle oscillations between order and chaos, which is implied in *Erläuterungen zu Hölderlins Dichtung*, therefore resembles to a certain extent the way in which Deleuze and Guattari speak of the schizophrenic and paranoid tendencies of life. For it is clear that these two tendencies are never quite apart, but that they rather incessantly confront, change and incite each other; however mutually contradictory, they are to be understood as equally primordial. Although the schizophrenic tendency is characterized as revolutionary whereas the paranoid one as reactionary, they don't confront each other as the positive and the negative pole, but both have their own sense and value that render them indispensable for life (even though it may not seem so in *L'Anti-Œdipe*, in *Milles plateaux* it is quite evident).[5]

As long as the paranoid side of experience has predominance, what is brought to the fore is the need for self-preservation and maintenance of the *status quo*; the schizophrenic side of experience, on the other hand, harbors the possibility of self-overcoming, of ecstatic advancement out of oneself as well as the possibility of the escape from the given situation. Insofar as the schizophrenic process shatters both the establish order of experience and the integrity of individual being, the paranoid process resists chaos and prevents the integral unity of experience and individual being from disintegrating.

Both processes, however, have their own risks and perils. The very fact that Deleuze and Guattari use notions adopted from the realm of psychiatry implies that the schizophrenic tendency becomes destructive once isolated, turned into a goal in itself and driven to the extreme, which also, though in a different form, applies to the paranoid tendency. Whereas in the first case the schizophrenic breakdown of the established structures of thought, perception and action threatens to turn into a total collapse into chaos, in the other case one must take into account the risk that the paranoid need for self-preservation may lead to hatred of any change and to the wish to destroy everything that might cause a change.

What needs to be added to the realization of all the risks bound with the schizo-phrenic and paranoid processes is how these processes relate to the territory as to the familiar, inhabited world. Territory, according to Deleuze and Guattari, is not a static given, but rather the result of a contradictory effect of deterritorialization and reterritorialization. These two movements form the fundamental dynamic moments of life, where deterritorialization is connected with the schizophrenic tendency, whereas reterritorialization is bound with the paranoid tendency. While the schizo-phrenic tendency involves the deterritorialization, within whose framework the inhabited territory is abandoned and experience opens itself to chaos, the paranoid tendency concentrates on the movement of reterritorialization which resists chaos in that it creates and maintains an inhabited territory where chaos is vanquished by order and stability. Territory guarantees the prevalence of order over chaos, and its abandonment therefore makes the habitual familiar order dissipate in chaos.

It is therefore understandable that the inner peril of the paranoid tendency lies in the fossilization and stagnation within the frame of a hermetically closed territory; the risk run by the schizophrenic tendency is, on the contrary, an all too radical or sudden deterritorialization, which instead of the liberation of the repressed desire for the new ends in pure self-destruction.

In order for both these risks to be clearly nameable, schizoanalysis, as Deleuze and Guattari call their conception, distinguishes between relative and absolute

---

[5] Deleuze, and Guattari. *Mille plateaux*, 503.

deterritorialization. As long as deterritorialization presents an escape from the given situation, relative deterritorialization is an escape which in no way disturbs the integrated order of experience and the integral unity of individual being, whereas absolute deterritorialization means such a process of escaping the closed territory by which the order of experience and the unity of individual being completely disintegrate. During absolute deterritorialization, the intentional unity of consciousness collapses, and experience opens itself to chaos, to its endless mutations and multitudes. This requires that there should be individuation in the sense of conglomeration and sedimentation of the shattered singular components taking place along with absolute deterritorialization. This individuation is the germ of reterritorialization that must proceed in parallel with absolute deterritorialization, unless a schizophrenic breakdown is to occur.

Reterritorialization is thus no mere return to the original territory, but rather a reconfiguration of singular elements that forms new relations among them, and thus a new shape of territory.[6] In other words, reterritorialization that accompanies absolute deterritorialization creates a new territory, or at least modifies the old one. Home-coming is here possible only as a creation of a new home. In this sense, Deleuze and Guattari go further than Heidegger in his *Erläuterungen zu Hölderlins Dichtung* where he presupposes that the poet coming home from abroad finds the *same* home he has left.

In order to understand how it is possible that absolute deterritorialization shatters not only the unity of individual being, but also the firm structure of territory which could be re-created, but shall never be the same as before, we must take into account the difference between the macroscopic and microscopic levels of utterance, which is a sort of alternative to Heidegger's ontico-ontological difference. Deleuze and Guattari do not settle for the difference between the state of things and chaos in which order arises, but also work with the conceptual distinction between the molar and molecular structures. A first step to an understanding of this distinction might be what R. D. Laing says about the molar and molecular split of personality.[7] Insofar as the molar split of personality lies in the enactment of a certain role, as in the case of a "hysteric" who forgets himself and "loses control" over himself, the molecular break-up of personality essentially prevents any role from being played. This occurs, according to Laing, especially in schizophrenia, where the line of actions and gestures is often fragmented in such a way as to give the impression that no one at all acts in them. Moreover, the molecular disintegration of personality leads not only to the disintegration of the complex whole of perception and action, but also to the disintegration of grammatical structures and verbal coherence.

If we remain on the level of human experience we can therefore say that the schizophrenic tendency, which gets fulfilled in absolute deterritorialization, reveals molecular structures, whereas the paranoid tendency holds on to molar structures such as constant personal integrity, the firm grip of social bonds and the unalterable identity of things that appear within territory. However, all these molar structures

---

[6] Deleuze, and Guattari. *Mille plateaux*, 635.
[7] Laing. *The Divided Self*, 210.

fall apart once they have become absolutely deterritorialized. Since absolute deterritorialization, unlike relative deterritorialization, opens up space for chaos which leaves no stone unturned, there would remain nothing of molar structures, if there were no parallel process of reterritorialization.

When, on the contrary, the poet in *Erläuterungen zu Hölderlins Dichtung* abandons the world of familiar beings where he is at home, and sets out for a journey into the unknown, his home is in no way affected by this. The question thus remains: what happens when the poet in his confrontation with chaos finds new order? Does he return home to the familiar things and people, or does he gain a new home? This problem alone implies that although Heidegger in *Erläuterungen zu Hölderlins Dichtung* does to a considerable extent abandon the romantic orientation, his philosophical conception still does not overcome all that separates it from schizoanalysis developed by Deleuze and Guattari.

By way of conclusion, let us thus give voice to a long-suppressed objection: is not the abyss between schizoanalysis and ontological analysis of being-there too wide for it to be possible to interpret Heidegger through Deleuze and Guattari?[8] Is not the attempt to undertake the schizoanalytic re-description of the existential project of being-there doomed to failure from the very outset?

This objection must be accepted if we take into account that schizoanalysis is different from existential analysis not only due to its terminology, but also due to its method and its focus. While existential analysis of being-there aims, by means of analyzing individual existence, at revealing the *unified* ontological structure of being in openness and therein encompassed individual being, schizoanalysis examines the molar unity of personality in order to discover behind it the burgeoning of molecular multiplicities that undergo the process of consolidation and individuation. "The task of schizoanalysis is that of tirelessly taking apart egos and their presuppositions; liberating the pre-personal singularities they enclose and repress," claim Deleuze and Guattari.[9] Accordingly, their conception of analysis approaches the original sense of the Greek word ἀναλύειν, which means not only partitioning into pieces (as in Homer's *Odyssey*, where Penelope unweaves the cloth she has woven during the day), but also the untying of bonds and liberation from captivity. In schizoanalysis the act of liberation lies in the loosening of power-structures and mechanism of manipulation of today's capitalist society that turn man into an atomized individual. What is at stake is not to free "somebody" who cannot find his/her way through the general self-alienation and self-oblivion to himself/herself, but to free life from the captivity of individualism, to release it for the possibilities of experiment, rapture and ecstasy. On the contrary, existential analysis with its concept

---

[8] Note: One cannot pretend that Deleuze and Guattari's conception remains unaffected by this attempt. In its confrontation with the ontological analysis of being-there, schizoanalysis is re-interpreted at least as much as its counterpart.

[9] Deleuze, Gilles, and Guattari, Félix. 1972. *L'Anti-Oedipe. Capitalisme et schizophrénie*, 434. English edition: Deleuze, Gilles, and Guattari, Félix. 1983. *Anti-Oedipus: Capitalism and Schizophrenia* (trans: Hurley, Robert, Seem Mark, and Lane, Helen R.). Minneapolis: University of Minnesota Press, 362.

of self-oblivion and self-discovery can never overcome the barrier of individualism, since that is precisely its fundamental principle, which is reflected in the very statement that ontological analysis of being-there should not be "a reduction into elements, but the articulation of the (a priori) unity of a composite structure (*Strukturgefüge*)."[10] With this contention, Heidegger explicitly draws on the way in which *Kritik der reinen Vernunft* uses the notion of "analytic." Even though he does not subscribe to the philosophy of transcendental subjectivity as such, Heidegger holds that the sense of the analysis of being-there is derived from the sense which Kant attributes to analytic, which he understands as an examination of the powers of understanding that is meant to lead to the revelation of the unity of the objectivity of the objects of cognition. It follows from this that the analytic of being-there is in *Zollikoner Seminare* conceived of as a decomposition whose goal is to unveil the unified ontological composition of being in openness, upon which the unified structure of individual existence is grounded.

However, the above-mentioned objection can also be given a negative response, once we use – in all awareness of its irreducible peculiarity – schizoanalysis as a tool by means of which we can free Heidegger from out of the trap into which he let himself be caught in *Zollikoner Seminare*. If we position Deleuze and Guattari against Heidegger and Boss, it becomes clear that the privative conception of illness founded upon the opposition between the authentic and the inauthentic existence is not the only access path to the problem of mental disorder, but rather a dead end. Schizoanalysis can then provide us not only with an alternative view of the psychopathological problems, but also point to those possibilities of Heidegger's thought which the so-called therapeutic *Daseinsanalysis* failed to bring to attention. If we managed to map these possibilities at least partially, the goal of our work has been achieved.

References

1. Deleuze, Gilles, and Félix Guattari. 1972. *L'Anti-Oedipe: Capitalisme et schizophrénie*. Paris: Minuit. English edition: Deleuze, Gilles, and Félix Guattari. 1983. *Anti-Oedipus: Capitalism and Schizophrenia*. Trans. Robert Hurley, Mark Seem, and Helen R. Lane. Minneapolis: University of Minnesota Press.
2. Deleuze, Gilles, and Félix Guattari. 1980. *Mille plateaux: Capitalisme et schizophrénie*. Paris: Minuit. English edition: Deleuze, Gilles, and Félix Guattari. 1987. *Thousand Plateaus*. Trans. Brian Massumi. Minneapolis: Minnesota University Press.
3. Heidegger, Martin. 1951. *Erläuterungen zu Hölderlins Dichtung*. Frankfurt am Main: Vittorio Klostermann. English edition: Heidegger, Martin. 2000. *Elucidations of Hölderlin's Poetry*. Trans. Keith Hoeller. New York: Humanity Books.
4. Heidegger, Martin. 1987. *Zollikoner Seminare. Protokolle, Gespräche, Briefe*. ed. Medard Boss. Frankfurt am Main: Vittorio Klostermann. English edition: Heidegger, Martin. 2001. *Zollikon Seminars*. Trans. Franz Mayr and Richard Askay. Evanston: Northwestern University Press.

---

[10] Heidegger. *Zollikoner Seminare*, 148–50.

5. Heidegger, Martin. 1993. *Sein und Zeit*, 17th ed. Tübingen: Niemeyer. English edition:Heidegger, Martin. 1996. *Being and Time*. Trans. Stambaugh, Joan. Albany: SUNY Press.
6. Laing, Ronald D. 1960. *The divided self*. London: Tavistock Publications.
7. Nietzsche, Friedrich. 1994. *On the Genealogy of Morality*. Trans. Carol Diethe. London: Cambridge University Press.

Bibliography

1. Alleman, Beda. 1954. *Hölderlin und Heidegger*. Zurich: Atlantis Verlag.
2. Aristotle. 1984. *Metaphysics*, ed. Jonathan Barnes. Oxford: Princeton University Press.
3. Binswanger, Ludwig. 1949. *Henrik Ibsen und das Problem der Selbstrealisation in der Kunst*. Heidelberg: Verlag Lambert Schneider.
4. Binswanger, Ludwig. 1955. *Ausgewählte Vorträge und Aufsätze, Bd. II: Zur Problematik der psychiatrischen Forschung und zum Problem der Psychiatrie*. Bern: Francke.
5. Binswanger, Ludwig. 1957. *Schizophrenie*. Pfullingen: Neske.
6. Binswanger, Ludwig. 1957. *Der Mensch in der Psychiatrie*. Pfullingen: Neske.
7. Binswanger, Ludwig. 1958. The case of Ellen West: An anthropological-clinical study. In *Existence: A New Dimension in Psychiatry and Psychology*. Werner M. Mendel (Trans.), Joseph Lyons (Trans.), Rollo May (ed.), Ernest Angel (ed.), Henri F. Ellenberger (ed.). New York: Basic Books.
8. Binswanger, Ludwig. 1964. *Grundformen und Erkenntnis menschlichen Daseins*, 4th ed. München/Basel: Ernst Reinhardt Verlag.
9. Binswanger, Ludwig. 1965. *Wahn. Beiträge zu seiner phaenomenologischen und daseinsanalytischen Erforschung*. Pfullingen: Neske.
10. Blanchot, Maurice. 1955. *L'Espace littéraire*. Paris: Gallimard.
11. Blankenburg, Wolfgang. 1971. *Der Verlust der natürlichen Selbstverständlichkeit. Ein Beitrag zur Psychopatologie symptomarmer Schizophrenien*. Stuttgart: Ferdinand Enke Verlag.
12. Blankenburg, Wolfgang. 1984. Angst und Hoffnung – Grundperspektiven der Welt-und Selbst-auslegung psychisch Kranker. In *Angst und Hoffnung. Grundperspektiven der Weltauslegung*, ed. Günter Eifler, Otto Saame, and Peter Schneider. Mainz: Johannes Guttenberg-Universität.
13. Blankenburg, Wolfgang. 1991. Pespektivität und Wahn. In *Wahn und Perspektivität. Störungen im Realitätsbezug des Menschen und ihre Therapie*, ed. Wolfgang Blankenburg. Stuttgart: Ferdinand Enke Verlag.
14. Boque, Ronald. 1989. *Deleuze and Guattari*. London/New York: Routledge.
15. Boque, Ronald. 1999. Art and territory. In *A Deleuzian century?* ed. Ian Buchanan. Durham/London: Duke University Press.
16. Boss, Medard. 1975. *Es träume mich vergangene Nacht*. Bern: Verlag Hans Huber.
17. Boss, Medard. 1975. *Grundriss der Medizin und der Psychologie*. Bern/Stuttgart/Wien: Verlag Hans Huber.
18. Boss, Medard. 1979. *Von der Psychoanalyse zur Daseinsanalyse*. Wien: Europa Verlag.
19. Canguilhem, Georges. 1966. *Le normal et le pathologique*. Paris: P.U.F.
20. Canguilhem, Georges. 2002. *Écrits sur la médecine*. Paris: Édition du seuil.

© Springer International Publishing Switzerland 2015
P. Kouba, *The Phenomenon of Mental Disorder*, Contributions
to Phenomenology 75, DOI 10.1007/978-3-319-10323-5

21. Caputo, John D. 1987. *Radical Hermeneutics. Repetition, deconstruction and the hermeneutic project.* Bloomington/Indianapolis: Indiana University Press.
22. Caputo, John D. 2000. *More radical hermeneutics: On not knowing who we are.* Bloomington/ Indianapolis: Indiana University Press.
23. Charbonneau, Georges. 1995. Selbstheit und Psychose. In *2. Forum für Daseinsanalyse.* Basel: Karger AG.
24. Condrau, Gion. 1962. *Angst und Schuld als Grundprobleme der Psychotherapie.* Bern und Stuttgart: Verlag Hans Huber.
25. Condrau, Gion. 1992. *Sigmund Freud und Martin Heidegger.* Bern/Stuttgart: Verlag Hans Huber.
26. Condrau, Gion. 1998. *Daseinsanalyse: philosophische und anthropologische Grundlagen: die Bedeutung der Sprache: Psychotherapieforschung aus daseinsanalytischer Sicht.* Dettelbach: Röll.
27. Condrau, Gion. 1998. *Martin Heidegger's impact on psychotherapy.* Dublin: Edition Mosaic.
28. Dastur, Françoise. 1995. Phänomenologie und Antropologie. In *2. Forum für Daseinsanalyse.* Basel: Karger AG.
29. de Waelhens, Alphonse. 1972. *La psychose. Essai d'interprétation analytique et existentiale.* Louvain: Éditions NAUWELAERTS.
30. Deleuze, Gilles. 1962. *Nietzsche et la philosophie.* Paris: PUF.
31. Deleuze, Gilles. 1963. *La Philosophie critique de Kant.* Paris: PUF.
32. Deleuze, Gilles. 1967. *Présentation de Sacher-Masoch: le froid et le cruel.* Avec le texte intégral de *La Vénus à la fourrure.* Paris: Minuit.
33. Deleuze, Gilles. 1986. *Foucault.* Paris: Minuit.
34. Deleuze, Gilles. 1990. *Pourparlers.* Paris: Minuit.
35. Deleuze, Gilles. 1993. *Critique et Clinique.* Paris: Minuit.
36. Deleuze, Gilles. 1996. *Proust et les signes.* Paris: PUF.
37. Deleuze, Gilles. 1968. *Différence et répétition.* Paris: PUF. English edition: Deleuze, Gilles. 1995. *Difference and Repetition.* Trans. Paul Patton. New York: Columbia University Press.
38. Deleuze, Gilles, and Félix Guattari. 1975. *Kafka. Pour une littérature mineure.* Paris: Minuit.
39. Deleuze, Gilles, and Félix Guattari. 1972. *L'Anti-Oedipe: Capitalisme et schizophrénie,* Paris: Minuit. English edition: Deleuze, Gilles, and Guattari, Félix. 1983. *Anti-Oedipus: Capitalism and Schizophrenia.* Trans. Robert Hurley, Mark Seem, and Helen R. Lane. Minneapolis: University of Minnesota Press.
40. Deleuze, Gilles, and Félix Guattari. 1980. *Mille plateaux: Capitalisme et schizophrénie.* Paris: Minuit. English edition: Deleuze, Gilles, and Félix Guattari. 1987. *Thousand Plateaus.* Trans. Brian Massumi. Minneapolis: Minnesota University Press.
41. Deleuze, Gilles, and Félix Guattari. 1991. *Qu'est- ce que la philosophie?* Paris: Minuit. English edition: Deleuze, Gilles, and Félix Guattari. 1994. *What is Philosophy?* Trans. Hugh Tomlison and Graham Burchill. New York: Columbia University Press.
42. Deleuze, Gilles, and Claire Parnet. 1977. *Dialogues.* Paris: Flammarion.
43. De Man, Paul. 1983. *Blindness and insight. Essays in the rhetoric of contemporary criticism.* Minneapolis: University of Minnesota Press.
44. Descartes, René. 1908. *Discours de la métode.* In *Oeuvres de Descartes,* IX Vols. Paris: Ch. Adam et P. Tannery.
45. Descombes, Vincent. 1979. *Le même et l'autre.* Paris: Minuit.
46. Ebeling, Hans. 1991. *Philosophie und Ideologie.* Reinbek bei Hamburg: Rowohlt.
47. Figal, Günter. 1994. *Für eine Philosophie von Freiheit und Streit: Politik – Ästhetik – Metaphysik.* Stuttgart und Weimar: Metzler.
48. Foucault, Michel. 1963. *Naissance de la Clinique.* Paris: PUF. English edition: Foucault, Michel. 1973. *The Birth of the Clinic.* Trans. A.M. Sheridan. London: Tavistock Publications Limited.
49. Foucault, Michel. 1964. *L'histoire de la folie à l'âge classique.* Paris: Gallimard.
50. Foucault, Michel. 1966. *Maladie mentale et psychologie.* Paris: PUF.
51. Foucault, Michel. 1971. *L'Ordre du discours.* Paris: Gallimard.

52. Foucault, Michel. 1971. Nietzsche, la généalogie, l'histoire. In *Hommage à Jean Hyppolite*. Paris: PUF.
53. Foucault, Michel. 1970. *The order of things*, ed. Ronald D. Laing. London: Tavistock Publications Ltd.
54. Foucault, Michel. 1994. *Dits et écrits 1954–1988 par Michel Foucault*, ed. Daniel Defert and Francois Ewald. Paris: Gallimard.
55. Frank, Manfred. 1984. *Was ist Neostrukturalismus?* Frankfurt am Main: Suhrkamp.
56. Goldstein, Kurt. 2000. *The organism. A holistic approach to biology derived from pathological data in man*. New York: ZONE Books.
57. Goodchild, Philip. 1996. *Deleuze and Guattari*. London: SAGE Publications.
58. Gosetti-Ferencei, Jennifer Anna. 2004. *Heidegger and the subject of poetic language. Toward a new poetics of Dasein*. New York: Fordham University Press.
59. Grimsley, Ronald. 1955. *Existentialist thought*. Cardiff: University of Wales Press.
60. Grondin, Jean. 1991. *Einführung in die philosophische Hermeneutik*. Darmstadt: Wissenschaftliche Buchgesellschaft.
61. Guattari, Félix. 1972. *Psychoanalyse et transversalité*. Paris: Maspero.
62. Guattari, Félix. 1977. *La Révolution moléculaire*, Séries 'Encre'. Paris: Éditions Recherches.
63. Heidegger, Martin. 1947. *Über den Humanismus*. Frankfurt am Main: Vittorio Klostermann.
64. Heidegger, Martin. 1949. *Vom Wesen des Grundes*. Frankfurt am Main: Vittorio Klostermann.
65. Heidegger, Martin. 1950. *Holzwege*. Frankfurt am Main: Vittorio Klostermann.
66. Heidegger, Martin. 1951. *Erläuterungen zu Hölderlins Dichtung*. Frankfurt am Main: Vittorio Klostermann. English edition: Heidegger, Martin. 2000. *Elucidations of Hölderlin's Poetry*. Trans. Keith Hoeller. New York: Humanity Books.
67. Heidegger, Martin. 1954. *Vom Wesen der Wahrheit*. Frankfurt am Main: Vittorio Klostermann.
68. Heidegger, Martin. 1954. *Vorträge und Aufsätze*. Pfullingen: Günter Neske.
69. Heidegger, Martin. 1954. *Was heisst DeLken?* Tübingen: Max Niemeyer Verlag.
70. Heidegger, Martin. 1956. *Was ist das – die Philosophie?* Pfullingen: Günter Neske.
71. Heidegger, Martin. 1957. *Hebel- der Hausfreund*. Pfullingen: Günter Neske.
72. Heidegger, Martin. 1958. *Grundsätze des Denkens*. Pfullingen: Günter Neske.
73. Heidegger, Martin. 1959. *Unterwegs zur Sprache*. Pfullingen: Günter Neske.
74. Heidegger, Martin. 1962. *Die Frage nach dem Ding*. Tübingen: Niemeyer.
75. Heidegger, Martin. 1965. *Der Ursprung des Kunstwerkes*. Stuttgart: Ph. Reclam Jun.
76. Heidegger, Maptin. 1969. *Zur Sache des Denkens*. Tübingen: Max Niemeyer.
77. Heidegger, Martin. 1971. *Schellings A'handlung Über das Wesen der menwchlichen Freiheit (1809)*, ed. Hildegard Feick. Tübingen: Max Niemeyer Verlag.
78. Heidegger, Martin. 1976. *Wegmarken*. Frankfurt am Main: Vittorio Klostermann. English edition: Heidegger, Martin. 1998. *Pathmarks*. Trans. William McNeill. Cambridge: Cambridge University Press.
79. Heidegger, Martin. 1983. *Die Grundbegriffe der Metaphysik: Welt, Endlichkeit, Einsamkeit*. Frankfurt am Main: Vittorio Klostermann. English edition: Heidegger, Martin. 1995. *The Fundamental Concepts of Metaphysics. World, Finitude, Solitude*. Trans. William McNeill and Nicholas Walker. Bloomington: Indiana University Press.
80. Heidegger, Martin. 1987. *Zollikoner Seminare. Protokolle, Gespräche, Briefe*. ed. Medard Boss. Frankfurt am Main: Vittorio Klostermann. English edition: Heidegger, Martin. 2001. *Zollikon Seminars*. Trans. Franz Mayr and Richard Askay. Evanston: Northwestern University Press.
81. Heidegger, Martin. 1989. *Der Begriff der Zeit*. Tübingen: Max Niemeyer Verlag.
82. Heidegger, Bartin. 1989. *Beiträge zur Philosophie (vom Ereignis)*. Frankfurt am Mein: Vittorio Klostermann. English edition: Heidegger, Martin. 1999. *Contributions to Philosophy (From Enowning)*. Trans. Parvis Emad and Kenneth Maly. Bloomington: Indiana University Press.
83. Heidegger, Martin. 1990. *Die Selbstbehauptung der deutschen UniVersität.Das Rektorat 1933/34*, 2nd ed. Frankfurt am Main: Vittorio Klostermann.
84. Heidegger, Martin. 1993. *Sein und Zeit*, 17th ed. Tübingen: Niemeyer. English edition: Heidegger, Martin. 1996. *Being and Time*. Trans. Joan Stambaugh. Albany: SUNY Press.

85. Heidegger, Martin. 1993. *Europa und die Philosophie*. Frankfurt am Main: Vittorio Klostermann.
86. Helting, Holger. 1999. *Einführung in die philosophischen Dimensionen der psychotherapeutischen Daseinsanalyse*. Aachen: Shaker Verlag.
87. Hoeller, Keith (ed.). 1988. *Heidegger and psychology. A special issue from the review of existential psychology and psychiatry*. Seattle: Promethean Press.
88. Holland, Eugene W. 1999. *Deleuze and Guattari's Anti-Oedipus. Introduction to schizoanalysis*. London/New York: Routledge.
89. Holzhey-Kunz, Alice. 1986. Todestrieb und Sein-zum-Tode. *Daseinsanalyse* 3: 98–109.
90. Holzhey-Kunz, Alice. 1987. Der Wunsch daseinsanalytisch wiederentdeckt. *Daseinsanalyse* 4: 51–64.
91. Holzhey-Kunz, Alice. 1988. Die zweideutigkeit seelischen Leidens. *Daseinsanalyse* 5: 81–95.
92. Holzhey-Kunz, Alice. 1992. Psychotherapie und Philosophie. *Daseinsanalyse* 9: 153–162.
93. Holzhey-Kunz, Alice. 1994. *Leiden am Dasein: die Daseinsanalyse und die Aufgabe einer Hermeneutik psychopathologischer Phänomene*. Wien: Passagen-Verlag.
94. Holzhey-Kunz, Alice. 1995. Ist die Analyse ein philosophischer Prozess?. In *2. Forum für Daseinsanalyse*. Basel: Karger AG.
95. Holzhey-Kunz, Alice. 1999. Die Daseinsanalytik von *Sein und Zeit* als Grundlage einer hermeneutischen Psychopathologie. In *Siebzig Jahre Sein und Zeit. Wiener Tagungen zur Phänomenologie*, ed. Helmuth Vetter. Frankfut am Mein: Lang – Verlag.
96. Janke, Wolfgang. 1982. *Existenzphilosophie*. Berlin/New York: Walter de Gruyter & Co.
97. Karall, Kristina. 1995. Die Geburt der Psychoanalyse im Lichte von Heideggers Daseinsanalytik. In *2. Forum für Daseinsanalyse*. Basel: Karger AG.
98. King, Magda. 1964. *Heidegger's philosophy – A guide to his basic thought*. New York/London: The Macmillan Company/Collier-Macmillan Limited.
99. Kühn, Rolf. 1991. Zeitlichkeit und die Situation. Zu Heideggers Begriff der Geworfenheit. *Daseinsanalyse* 8: 241–251.
100. Kühn, Rolf. 1991. Zum Verhältnis von Leben und Dasein. *Daseinsanalyse* 8: 184–198.
101. Lacue-Labarthe, Phillippe. 2007. *Heidegger and the Politics of Poetry*. Trans. Jeff Fort. Urbana/Chicago: University of Illinois Press.
102. Laing, Ronald D. 1960. *The divided self*. London: Tavistock Publications.
103. Laing, Ronald D. 1971. *The politics of experience*. Harmondsworth: Penguin Books.
104. Laing, Ronald D. 1998. *Wisdom, madness and folly. The making of a psychiatrist 1927–57*. Edinburgh: Canongate Classics.
105. Le Blanc, Guillaume. 1998. *Canguilhem et les normes*. Paris: PUF.
106. Lotz, Johannes B. 1975. *Martin Heidegger und Thomas von Aquin*. Stuttgart: Verlag Günter Neske.
107. Lyotard, Jean-François. 1954. *La Phénomenologie*. Paris: PUF.
108. Macann, Christopher. 1993. *Four pheomenological philosophers*. London/New York: Routledge.
109. Maldiney, Henri. 1991. *Penser l'homme et la folie*. Grenoble: Editions Jérôme Millon.
110. Massumi, Brian. 1992. *A User's Guide to Capitalism and Schizophrenia. Deviations from Deleuze and Guattari*. Cambridge, MA: MIT Press.
111. Merleau-Ponty, Maurice. 1945. *Phénoménologie de la perception*. Paris: Gallimard.
112. Mullarkey, John. 1999. Deleuze and materialism: One or several matters? In *A Deleuzian century?* ed. Ian Buchanan. Durham/London: Duke University Press.
113. Němec, Jan, Jan Patočka, and Petr Rezek. 1976. *Vybrané filosofické problémy psychopatologie a normality*. Prague: Archiv Jana Patočky.
114. Nietzsche, Friedrich. 1994. *On the Genealogy of Morality*. Trans. Carol Diethe. London: Cambridge University Press.
115. Schüssler, Ingeborg. 1989. Dasein und Sein bei Martin Heidegger. *Daseinsanalyse* 4: 278–313.

116. Padrutt, Hanspeter. 1988. Der Sinn des in *Sein und Zeit* genannten Verfallens. *Daseinsanalyse* 5: 310–331.
117. Patočka, Jan. 1993. *Úvod do fenomenologické filosofie*. Prague: OIKOYMENH.
118. Patočka, Jan. 1995. *Tělo, společenství, jazyk, svět*. Prague: OIKOYMENH.
119. Patton, Paul. 2000. *Deleuze & the political*. London/New York: Routledge.
120. Plato. 1921. VII, *Theaethetus, Sophist* (Loeb Classical Library). Trans. Harold North Fowler. Cambridge, MA: Harvard University Press.
121. Reinholdt, Kurt F. 1960. *Existentialist revolt*. New Enlarged Edition with an Appendix on Existentialist Psychotherapy. New York: Frederick Ungar Publishing Co.
122. Richardson, William J. 1963. *Heidegger: Through phenomenology to thought*. The Hague: Martinus Nijhoff.
123. Richardson, William J. 1993. Heidegger among the Doctors. In *Reading Heidegger: Commemorations*. Bloomington/Indianapolis: Indiana University Press.
124. Torno, Timothy. 1995. *Finding time. Reading for temporality in Hölderlin and Heidegger*. New York: Peter Lang.
125. von Uslar, Detlef. 2001. Heidegger und Hölderlin. Philosophie in der Dichtung. *Daseinsanalyse* 17: 155–169.
126. Vattimo, Gianni. 1993. *The Adventure of Difference, Philosophy after Nietzsche and Heidegger*. Trans. Cyprian Blamires. Baltimore: The Johns Hopkins University Press.
127. Vetter, Helmuth. 1993. Es gibt keine unmittelbare Gesundheit des Geistes. *Daseinsanalyse* 10: 65–79.
128. Vetter, Helmuth. 1995. Phänomenologie und Hermeneutik als Grundlage der daseinsanalytischen Psychtherapie. In *2. Forum für Daseinsanalyse*. Basel: Karger AG.
129. Vogt, Norbert. 1995. Phänomenologie und Postmoderne. In *2. Forum für Daseinsanalyse*. Basel: Karger AG.
130. von Herrmann, Friedrich-Wilhelm. 1985. *Subjekt und Dasein*. Frankfurt am Main: Vittorio Klostermann.
131. von Herrmann, Friedrich-Wilhelm. 1988. Der Humanismus und die Frage nach dem Wesen des Menschen. *Daseinsanalyse* 5: 259–281.
132. von Herrmann, Friedrich-Wilhelm. 1995. Daseinsanalyse und Ereignisdenken'. In *2. Forum für Daseinsanalyse*. Basel: Karger AG.
133. Wucherer-Huldenfeld, Augustinus Karl. 1995. Zum Verständnis der Zeitlichkeit in Psychoanalyse und Daseinsanalytik. In *2. Forum für Daseinsanalyse*. Basel: Karger AG.
134. Žižek, Slavoj. 1989. *The sublime object of ideology*. London/New York: Verso.
135. Žižek, Slavoj. 1996. *The indivisible reminder. An essay on Schelling and related matters*. London/New York: VERSO.

Index

A

Aging, 18, 25, 168, 191
Alleman, Beda, 140
Analytics, 22
Anxiety, 32–41, 44, 59, 65–69, 73, 75–77, 80, 81, 84–89, 101–103, 115, 116, 148, 155, 158, 180
Aristotle, 91, 96, 97
Arrangement, 12, 16, 19, 20, 39, 73, 74, 87, 88, 140, 154, 165, 182
Authentic existence, 40, 68–73, 75, 76, 80, 82–84, 89, 91, 100, 101, 109–111, 116, 117, 125, 146, 193, 196, 198

B

Being, 1, 11, 59, 91, 129, 139, 169, 193
Being-ahead-of-itself, 72, 77, 82, 85
Being-already-in, 72, 77, 82
Being-at-home, 67, 74, 116, 117, 122, 124, 143, 146, 147
Being-away, 129–137, 139
Being-beyond-the-world, 42–44, 46, 177
Being-free, 48, 66, 75, 101, 120
Being-guilty, 67, 68
Being-in-the-world, 2–7, 9, 22–24, 26, 27, 30–35, 37–44, 46, 47, 49–52, 60, 62–74, 77, 79–81, 83, 85, 87, 92–101, 103–118, 120–124, 170, 172, 181, 184, 185, 187, 189
Being of beings, 18–21, 46, 47, 50, 119, 132
Being present-at-hand, 130, 132
Being ready-to-hand, 150
Being-there, 47, 48, 52, 54, 78, 92, 93, 103, 119, 123, 132, 133, 136
Being-together-with, 38, 71, 72, 76–78, 82–87, 89, 146, 147, 154, 173
Being-toward-death, 40, 41, 46, 79–82, 115, 116, 135, 136, 191
Binswanger, Ludwig, 1, 44
Bipolar affective disorder, 100, 107, 109, 175
Blanchot, Maurice, 88
Blankenburg, Wolfgang, 172
Body, 3, 9, 15, 18, 22–24, 26, 30, 64, 66, 67, 95, 105–107, 114, 118, 119, 188–191
Boss, Medard, 1, 103

C

Calculability, 11, 14, 19
Caputo, John D., 170, 175
Care, 40–42, 46, 69–77, 79, 80, 144, 164, 176, 179
Chaos, 153, 155, 156, 160, 162, 164, 167, 176, 179, 180, 189–191, 194–196, 198, 199
Chaotic nonentity, 183–185, 187
Clearing of being, 48, 91, 97, 98, 103, 105, 108, 109, 118, 119, 132–136, 143–159, 164–168, 179, 190, 193

D

Daseinsanalysis, 26, 27, 30, 32, 33, 37, 39, 40, 43, 46–51, 102–104, 111–113, 116, 202
Deficiency, 4, 29, 33, 38, 52, 97, 99
Deleuze, 7, 55, 62
Deleuze, Gilles, 7, 74

© Springer International Publishing Switzerland 2015
P. Kouba, *The Phenomenon of Mental Disorder*, Contributions
to Phenomenology 75, DOI 10.1007/978-3-319-10323-5

CPSIA information can be obtained
at www.ICGtesting.com
Printed in the USA
LVHW051350080322
712915LV00011B/406